# Testing and Analysis of GMO-containing Foods and Feed

# Food Analysis & Properties

*Series Editor:*
Leo M. L. Nollet
*University College Ghent, Belgium*

Phenolic Compounds in Food: Characterization and Analysis (2018)
*Edited by Leo M.L. Nollet, Janet Alejandra Gutierrez-Uribe*

Spectroscopic Methods in Food Analysis (2018)
*Edited by Adriana S. Franca and Leo M.L. Nollet*

Multiresidue Methods for the Analysis of Pesticide Residues in Food (2017)
*Edited by Horacio Heinzen, Leo M.L. Nollet, and Amadeo R. Fernandez-Alba*

Marine Microorganisms: Extraction and Analysis of (2016) Bioactive Compounds
*Edited by Leo M. L. Nollet*

Flow Injection Analysis of Food Additives (2015)
*Edited by Claudia Ruiz-Capillas and Leo M. L. Nolle*

Testing and Analysis of GMO-containing Foods and Feed
*Edited by Salah E. O. Mahgoub and Leo M. L. Nollet*

For more information, please visit the Series Page: https://www.crcpress.com/Food-Analysis--Properties/book-series/CRCFOODANPRO

# Testing and Analysis of GMO-containing Foods and Feed

Edited by
Salah E. O. Mahgoub and Leo M. L. Nollet

CRC Press
Taylor & Francis Group
Boca Raton London New York

CRC Press is an imprint of the
Taylor & Francis Group, an **informa** business

CRC Press
Taylor & Francis Group
6000 Broken Sound Parkway NW, Suite 300
Boca Raton, FL 33487-2742



Printed on acid-free paper

International Standard Book Number-13: 978-1-138-03638-3 (Hardback)



**Library of Congress Cataloging-in-Publication Data**

Names: Mahgoub, Sala E. O. (Salah Eldin Osman), editor.
Title: Testing and analysis of GMO-containing foods and feed / edited by Salah E.O. Mahgoub & Leo M.L. Nollet.
Description: Boca Raton, Florida : CRC Press, [2019] | Includes bibliographical references and index.
Identifiers: LCCN 2018023407 | ISBN 9781138036383 (hardback : alk. paper) | ISBN 9781315178592 (ebook)
Subjects: LCSH: Genetically modified foods—Testing. | Genetically modified foods—Analysis.
Classification: LCC TP248.65.F66 T46 2019 | DDC 664—dc23
LC record available at https://lccn.loc.gov/2018023407

**Visit the Taylor & Francis Web site at**
**http://www.taylorandfrancis.com**

**and the CRC Press Web site at**
**http://www.crcpress.com**

*I would like to dedicate this work to my family. To my sincere, wonderful wife, Sumia, for her unlimited support, encouragement, and patience during my involvement in the manuscript preparation. To my son, Amar, and my daughters, Sali, Eman, and Umnia, for their continued support and follow-up on daily basis. They have all created a conducive environment that enabled me to research and collect relevant information for the book. To all of them I say "thank you," and may "Allah" bless them all.*

*I present this work to all readers with interest in obtaining new information on contemporary issues that affect their lives.*

# Contents

# Preface

An increasing number of genetically modified organisms (GMOs) and transgenic plants continues to be produced every day. One of the main applications and use of GMOs addresses the challenges faced by global agriculture and food. A significant portion of these GMOs have already been approved, or are under approval for use. The development of GMOs and their incorporation in foods and feed proved to be a highly contentious and controversial issue and raised many concerns. In response to these concerns, many national and international authorities have enacted guidelines and regulations to govern and control the use and transport of GMOs and their products. These regulations necessitated the design of methods that can detect and analyze the presence of GMOs or their products in agriculture produce, food, and feed production chains. It is important and helpful to be able to analyze the presence of GMO and non-GMO components and ingredients in food and feed. Design of techniques and instruments that would detect, identify, and quantify GM ingredients in food and feed will help inspection authorities to relay reliable information to consumers who might be concerned about the presence of GM ingredients. Information generated by detection of GMOs in food and feed would be helpful for setting regulations that govern the use of GM components as well as for labeling purposes.

A number of analytical methods for the analysis of GMOs have been developed and are reported in the literature. Marmiroli et al. (2008) have reviewed the different aspects and the analytical methods related to detection, identification, and quantification of GM material within the food and feed chain. Dong et al. (2008) compiled a "GMO Detection Method Database" (GMDD) covering almost all the previously developed and reported GMOs detection methods grouped by different strategies as well as a user-friendly search service of the detection methods.

Qualitative detection methods of GM-DNA sequences in foods and feeds have evolved fast during the past few years (Schreiber 1999). The recent book on genetically modified foods (Mahgoub 2016) includes a section summarizing the methods used for detection, identification, and quantification of GMOs in food and feed. There is a continuous need for the development of more advanced multi-detection systems and for periodic updates of the databases related to these systems. The present publication aims at presenting updates and comprehensive views on the various methods and techniques in use today for the detection, identification, and quantification of GMOs in foods and feed. The methods need to be reliable, standardized, and accurate, so that they are suitable for use under different circumstances.

Chapter 1 gives a comprehensive overview of GMOs. It aims to highlight the basic aspects related to GMOs before going into details of the methods and techniques adopted for their detection, identification, and quantification. The chapter starts by defining GMOs and explains the relationships and links between GMOs and biotechnology.

Other topics covered in the chapter include the techniques followed to produce GMOs, the various ways by which GMOs are used, the controversy surrounding them, and the guidelines and laws governing their regulations. The chapter ends by giving a picture of the perception of consumers and the public awareness on GMOs and products containing them. Recent developments and up-to-date information on GMOs are also included at the end of the chapter.

It is important to realize that in any type of experiment, following the correct steps of sampling is crucial and critical to obtain the accurate and credible results. This needs to be taken into consideration when sampling for GMO testing. A specific sampling plan needs to be designed and followed, depending on the nature of GMO product to be tested, for example, seeds, food, and food ingredient. Chapter 2 deals with the first step of GMO analysis, namely, sampling and sample preparation. The chapter information is drawn from a technical report published by the "European Commission Joint Research Centre, Institute for Health and Consumer Protection" (European Union 2014). This document provides guidelines for a correct sample preparation in GMO analysis on food, feed, seed, plants, and propagating material samples. These guidelines cover the key steps of the sample preparation, i.e., the size of the laboratory sample, the mass reduction techniques, and techniques for comminution and mixing; considerations about the test portion are included and some performance tests to be applied at different steps of the process are provided.

Chapter 3 discusses immunoassays (protein-based) methods commonly used in GMO analysis. These methods are employed for both qualitative (detection) and quantitative (amount) of new foreign proteins added through genetic modification of plants. Immunoassays use antibodies of high level of specificity for the target molecule. There are many different immunoassay formats, and the choice of format is dependent on the target proteins and application. A number of immunoassay techniques are in use. These include Enzyme-Linked Immunosorbent Assay (ELISA), dipstick strip assay, immuno-PCR, Western blot, and dot immuno-binding assay. Details on these methods are covered in the chapter.

Among the various techniques used in GMOs analysis, PCR is the most commonly and widely utilized technique. It acts as a genetic amplification technique that is employed in GMO analysis. Chapter 4 discusses the PCR technique. The author gives detailed information on the application of this technique and of its various formats used for both qualitative and quantitative detection and analysis of GMOs in different plant species and GM derived products.

Chapter 5 deals with sensors, specifically biosensors, in relation to GMO analysis. Biosensors are considered as a cutting-edge technology, as they allow the development of fast and inexpensive analytical methods with desirable properties, such as specificity, sensitivity, reliability, portability, real-time analysis, ease of automation, and simplicity of operation. Following a detailed discussion of the different types of biosensors, the author explains how they can be used as platforms for GMO detection. Schematic illustrations, which help understand how the different formats operate, are included in the chapter.

In Chapter 6, the application of nucleic acid microarrays to the detection of GMOs is discussed. It has been observed that while the real-time PCR assays remain the most widely used technology for GMO monitoring, they are limited to detecting one or a few genetic elements in each assay. Testing for such a large number of different GM crops by single or multiplex real-time PCR is rapidly becoming prohibitively expensive. Therefore, search for other methods that allow high-throughput screening of numerous specific DNA sequences for GMO monitoring continued. One approach that has generated considerable research interest is microarray technology. Microarray technology, also known as DNA chip-technology or biochip, has been developed and used for automated rapid screening of gene expression and sequence variation of large number of samples. It measures the expression levels of large numbers of genes at the same time. Microarrays provide a platform on which anywhere from a few to tens of thousands of specific biomolecules can be detected simultaneously. As a result, significant research efforts have been put into developing microarray-based methods for GMO detection, to overcome the multiplexing limitations of real-time PCR. In this chapter, the essential features of microarrays used for DNA detection are reviewed, the different GMO-specific microarrays that have been developed are compared, and the prospects for the use of this technology in the future are discussed.

Following the detailed discussion of the various GMO detection and analysis methods in use today, Chapter 7 concludes the section by highlighting up-to-date information on recent developments in those methods. The author discusses the results of some recent publications on new developments related to GMO detection and analysis.

Chapter 8 is a guidance document (European Union 2011) on validation and standardization methods for GMO testing, prepared by the European Network of GMO laboratories (ENGL). Any new analytical method evolves through a number of steps. After the initial development and optimization phases, the developing laboratory performs an in-house validation on the method to ensure that the method is fit for the intended purpose. Before the method can be accepted as an International Standard, it needs to be validated in a number of laboratories (European Union 2011). Validation of methods is the process of showing that the combined procedures of sample extraction, preparation, and analysis will yield acceptably accurate, reliable, and reproducible results for a given analysis in a specified matrix. The document covers definitions of the different terms related to validation, for example, verification, precision, laboratory sample, analytical sample, limit of quantification, limit of detection, and describes the steps followed in the validation procedure.

Chapter 9 discusses various aspects related to reference materials used in GMO testing and analysis. The author indicates that the information in the chapter has been extracted from documents published by the European Commission on *Reference Materials for GMO analysis*. Reference material is usually used for calibration or to evaluate and validate the performance of a test method. The reference material has to have a reasonable stability and a homogeneous nature in order to be suitable for application. Different GMOs require different reference materials. The relevant and appropriate reference material needs to be used alongside the test sample under the same conditions. This chapter presents information on certified reference materials, types of available reference materials used in GMO testing, the development of GMO reference materials, and the use of GMO reference materials.

Chapter 10 lists and describes some of the ISO standards designed for identifying and detecting the presence of GM material in foods. These standards are expected to add some degree of transparency to the widely controversial issue of genetic modification particularly when it comes to food and health. Some of the ISO standards presented in the chapter include the following:

- ISO 21569: 2005—Foodstuffs—Methods of analysis for the detection of GMOs and derived products—Qualitative nucleic acid based methods.
- ISO/TS 21569-2:2012—Horizontal methods for molecular biomarker analysis.
- ISO/TS 21569-3:2015—Horizontal methods for molecular biomarker analysis—Methods of analysis for the detection of genetically modified organisms and derived products.
- ISO/TS 21569-5:2016—Horizontal methods for molecular biomarker analysis.

- ISO/TS 21098:2005—Foodstuffs—Nucleic acid based methods of analysis of genetically modified organisms and derived products.
- ISO 21570:2005—Foodstuffs—Methods of analysis for the detection of genetically modified organisms and derived products—Quantitative nucleic acid based methods.
- ISO 21571:2005—Foodstuffs—Methods of analysis for the detection of genetically modified organisms and derived products—Nucleic acid extraction.
- ISO 21572:2013—Foodstuffs—Molecular biomarker analysis—Protein-based methods.
- ISO/AWI 22753—Molecular biomarker analysis—Methods of analysis for the detection of genetically modified organisms.
- ISO 24333:2009—Cereals and cereal products—Sampling.

These standards are usually revised and updated by ISO and the updated versions are published.

Chapter 11 discusses the reference methods used in GMO analysis. For reference methods to be approved for use, they have to be validated through collaborative trials and according to known principles and requirements, for example, ISO, IUPAC, and also they have to be verified by an authorized body, for example, EU-RL GMFF in the context of compliance with a set legislative act. The chapter cites the "EU Database of Reference Methods for GMO Analysis" as one example of the various databases that describe reference methods developed for GMO testing and analysis.

Salah E. O. Mahgoub
*Bay Path University*
*Longmeadow, Massachusetts*

## REFERENCES

Dong, W., Yang, L., Shen, K., et al. 2008. Database GMDD: a database of GMO detection methods. *BMC Bioinformatics*, 9:260, doi: 10.1186/1471-2105-9-260 (pdf). (Also available from: www.biomedcentral.com/1471-2105/9/260 (accessed February 26, 2018).

European Union. 2011. Verification of analytical methods for GMO testing when implementing interlaboratory validated methods. Guidance document from the European Network of GMO laboratories (ENGL), prepared by the ENGL working group on "Method Verification". JRC Scientific and Technical Reports. European Commission Joint Research Centre, Institute for Health and Consumer Protection Report. EUR 24790 EN – 2011.

European Union. 2014. Guidelines for sample preparation procedures in GMO analysis. JRC Technical Report. European Commission Joint Research Centre, Institute for Health and Consumer Protection Report EUR 27021 EN.

Mahgoub, S.E.O. 2016. *Genetically Modified Foods: Basics, Applications, and Controversy*. CRC Press, Taylor & Francis Group, Boca Raton, FL.

Marmiroli, N., Maestri, E., Gullì, M., et al. 2008. Methods for detection of GMOs in food and feed. *Analytical and Bioanalytical Chemistry* 392:369–384.

Schreiber, G.A. 1999. Challenges for methods to detect genetically modified DNA in foods. *Food Control* 10(6):351–352.

# Editors

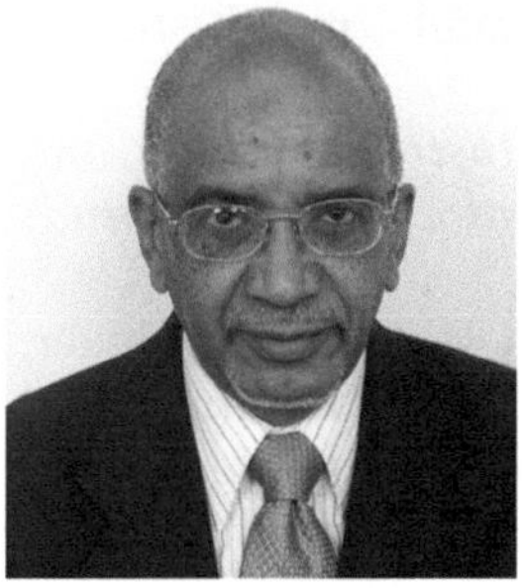

**Salah E. O. Mahgoub** is a Certified Food Scientist (CFS), Professional member of the Institute of Food Technologists (IFT, USA), and Fulbright scholar at Iowa State University, Ames, Iowa, USA. He has a wide international work experience. He has been a professor in the University of Botswana, Botswana, University of Khartoum, Sudan, and an adjunct professor at Kaplan University, and Bay Path University, USA. Mahgoub is a critical thinker with proven experience in food science, food processing, genetically modified foods, functional foods, and nutrition in relation to various consumer issues. Additionally, Mahgoub is an experienced researcher, a team leader, and an effective team player with proven track on developing products from the concept to the shelf and the impact on consumer preferences. Salah E. O. Mahgoub worked as a consultant for FAO, UNICEF, and ministries of health and agriculture in Sudan. He has published a book on GM foods, book chapters, 40 articles and conference proceedings in peer reviewed journals, and presented and participated in 42 conferences and workshops globally.

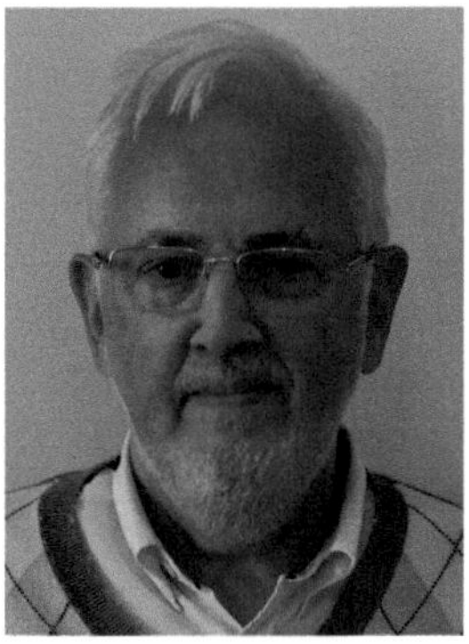

**Leo M. L. Nollet, PhD,** received an MS (1973) and PhD (1978) in biology from the Katholieke Universiteit Leuven, Belgium. He is an editor and associate editor of numerous books. He edited for M. Dekker, New York—now CRC Press of Taylor & Francis—the first, second, and third editions of the books entilted *Food Analysis by HPLC* and *Handbook of Food Analysis*. The last edition is a two-volume book. He also edited the *Handbook of Water Analysis* (first, second, and third editions) and *Chromatographic Analysis of the Environment*, Third and Fourth Edition (CRC Press).

With F. Toldrá he coedited two books published in 2006 and 2007, and 2017: *Advanced Technologies for Meat Processing* (CRC Press) and *Advances in Food Diagnostics* (Blackwell Publishing—now Wiley). With M. Poschl he coedited the book *Radionuclide Concentrations in Foods and the Environment* also published in 2006 (CRC Press).

Dr. Nollet has also coedited several books with Y. H. Hui and other colleagues: *Handbook of Food Product Manufacturing* (Wiley, 2007), *Handbook of Food Science, Technology, and Engineering* (CRC Press, 2005), *Food Biochemistry and Food Processing* (first and second editions; Blackwell Publishing—now Wiley—2006 and 2012), and the *Handbook of Fruits and Vegetable Flavors* (Wiley, 2010).

In addition, he edited the *Handbook of Meat, Poultry and Seafood Quality*, first and second editions, (Blackwell Publishing—now Wiley—2007 and 2012).

From 2008 to 2011, he published five volumes on animal product-related books with F. Toldrá, namely, the *Handbook of Muscle Foods Analysis*, the *Handbook of Processed Meats and Poultry Analysis*, the *Handbook of Seafood and Seafood Products Analysis*, the *Handbook of Dairy Foods Analysis*, and the *Handbook of Analysis of Edible Animal By-Products*. Also in 2011, he coedited two volumes with F. Toldrá for CRC Press: *Safety Analysis of Foods of Animal Origin and Sensory Analysis of Foods of Animal Origin*. In 2012, they both published the *Handbook of Analysis of Active Compounds in Functional Foods*.

In a coedition with Hamir Rathore, the book *Handbook of Pesticides: Methods of Pesticides Residues Analysis* was marketed in 2009, *Pesticides: Evaluation of Environmental Pollution* in 2012, *Biopesticides Handbook* in 2015 and *Green Pesticides Handbook: Essential Oils for Pest Control* in 2017.

Other finished book projects include *Food Allergens: Analysis, Instrumentation, and Methods* (with A. van Hengel; CRC Press, 2011) and *Analysis of Endocrine Compounds in Food* (Wiley-Blackwell, 2011).

Dr. Nollet's recent projects include *Proteomics in Foods* with F. Toldrá (Springer, 2013) and *Transformation Products of Emerging Contaminants in the Environment: Analysis, Processes, Occurrence, Effects and Risks* with D. Lambropoulou (Wiley, 2014).

In the series, Food Analysis & Properties, he edited with C. Ruiz-Capillas, *Flow Injection Analysis of Food Additives* (CRC Press, 2015), *Marine Microorganisms: Extraction and Analysis of Bioactive Compounds* (CRC Press, 2016), with A.S. Franca, *Spectroscopic Methods in Food Analysis* (CRC Press, 2017), with Horacio Heinzen and Amadeo R. Fernandez-Alba, *Multiresidue Methods for the Analysis of Pesticide Residues in Food* (CRC Press, 2017) and with Janet Alejandra Gutierréz Ulrinbe, *Phenolic Compounds in Food: Characterization and Analysis* (CRC Press, 2018).

# List of Contributors

**Gilbert Berben**
Walloon Agricultural Research Center (CRA-W)
Department Valorization of Agricultural Products
Unit Authentication and Traceability
Gembloux, Belgium

**Frédéric Debode**
Walloon Agricultural Research Center (CRA-W)
Department Valorization of Agricultural Products
Unit Authentication and Traceability
Gembloux, Belgium

**Francesco Gatto**
Joint Research Centre
Brussels, Belgium

**O. Goerlich**
Joint Research Centre
Brussels, Belgium

**Lutz Grohmann**
Joint Research Centre
Brussels, Belgium

**Lotte Hougs**
Joint Research Centre
Brussels, Belgium

**Rajesh Kumar**
Department of Genetics and Plant Breeding
Institute of Agricultural Sciences, RGSC
Banaras Hindu University
Mirzapur, India

**K. Lieske**
Joint Research Centre
Brussels, Belgium

**Stuart J. Lucas**
Sabanci University Nanotechnology Research and Application Center (SUNUM)
Sabanci University
Istanbul, Turkey

**Marta Sánchez-Paniagua López**
Department of Chemistry in Pharmaceutical Sciences
Analytical Chemistry Teaching Unit
Pharmacy Faculty
Complutense University of Madrid
Madrid, Spain

**Beatriz López-Ruiz**
Department of Chemistry in Pharmaceutical Sciences
Analytical Chemistry Teaching Unit
Pharmacy Faculty
Complutense University of Madrid
Madrid, Spain

**Salah E. O. Mahgoub**
Bay Path University
Longmeadow, MA, United States of America

**Carmen Lorena Manzanares-Palenzuela**
Department of Inorganic Chemistry
University of Chemistry and Technology Prague
Prague, Czech Republic

**Marco Mazzara**
Joint Research Centre
Brussels, Belgium

**Frank Narendja**
Joint Research Centre
Brussels, Belgium

**Leo M. L. Nollet**
University College Ghent
Gent, Belgium

**J. Ovesna**
Joint Research Centre
Brussels, Belgium

**Nina Papazova**
Joint Research Centre
Brussels, Belgium

**I.M.J. Scholtens**
Joint Research Centre
Brussels, Belgium

**Vishal Srivashtav**
Department of Genetics and Plant Breeding
Institute of Agricultural Sciences, RGSC
Banaras Hindu University
Mirzapur, India

**Abhilasha Tripathi**
Department of Neurology
Sanjay Gandhi Postgraduate Institute of Medical Sciences
Lucknow, India

**Jana Zel**
Joint Research Centre
Brussels, Belgium

# SECTION 1

# GMOs

# CHAPTER 1

# Genetically Modified Organisms

*Salah E. O. Mahgoub*
Bay Path University

CONTENTS



## 1.1 WHAT ARE GENETICALLY MODIFIED ORGANISMS?

Genetically modified organisms (GMOs) continue to come in the news every day and being debated for a long time between supporters and opposers. The first question that needs an answer is "what are GMOs." GMOs is an acronym for "genetically modified organisms." Although a number of alternate terms, which include genetically altered organisms and genetically engineered organisms (GEOs), are sometimes used, clear differences can be drawn among these terms. The term "genetically altered" or "genetically modified organisms" can be used to mean changing the genetic makeup of a living organism using traditional (e.g., crossbreeding) or new methods (transgenesis). On the other hand, the term "genetically engineered organisms" refers to a very precise method of transferring genes among living organisms to achieve a defined goal. Generally, we find that genetic modification (GM) and genetic engineering (GE) are used synonymously.

A number of definitions have been presented for the term "genetically modified organisms," depending on the level of details included in the definition. According to the World Health Organization (WHO 2014), GMOs can be defined as "organisms in which the genetic material (DNA) has been altered in a way that does not occur naturally." GMOs are plants, animals, or microorganisms that have their genetic structure modified. They are produced because they can add some advantages such as lower price, longer durability or higher nutritional value, or both. Any organism in which the genetic material has been changed in a manner that does not occur naturally by mating and/or natural recombination would be regarded as a GMO. Generally, any living thing that has been genetically modified would be referred to as GMO.

The "Health and Safety Executive" website (2017) defines GMOs as organisms whose genes have been artificially altered to modify their characteristics in some way or another. It elaborates on the process of GM stating that it is the process of altering the genetic material of an organism by using a method that does not occur in nature. Often GM involves isolating and removing the DNA encoding a single gene from one organism, manipulating it outside the cell (in a laboratory) and reinserting it into the same organism or into the genetic material of another organism. The aim of GM is often to introduce a new or altered characteristic to the target organism.

The NON GMO Project (2017) defines a GMO as any living organism (plant, animal, and microorganism) in which the genetic makeup has been modified using recombinant DNA methods (also called gene splicing), gene modification, or transgenic technology. This definition more or less describes genetic engineering, which is considered as one type of GM. GM can be used to refer to "changing of a specific gene in an organism," whereas GE can be used to denote "transfer of genes from one living organism to another living organism." The term GMO does not always imply, but can include, targeted insertions of genes from one organism into another described as GE. GE is a more specifically defined type of GM that leads to the development of a GMO designated as a "transgenic organism." This is an organism whose genetic makeup has been altered by the addition of genetic material from an unrelated organism.

The Cartagena Protocol (Husby 2007) gives some related definitions. It defines living organism (LO) as any biological entity capable of transferring or replicating genetic material, including sterile organisms, viruses, and viroids, and living modified organism (LMO) as any living organism that possesses a novel combination of genetic material obtained through the use of modern biotechnology. On the other hand, the European Union (EU) Directive 2001/18/EC, Article 2, 1) 2, 2a, 2b, and article 3 defines "organism" as any biological entity capable of replicating or transferring genetic material, and GMO as an organism, with the exception of human beings, in which the genetic material has been altered in a way that does not occur naturally by mating and/or natural recombination.

As stated earlier, GMOs can be plants, animals, or (most commonly) microorganisms. If the GMO is a microorganism, it is typically referred to as a genetically modified microorganism (GMM). Although humans may undergo GM, for example, during gene therapy, they are not legally regarded as GMOs. A GMO that is a plant or an animal can be referred to as a larger GMO (LGMO) (Health and Safety Executive 2017).

The Penn State College of Agricultural Sciences (2015) summarizes the sequence of events that lead to the introduction of GM. The process of evolution, which involves natural change in living organisms, takes place over time. This natural process usually takes a long time to happen. This prompted interested observers to intervene to speed up, direct, and control the process of evolution to improve the traits of living organisms. Individual organisms that showed desirable characteristics were selected and crossed with organisms with similar traits. This process represented the early human intervention to manipulate the genetic makeup of living organisms, which continued to develop and improve over time until it reached the genetic engineering stage used today. To achieve outcomes that once took thousands of years and countless failures, scientists are now turning to genetic engineering techniques, which enable them to speed up the process of evolution and fine-tune it to create precise changes in the physical attributes of organisms to achieve certain benefits.

It is important to have some control measures to manage and limit contact between GMOs and humans and the surrounding environment. This is needed to provide and guarantee a high level of safety: an issue very much geared to the production of GMOs. The term "contained use" has been introduced to cover any activity involving GMOs where physical, chemical, or biological barriers are used as control measures to limit contact between GMOs and humans or the environment and provide a high level of safety. It relates to the actual process of GM and also to the use, storage, transport and destruction of GMOs (Health and Safety Executive 2017).

"NON GMO" is an opposing term to GMO introduced by the "NON GMO Project." The NON-GMO Project Standard sets detailed specifications to define a non-GMO ingredient, which states: "an ingredient can be classified as high risk if it is derived from, contains derivatives of, or is produced through a process involving organisms that are known to be genetically modified and commercially produced" (NON GMO Project 2017). Animal-derived food products, such as meat, eggs, dairy, and honey, are considered to fall under the high-risk category set by the non-GMO Project. This is due to the incorporation of high levels of GMOs in animal feed.

## 1.2 GMOs AND BIOTECHNOLOGY

Many people think that biotechnology is a relatively new discipline that is getting a lot of attention only recently and that it involves only new sophisticated processes. For many, "biotechnology" is synonymous with the production of GMOs (also known as transgenics). It is important to differentiate between "biotechnology" and "GMOs" and explain the relationship that exists between them. Biotechnology is a term that encompasses all the technologies that deal with living organisms. It is derived from the two words "biological" and "technology." The word "biotechnology" originated from a cross between two Greek words, namely, "bios" (which refers to everything to do with life) and "technikos" (meaning involving human knowledge and skills) (EuropaBio 2017). Biotechnology could be viewed as a multidisciplinary area of study since it is based on, and linked to, other basic biological sciences, such as genetics, cell biology, microbiology, biochemistry, molecular biology, and tissue culture. Biotechnology is a collective term for a group of technologies that use biological matter or processes to generate new and useful products and processes. As such, it ranges in complexity and maturity from ancient brewing and bread-making techniques to GM through hybridization and interbreeding of plants and animals, as well as the manipulation of individual genes in humans, animals, plants, and microorganisms (UNCTAD Secretariat 2002).

Mahgoub (2016) has summarized the historical developments in biotechnology. The biotechnology timeline indicates that biotechnology applications go back to about thousands of years BC. The timeline covers up-to-date applications of biotechnology.

The diversity in the use of biotechnology as a tool in the scientific and industrial arenas has made it necessary to have a system to classify biotechnology applications based on common features or final purpose. Five main groups in biotechnological applications have been identified by a color system (Martínez 2011). They are designated as red, white, green, gray, and blue biotechnologies. The red biotechnology is used to define the various biotechnologies used in, or related to, medicine; white biotechnology, also referred to as "industrial biotechnology," encompasses all the biotechnology applications related to industrial processes; the green biotechnology focuses on agriculture; gray biotechnology is used to describe all applications of biotechnology that are directly related to the environment; and blue biotechnology describes technologies applied for marine and aquatic resources (Mahgoub 2016).

Biotechnology is considered as a key technology for the new millennium. It has an immense range of applications in agriculture, medicine, food processing, environmental protection, mining, and even nanoelectronics (UNCTAD Secretariat 2002). The range of applications that benefit from biotechnology spans from traditional uses such as production of bread, alcohol, and cheese to more modern applications such as its use in the production of GMOs. In that sense, GMOs production falls under the umbrella of biotechnology, being one of the modern applications of biotechnology. Various tools of biotechnology are used to produce GMOs. Some of the areas, under the disciplines of agriculture, pharmacology, and medicine, that utilize biotechnology are molecular biology, microbiology, embryology, cell and tissue culture, and genetic engineering. In the field of health, biotechnology has been widely used for the development and production of drugs, vaccines, and diagnostics. Biotechnology has also been used in pharmocogenomics, which deals with individual response to drugs based on genetic makeup. Gene therapy, which involves the genetic engineering of a patient's genetic code to remove or replace a mutant gene that is causing disease, is yet another area where biotechnology is applied. Another area in which biotechnology is being recently utilized is the "Human Genome Project" (UNCTAD Secretariat 2002).

"Genetic modification" is a general term that encompasses both old and new biotechnologies. Broadly, biotechnology can be divided into two major branches (Shrestha 2010):

- Non-gene biotechnology (old biotechnology)—processes and procedures that deal with whole cells, tissues, or even individual organisms.
- Gene biotechnology (new biotechnology)—techniques that involve gene manipulation, cloning, and similar processes.

GM, sometimes known as "transgenic technology" and "genetic engineering," is a type of modern biotechnology that comprises a set of techniques used to manipulate, change, or engineer the genetic material, DNA, of a living organism. These techniques enable scientists to cut and join, mutate, copy and multiply genes, and subsequently, isolate and transfer them from one organism to another, resulting in what is known as a "genetically modified organism".

GE and GM are often used interchangeably when referring to varieties of crops developed by means other than traditional breeding. GM refers to a range of methods (such as selection, hybridization, and induced mutation) used to alter the genetic composition of domesticated plants and animals to achieve a desired result. GE is one type of GM that involves the intentional introduction of a targeted change in a plant, animal, or microbial gene sequence to achieve a specific result (NC State Extension 2017). It can thus be said that GE describes more precisely the modern technique of transgenesis. It seems that this confusion came from the usage by popular media and became the norm even by scientists.

GE is considered as one of the modern applications of biotechnology. It is a biotechnological application where the DNA or genes of organisms are manipulated according to a specific requirement. An identified gene of other organisms that are responsible for a certain function is isolated, and it is introduced into another organism, let the gene express, and benefit from it (Naveen 2012). The organism to whom the gene has been introduced is called the GMO or GEO.

## 1.3 HOW ARE GMOs PRODUCED?

It was explained earlier that GM falls under the umbrella of biotechnology. Both conventional and modern biotechnological techniques are used to produce GMOs. The conventional biotechnology techniques used in agriculture, which are also referred to as non-GE techniques or old biotechnology techniques, include the following types (Mahgoub 2016):

- Simple selection
- Marker-assisted selection
- Crossing
- Interspecies crossing
- Embryo rescue
- Somatic hybridization
- Somaclonal variation
- Mutation breeding
- Plant tissue culture and micropropagation

These techniques have been in use in agriculture for a long time and have resulted in plants that did not exist naturally.

The modern biotechnological techniques usually describe the techniques used in GE. The following methods represent some of the GE techniques applied today to induce desired changes in the genetic makeup of agricultural crops:

- Microbial vectors (including bacterial carriers and viral carriers)
- Electorporation
- Microinjection
- Microprojectile bombardment
- Gene splicing
- Gene silencing
- Calcium phosphate precipitation
- Lipofection

The discovery of the transfer of DNA from one living organism to another came in the year 1946. The first genetically engineered plant—an antibiotic-resistant tobacco plant—was developed in 1983. One of the first food-related GMOs developed through GE was the Flavr Savr tomato. The California-based Calgene company produced it from tomato seeds genetically modified to contain the ACC synthase gene, which delays ripening until after picking (Takepart 2017). The production of Flavr Savr tomato helped the initiation of further work to produce GE crops, which led to the production of *Bacillus thuringiensis* (Bt) crops including canola, corn, soybean, potatoes, and squash. Some of the traits achieved by GE include ability of the plant to produce its own pesticide, resistance to herbicides, and resistance to viruses. Another positive property achieved by GE is the enhancement of nutrients in food crops. In the year 2000, scientists genetically modified rice to increase its vitamin A content, marking the first time the technology was used to increase food's nutrient content (Takepart 2017).

The process of GE involves the following basic steps: identifying a trait of interest, isolating that genetic trait, inserting that trait into the genome of a desired organism, and then growing the engineered organism (Powell 2015).

Following are details of the steps followed in GE:

Step 1: Nucleic acid (DNA/RNA) Extraction

In any isolation procedure, the initial step is the disruption of the cell in order to break the cell wall of the organism containing the desired trait, which may be viral, bacterial, or plant cells. This helps the extraction of the nucleic acid.

Step 2: Gene Cloning

The cloning process involves four stages: generation of DNA fragments, joining to a vector, propagation in a host cell, and selection of the required sequence.

Step 3: Gene Design and Packaging

Once the desired gene has been cloned, it has to be linked to pieces of DNA that will control its expression inside the plant cell

Step 4: Transformation (Gene insertion)

Step 5: Backcross Breeding

This process involves crossing the transgenic plants produced with elite breeding lines or commercial varieties that already have the desired agronomic traits but lack the trait of the transgene.

Those steps are started in the biotechnology lab, then transferred to the green house for initial growth and finally taken to the field where the crop develops to its maturity.

## 1.4 THE CONTROVERSY ABOUT GMOs

In recent history, there are a few issues that have received more attention and wider debate than the use of biotechnology, specifically GE, to produce GMOs and GM foods. I believe that the world population may be viewed as belonging to one of three groups with regard to GMOs and GM foods production and use: proponents, opponents, and the confused. Beliefs concerning GMOs tend to be dominated by two opposing narratives: GMO critics despise corporate control and greed, and fear the unnatural, while GMO advocates see this technology as an example of the triumph of human ingenuity and science (Novella 2014).

The debate on the various issues related to GMOs and GM foods, for example, production, labeling, consumption, safety, ethics, and socioeconomics, has mounted to a seemingly level of a war. It seems to be a war of words and exchange of views rather than an exchange of facts and credible information (Mahgoub 2016).

There is wide controversy over GMOs, especially with regard to their use in producing food. The dispute involves different parties including buyers, biotechnology companies, governmental regulators, nongovernmental organizations, and scientists.

The main areas of debate and controversy encompass the actual and potential effects of GM crops and GM foods on human and animal health and on the environment, the effect on pesticide resistance, the credibility, and objectivity of conducted and published research on gene technology and GM foods, whether GM food should be labeled, the impact of gene technology and GM crops on farmers, the expected role of government regulators, the conflict of interest among biotechnology companies, researchers, and government regulators, and the possible role of GM foods in feeding the world population and helping to reduce food insecurity worldwide.

The key issues of concern surrounding production and use of GMOs, which prompted the controversy surrounding them, have been discussed by Mahgoub (2016) and include:

- Concerns about food safety and human health
- Environmental concerns
- Ethical concerns
- Regulatory and legal concerns
- Economic concerns
- Animal health and welfare
- Consumer choice
- Concerns about bias in scientific publishing

### 1.4.1 Proponents and Opponents of the GM Technology

Examples of supporters of the GM technology include its developers and users, some governments, and governments' institutions, such as regulators, United Nations (UN) organizations, for example, Food and Agricultural Organization (FAO), World Health Organization (WHO), and some consumers. On the opposing side, there are a number of international groups and institutions that are against production of GM foods. Some examples include the Greenpeace, Friends of the Earth, the Christian Aid, the Institute for Food and Development Policy, and some consumers. The following lists reflect examples of the two groups:

- Proponents (Supporters):
  - International bodies and governments of some countries
    - UN and other international bodies, for example, Food and Agriculture Organization (FAO), World Health Organization (WHO), Consultative Group on International Agricultural Research (CGIAR), World Trade Organization (WTO), World Food Programme (WFP), World Bank and International Monetary Fund (IMF), and Organization for Economic Co-operation and Development (OECD)
    - U.S. government departments, for example, Food and Drug Administration (FDA), U.S. Department of Agriculture (USDA), and U.S. Agency for International Development (USAID).
    - U.K. bodies, for example, Department of Environment, Food, and Rural Affairs (DEFRA), Food Standards Agency (FSA), Advisory Committee on Releases to the Environment (ACRE), Advisory Committee on Novel Foods and Processes (ACNFP), Biotechnology and Biological Sciences Research Council (BBSRC), Department for International Development (DFID), National Farmers' Union (NFU), John Innes Centre (JIC), and The Royal Society (RS)

- Biotech, agrochemical, and associated companies, including
  - Monsanto
  - Syngenta
  - Bayer
  - DuPont/Pioneer Hi-Bred
  - Cargill
  - Advanta
  - Dow
- Pro-GM lobby groups
  - International Service for the Acquisition of Agri-Biotech Applications (ISAAA)
  - International Food Information Council Foundation
  - Biotechnology Industry Organization (BIO)
  - The American Association for the Advancement of Science (AAAS)
  - American Soybean Association (ASA)
  - National Corn Growers Association (NCGA)
  - European Association for Bioindustries (EuropaBio)
  - AfricaBio
  - AusBiotech Ltd
  - Agricultural Biotechnology Council (ABC)
  - CropGen
  - Crop Protection Association (CPA)
  - Sense About Science (SAS)
  - The Grocery Manufacturers Association (GMA)
  - Food and Drink Federation (FDF)
  - Institute of Ideas (IoI)
  - Science Media Centre (SMC)
  - Scientific Alliance (SA)
  - International Policy Network (IPN)
  - Global network of pro-corporate activists

- Opponents (Critics)
  - In the United States
    - Californians for GE-Free Agriculture
    - Campaign to Label Genetically Engineered Food
    - Center for Food Safety (CFS)
    - Council for Responsible Genetics (CRG)
    - Earth Liberation Front
    - Farmer to Farmer Campaign on Genetic Engineering
    - Friends of the Earth, (FoE)
    - GE Food Alert
    - Genetic Engineering Action Network (GEAN)
    - Greenpeace
    - Food First (Institute for Food and Development Policy)
    - Institute for Responsible Technologies
    - Keep Nature Natural
    - Northeast Resistance Against Genetic Engineering, (neRAGE)
    - Northwest Resistance Against Genetic Engineering (NW RAGE)
    - Organic Consumers Association
    - Rural Advancement Foundation International (RAFI)

- Sierra Club
- True Food Network
- The Union of Concerned Scientists
- The American Academy of Environmental Medicine (AAEM)

• In Europe
- ActionAid
- Blueridge Institute, Switzerland
- Christian Aid, United Kingdom
- Confederation Paysanne, Via Campesina, France
- Five Year Freeze
- Foundation for Organic and biodynamic research (FIRAB), Italy
- Friends of the Earth Europe
- Friends of the Earth, United Kingdom
- Genetics Forum
- GeneWatch
- Greenpeace EU
- Greenpeace, United Kingdom
- HDRA, United Kingdom
- Institute of Science in Society (ISIS)
- International Coalition to Protect the Polish Countryside (ICPPC), Poland
- Italian Association for Organic Agriculture (AIAB), Italy
- National Trust, United Kingdom
- Navdanya International
- NGIN/GM Watch
- Oxfam
- Pesticide Action Network
- Save our Seeds (SOS), Germany
- Scientists for global responsibility, United Kingdom
- Soil Association, United Kingdom
- The Green Alliance, United Kingdom
- The Green Party, United Kingdom
- VAS (Verdi Amviente e Societa Onlus)—Italia Green Environment and Society Italy
- Vegetarian Society, United Kingdom
- Wildlife Trusts
- Women's Environmental Network
- Women's Institute
- World Development Movement, United Kingdom
- World Peace Culture Fund Genetic Resources Conservation, Russia

• In Canada, Australia, and New Zealand
- Earthsave Canada
- Greenpeace Australia
- Gene Ethics, Australia
- Madge, Australia (Mothers are Demystifying Genetic Engineering)
- Greenpeace New Zealand

• In Africa
- African Biodiversity Network (ABN)
- African Centre for Biosafety

  - Biowatch South Africa
  - Earth Life Africa
  - Friends of the Earth, Africa. Friends of the Earth South Africa/groundwork
  - Gaia Foundation
- In Central and South America
  - Amigos della Tiera Uruguay (REDES)
  - Center of Studies for rural Change in Mexico (CECCAM) Mexico
  - Conservation Land Trust, Patagonia
  - Network for a GE Free Latin America (RALLT)
  - Sociedad Peruana de Derecho Ambiental (SPDA)
  - The Peruvian Environmental Law Society (Peru)
  - Uruguay Sustentable (Uruguay)
- In Asia
  - Navdanya, India
  - No! GMO Campaign, Japan

### 1.4.2 Arguments in Favor of GMOs and GM Foods

Supporters of GMOs production, and their applications in GM foods, present their case on the basis that these technologies have multiple benefits. The cited benefits include benefits for the farmers who grow crops using GM, benefits for the consumers, the economy, and the environment. There are other points stated by GMOs supporters that justify their claims. More details of their arguments are presented in the following sections.

Arguments presented by supporters are that GM could be used as a tool to improve characteristics of plants and animals, that it could help to reduce the extent of hunger and malnutrition worldwide, it could also reduce cost of production of plants and animals and hence helps food producers, and that there is no proven examples or cases of GM products adding health or environmental risks.

GMO advocates point out that GM technology is nothing new, and that it is simply an extension of the various technologies we have used for thousands of years to alter organisms. In any case, they claim that "the: it's not natural" argument is fallacious. Meanwhile, GMO should be looked upon as a powerful technology, and such technologies can have both powerfully good and powerfully bad consequences depending on how they are used. Pretty much all the food consumed by humans have already been extensively modified by human activity, for example through artificial selection or cross-pollination (Novella 2014).

The, US-based, Illinois Farm Bureau (IFB), which is a strong supporter of crop biotechnology, states "increased efforts through biotechnology to more rapidly develop traits which have recognized consumer benefits in order to: increase the marketability of our products, enhance the environment, increase net farm income, improve product quality, enhance U.S. agriculture's competitiveness in the world market and ensure worldwide consumers of stable, ample, safe, and nutritious U.S. products."(The Illinois Farm Bureau 2017).

Proponents of genetically modified foods say they are completely safe for human consumption and that no negative effect associated with their use has been found. They also say the cultivation of GE foods is necessary for increasing crop yields around the world and to dramatically cut back world hunger. Consumers around the world have been eating genetically modified foods for a long time, and purchasing them at cheaper prices (Takepart 2017).

The safety and the potential health effects of GMO food have been continuously investigated. Large volumes of research results show that existing GMOs are safe for human consumption and as animal feed. These conclusions have been endorsed by many renounced and credible professional bodies such as The American Association for the Advancement of Science (AAAS), The National Academies of Science (NAS), The World Health Organization (WHO). Critics claim there has not been enough testing (Novella 2014).

The "Health and Safety Executive" website (2017) states that the vast majority of work with GMOs in contained use is inherently safe. It is, therefore, very important to assess the risks of all activities and make sure that any necessary controls are put in place to protect people and the environment. It recommends that risk assessments for such work must be submitted to the regulatory authorities for approval before work can commence. The regulatory authorities are thus in a position to ensure that the work is carried out in facilities and equipment that contain the infectious materials during the work activities.

### 1.4.3 Arguments against GMOs and GM Foods

The basic argument presented by the opponents of GM technology is that there is no need for its application since there are better alternatives to it. The alternatives suggested include traditional breeding, non-GM biotechnology, and the use of organic agriculture.

One criticism of GM technology cited by its opponents is that, while it may be good for applications that require 1–2 genes to accomplish, some traits (like drought resistance) involve many genes. Traditional breeding techniques might therefore be better for such complex traits.

In their published report on "GMO Myths and Truths," Fagan et al. (2014), who are very strong opponents and critics of GMOs, claim that "there is no need to take risks with GM crops when effective, readily available, and sustainable solutions to the problems that GM technology is claimed to address already exist. Conventional plant breeding, in some cases helped by safe modern technologies like gene mapping and marker assisted selection, continues to outperform GM in producing high-yield, drought-tolerant, and pest- and disease-resistant crops that can meet our present and future food needs." They also believe that the quality and efficacy of our food production system depends only partly on crop genetics while the other part of the equation is farming methods. The report strongly crticized GM technology stating that "GM crops and foods are promoted on the basis of a range of far-reaching claims from the industry and its supporters." It included a long list of "myth" and "truth" under separate headings to refute the claims presented by GM technology supporters. The following headings were used:

- The genetic engineering technique
- Science and regulation
- Health hazards of GM foods
- Health hazards of Roundup and glyphosate
- GM crops—impacts on the farm and environment
- Feeding the world

The concerns raised against production of GM products are that consumption of GM foods may be a health hazard and that these foods may be unsafe for human consumption. Another concern raised is that GM may lead to a potential damage to the environment and undesirable changes and disruption to the entire ecosystem. The arguments presented to support these concerns are: the technology is unnatural and it may lead to unpredictable results, unexpected and unintended side effects; GM products are hazardous, their long-term use can produce ill effects on health; it degrades the environment, and erode biodiversity by spreading harmful genes leading to what is known as genetic pollution; it may cause allergies; it may lead to antibiotic resistance; GM might lead to elimination of indigenous agriculture and the loss of natural species; GM technology can lead to pollution and sterility of agricultural soil; GM may result in the extinction of seed varieties and lead to destruction of forest life; there are ethical and moral objections and that people are "messing with nature," raising the question "Do human beings have the right to view nature as their commodity, and alter the genetic structure of living things to correct what some perceive as their "deficiencies?" Critics also say the proliferation of genetically modified herbicide-resistant crops has led to the mutation of "superweeds" and "superpests" and insects that are impervious to herbicides and pesticides. This has led to an increase in the use of pesticides and herbicides since GE crops were introduced in U.S. agriculture. They claim that some farmers who grow and sell organic produce have experienced cross contamination from GE fields (Takepart 2017).

Three of the groups opposing GMOs and their use in GM foods, namely, The Organic Consumers Association (organicconsumers.org), The Union of Concerned Scientists (ucsusa.org), and Greenpeace (greenpeace.org), state that risks associated with GMOs have not been adequately identified and managed. They are also concerned about the objectivity of the work done by the regulatory authorities with regard to the safety of GMOs. Other concerns raised by these groups include the possible contamination of the non-GM food products, the potential damaging effects of GMOs on the environment, and the need for strict control of the food supply in companies that produce and market GMOs.

Opponents of GMOs also point to the fact that only a few powerful companies, like Monsanto, Syngenta, and Dow, control both the GM of seeds and the production of the pesticides and herbicides these crops are designed to withstand. GM has even led to the patenting of certain seeds, and Monsanto has sued farmers for saving and replanting seeds the company "owns" (Takepart 2017).

With regard to the issue of the safety of GMOs, critics say that there is no scientific consensus to support the claim that GMOs and products derived from them are safe for human or animal use. They indicate that results of many investigations show that GMOs cause harm to humans and animals when incorporated in food or animal feed.

Popular protests against GMOs and GM foods continue to be organized in different parts of the world, representing the voice of those opposing the production and use of GMOs. The rallies took place in different parts of the world, for example, Buenos Aires and other Argentinian cities, Portland, Oregon, and Los Angeles, USA and Kitchener, Ontario, Canada. The total number of protesters who took part and reported by different sources vary from hundreds of thousands (Hilbeck et al. 2015) to two million (Fusaro 2013). According to organizers, protesters in 436 cities and 52 countries took part in these protests (BBC News 2012; Sense About Science 2012).

Mahgoub (2016) reported some examples of those protests. In May 2012, a group called "Take the Flour Back" led by Gerald Miles protested against plans by a group from Rothamsted Experimental Station, based in Harpenden, Hertfordshire, England, to stage an experimental trial to use genetically modified wheat to repel aphids (Gaskell et al. 2010). On May 25, 2013, the "March Against Monsanto" movement held rallies in protest against companies that produce GM seed (Kopicki 2013). Sleenhoff and Osseweijer (2013) reported that more than two million people in fifty countries worldwide marched against Monsanto. The protest was ignited because of the adoption of what is now called the "Monsanto Protection Act." According to its critics, the act allows for the planting of unapproved GM crops in the United States, overruling previous court orders designed to protect the environment, people's health, and well-being.

Vandalism and threats by anti-GMO activists have also been reported in some rare cases. A few activist groups such as Earth Liberation Front and Greenpeace have vandalized GMO research in different parts of the world (CTV News Kitchener 2013; Harmon 2013; Quick 2013; Yahoo News AP. 2013). Some European countries including the United Kingdom witnessed the destruction of crop trials, belonging to academic or governmental research institutions, by protesters. Extreme cases of threats and violence against people and property were also reported (Pollack 2013). In the United States, anti-GMO groups burned the biotechnology laboratory of Michigan State University causing the destruction of property worth hundreds of thousands of dollars and the loss of research results (Experts 2014). Other incidents of violence and property damage against GMOs have also been reported in other parts of the globe, for example, in Australia in 2011 (CTV News Kitchener 2013; von Mogel 2013) and in Philippines in 2013 (Australian Broadcasting Corporation (ABC) News 2013; Science Daily 2013).

A more reasonable and prudent approach to deal with GMOs and GM foods would be to address the relevant facts and then conduct a robust and complete analysis of the appropriateness of a specific technology in relation to its intended target country or region. It is not objective to generalize that GE crops and GM foods are either unequivocally Frankenfoods or Miracle Crops. A rational approach would require judging GE crops on a case-by-case basis while considering all the costs, benefits, and risks estimated through robust assessments (Falck-Zepeda et al. 2013).

Both sides need to realize and express potential benefits and possible risks, hazards and threats of GM foods. It needs to be emphasized that no human activity is entirely risk-free, and that certainly no food, whether produced through GM or traditional techniques, is. This does not mean that we should believe in, or fully trust modern technologies, such as GM, without thorough study. Possible risks should be identified, evaluated and reduced as much as possible, to a safe level. There is an urgent need to emphasize that scientific findings are not expected to give clear-cut answers to pertinent questions on GM technology and GM foods, and should not be taken as the ultimate goal to end the debate surrounding GM foods.

GMOs are neither a panacea nor menace. GM is simply a powerful technology, and its impact will depend entirely on how it is used. In fact, it is difficult to talk about GMOs as if they are one thing, and when someone does they are likely speaking from an ideological position. Rather, each individual GMO needs to be assessed on its own risks and merits. Like many technologies, what matters most is how it is used (Novella 2014).

The Workshop Report published by the National Research Council of the National Academies (2008) recommends a more reasonable approach to the biotechnology and GE issue. The main focus of the report was on agricultural biotechnology, which relates more to GM crops and GM foods. The report states that the advent of agricultural biotechnology was marked by a wide array of debates inspired by concerns about safety. Those concerns were shaped by public perceptions that tended to emphasize the risks associated with agricultural biotechnology. It believes that the concerns were justified and had to be taken seriously, they tended to downplay the potential benefits of the technology. Moreover, much of the debate about agricultural biotechnology was shaped by advocacy efforts aimed at particular policy objectives. It suggests that careful and credible investigations on the potentials, the benefits, the opportunities, as well as the challenges related to the applications of biotechnology and its use in GE need to be conducted. Future considerations in realizing the global potential of agricultural biotechnology needs to be realized as well.

There is a need to identify important current and emerging global problems and then explore the possible application of biotechnology as one of many approaches to ease the problems, recognizing that all new technologies carry scientific and socioeconomic risks. Making use of the knowledge-based approaches to decision-making would be helpful in taking the appropriate decision and in addressing different issues amicably.

A more recent report published by the National Academies of Sciences, Engineering, and Medicine (2016) reflects yet another effort to present a more reasonable approach to the controversy around GE technology. The report covered GE crops through the year 2015 and focused on the agronomic and environmental effects of GE crops, the human health effects of GE crops, the social and economic effects of GE crops, the future GE technologies and GE crops, and the regulation of current and future GE crops. The stated goal of writing the report was to make available to the public, to researchers, and to policy-makers a comprehensive review of the evidence that has been used in the debates about GE crops and information on relevant studies that are rarely referred to in the debates. Information was solicited from various sources and different perspectives and an evaluation process was conducted to the gathered information. The report examined and analyzed the evidence regarding potential negative effects and benefits of currently commercialized GE crops and the potential benefits and negative effects of future GE crops. It came to the conclusion that available analyses were not complete and up-to-date and that an examination of the data on diverse biological and societal aspects of both current and future GE crops would therefore be useful.

In the end, it is my belief that the debate will, and should, continue. I consider the continuity of the debate a healthy sign, provided each debating side aims at arriving to factual conclusions. The debate will continue because some groups of both sides of the debate do not want to view the full picture of the GM technology and of the GM foods. Some GM technology supporters only focus on its benefits and on its positive aspects, while ignoring the possible risks. On the other side, GM technology and GM food critics highlight and try to magnify the potential risks to human health, the environment, and the whole ecosystem, without paying much attention to the positive aspects the technology has. Both sides need to realize and express potential benefits and possible risks, hazards, and threats of GM foods. The debate will also continue until researchers and scientists present credible results and interpretation of their work without being affected by external pressures to skew results or emphasize aspects that fulfill the goals of their research financers. The debate will continue and issues will remain controversial until consumers find out the facts, then give support or oppose accordingly and in an informed manner. Large sectors of consumers are confused because every day they find conflicting information and reports about GM foods. Each side of the debate tries to convince consumers that their arguments are truthful and that they represent the real picture. The technology supporters try to portray a rosy picture without mentioning the risks, while the opponents discuss the risks and threats of the GM technology. Most consumers are confused and do not know whom to trust. The debate should continue in a professional and objective manner and should put the welfare of the consumers at the heart of discussion agenda. The conversation can be a healthy one—exploring all the complex issues of the application of GM technology and how it can be used to lead to better practices and solutions and benefit the human race.

## 1.5 USES OF GMOs

GM has been widely used for the last two decades in a variety of industries (Wolfe 2013). Agriculture, medicine, pharmaceutical, and bioremediation represent some of the industries that benefited from the GM technologies.

### 1.5.1 Uses of GMOs in Agriculture

Agriculture is a major user of GMOs. Many plants have been modified to achieve specific attributes. One of the main areas that plant biotechnologists focused their research on is the enhancement of some agronomic traits of crops (Pew Initiative on Food and Biotechnology 2007). Some examples of the benefits attained by GE include increased crop yields, resistance to crop pests and diseases, reduced need for herbicides and pesticides, increased tolerance to drought, frost, other environmental stresses, salinity, and high levels of aluminum and boron, and improved nutrient profiles in food crops. Quick-maturing crops have also been genetically engineered. The quantitative and qualitative enhancement of agricultural crops would help to achieve food security and reduce costs of food and drugs. Other applications include the production of nonprotein (bioplastic) or nonindustrial (ornamental plant) products (Phillips 2008).

Examples of the currently followed herbicide-resistant cropping systems include RoundupReady (the active ingredient of which is glyphosate) used for soybean, corn, rapeseed, and cotton, and Liberty Link (the active ingredient of which is glufosinate) used in soybean, corn, canola, cotton, and sugar beet. RoundupReady is produced by Monsanto, while LibertyLink is produced by Bayer, two of the giant biotechnology companies worldwide.

Genuity®DroughtGard™ Hybrids are produced by Monsanto to help farmers mitigate the risk of yield loss when experiencing drought stress. The Western Great Plain farmers in the United States had the first opportunity to plant DroughtGard Hybrids on a commercial level (Mahgoub 2016).

The Monsanto corporation accounts for about 90 per cent of plant traits developed through transgenesis worldwide (Andrews 2013). The approved GM crops in the United States include: corn, soybean, canola, rice beet, flax and alfalfa (herbicide resistance); corn, cotton, potato and tomato (insect resistance); corn and chicory (sterile pollen); papaya, squash and plum (virus resistance); tomato (delayed ripening); canola, soybean (altered oil); corn (protein composition); and tobacco (reduced nicotine).

Although the enhancement of different agronomic traits in a number of crops has been achieved, improvement of products genetically modified to meet food processors or consumers needs seems to be limited. Efforts in that direction have been going on. More attention has been given to the production of GE crops with enhanced health and nutritional properties.

The enhancement of the nutritional quality of food crops has been a main concern and a goal for agriculturalists, food scientists and nutritionists. Different strategies have been developed and used to achieve that goal. Nutritional enhancement can be done at different stages of the food chain. It can be done at the crop production level and at the food processing level. With regard to the involvement of biotechnology, crop GE can be used to generate crop varieties with improved profiles for one or more nutrients. Enhancing the micronutrient (vitamin and mineral content) status of staple crops is considered to be one approach where crop biotechnology could generate crop varieties that could be used to strengthen food security and prevent malnutrition (FAO 2005). Different forms of malnutrition, for example protein-energy malnutrition (PEM) and micronutrient malnutrition can be managed through food crop enhancement using biotechnological techniques. Micronutrient malnutrition, especially lack of iron, zinc and vitamin A, currently affects more than half the world's population. Biotechnology can, thus, have a positive role in improving food and nutrition security worldwide.

Agricultural biotechnology has been used by scientists to develop GE foods with enhanced nutritional properties for the benefit of consumers. A group of food products aimed at consumers are those products with added health benefits (i.e., functional foods). Biotechnology has been successfully used to modify and improve the profiles of protein and amino-acids, vitamins, minerals, and edible oil and fatty acids.

Seed proteins of a number of major food crops, such as cereals and legumes, are naturally limiting in some amino acids, particularly the essential amino acids. Cereal grains are usually deficient in the amino acids lysine and tryptophan, while legumes are deficient in the sulfur amino acids methionine and cystine. The genes that encode seed proteins can be modified by GE to address the problem of nutritional quality in some staple crop varieties.

Vitamin profile can also be improved through GE. Vitamin A content of staple foods, which are naturally low in this vitamin, has been increased using GE. The highly-publicized, high pro-vitamin A transgenic rice, commonly known as "golden rice" is a typical example of the use of biotechnology to enhance vitamin profile in food crops.

Although most staple crops, such as rice, wheat, maize, sorghum, cassava, and beans, are not considered as important resources of mineral elements in human diets, yet minor increases in the mineral content of these staples would have a pronounced effect on human nutrition and health. This is due to the fact that large amounts of these staples are usually consumed in the diet. Both conventional and modern biotechnology techniques can be used to improve the nutritional quality of staple crops in terms of mineral content.

Edible oil content, characteristics, and fatty acid composition can be improved through GE. Plant sources of edible oil (i.e., seeds, nuts, and fruits) can be modified to achieve that goal. The fatty acid composition of an oil or fat can be modified in a way that suits the purpose for which it is going to be used. The ratio between saturated fatty acids and unsaturated fatty acids can be controlled through GE. An example of a functional food oil developed through biotechnology is Calgene's high lauric acid canola, Laurical™, which is modified to suit confectionery products and chocolates. Work on oil palm with low saturated fatty acids in Indonesia and Malaysia, and on coconut with high lauric acid in Philippines is also reported. Some of the aspects of edible oils and fats that can be improved through GE in order to enhance their nutritional, health and functionality characteristics include: reduction of saturated fatty acids, introduction of omega-3 polyunsaturated fatty acids, and enhancing the availability of novel fatty acids such as linoleic acid.

Another area where GM is used in agriculture is the production of biofertilizers. Biofertilizers refer to the soil nutrients made available to the plant through the use of living organisms, mainly bacteria and fungi. For many centuries, chemical fertilizers have been used in different cropping systems as agricultural inputs to increase and improve crop production. Concerns about tremendous harm from these chemicals to the environment have been expressed. It is believed that the use of biofertilizers, which are considered to be more friendly to the environment, and are cost effective, is the answer to this problem.

Soil nutrients can be depleted through continuous farming on the same piece of land without addition of nutrients from external sources. They might also be lost through other factors. This is when fertilization of the soil is needed and comes into effect. Phosphorus and nitrogen are two major nutrients needed by plants. They have important roles in plant quality, maturity, and to help the plant to withstand stress. Although these elements exist naturally in the environment, plants have a limited capacity to benefit from them by direct extraction from the environment. Plants are helped by the fungus *Penicillium bilaii* to benefit from the phosphate available in the soil. Through a series of chemical reactions, this fungus increases the phosphate availability to the plant. GE has been used to produce a biofertilizer from this fungus. It is done either by inoculating seeds with the fungus, or putting it directly in the soil where crops are planted. Biofertilizers advocates indicate that the use of this group of fertilizers will form part of the solution to the problems of increased soil salinity.

Naturally, plants have various relationships with microorganisms, particularly fungi, bacteria, and algae, the most common of which are *Mycorrhiza, Rhizobium, and Cyanophyceae.* Some of the observed benefits of these microbes include improvement of plant nutrition, disease resistance, and tolerance to biotic and abiotic conditions. These beneficial relationships have been used in a positive manner to develop biofertilizers. Biofertilizers such as *Rhizobium, Azotobacter, Azospirillum*, and blue-green algae (BGA) have been developed and used successfully for a long time. *Rhizobium* inoculant is usually applied for leguminous crops. *Azotobacter* can be used with crops like wheat, maize, mustard, cotton, potato, and other vegetable crops. *Azospirillum* inoculations are recommended mainly for sorghum, millets, maize, sugarcane, and wheat. BGA belonging to a general cyanobacteria genus, *Nostoc*, *Anabaena*, *Tolypothrix*, or *Aulosira*, fix atmospheric nitrogen and are used as inoculations for paddy crop grown both under upland and lowland conditions (Kiguli 2000).

The microorganisms in biofertilizers have the ability to retain and restore the soil's natural nutrient cycle. Both the plant and the soil thus benefit from biofertilzers application. Sometimes, the term "plant-growth promoting rhizobacteria" (PGPR) is used to describe biofertilizers denoting the several roles they play.

Some of the observed and reported of the benefits of biofertilizers include increase in crop yield, replacing chemical nitrogen and phosphorus, stimulation of plant growth, biological activation of the soil, restoring soil's natural fertility, and providing protection against drought and some soil-borne diseases.

Biotechnology has also been used for animals. A number of animals have been genetically engineered to increase yield and decrease susceptibility to disease. The application of scientific and engineering principles can be used in animal biotechnology to the processing or production of materials by animals or aquatic species to provide goods and services. Animal biotechnology encompasses the use of animal cells to generate valuable products through recombinant DNA technology, and the application of biotechnological approaches to rapidly multiply animals of desired genotype or to introduce specific changes in their genotype to achieve certain goals. Just like other assisted reproduction techniques such as artificial insemination, embryo transfer and in vitro fertilization, livestock cloning improves animal breeding programs allowing farmers and ranchers to produce healthier offspring, and therefore produce healthier, safer, and higher quality foods more consistently (Bio 2017). It includes both old (techniques that do not use GE) and modern (techniques that involve GE) types of biotechnologies.

Techniques that do not involve GE include domestication of wild animals, artificial selection, and assisted reproductive procedures (Mahgoub 2016). Spontaneous mutations can happen in domesticated animals leading to improvement of characteristics of the animals, whereas artificial selection involves the intervention of man. An example of the assisted reproductive procedures, which are used to alter animal characteristics, is what is known as Artificial Insemination (AI). AI involves collection of semen from select bulls with desired characteristics, for example the milk that their daughters produce, and using the semen to fertilize cows artificially. The select bulls are tested for fertility to ensure carry on of their genes during the AI process. It is anticipated that the AI technique will continue to be an integral component of the animal production systems.

A number of techniques that involve GE have been used to modify animal characteristics. The most notable examples of these techniques are: transgenics, gene Knock-Out technology, Somatic Cell Nuclear Transfer (Cloning), and the production of infertile aquatic species.

Transgenic principles involve the transfer of genes through different species. Methods to develop transgenic animals and transgenic aquatic species, for example fish, came into use since the early 1980s. Among transgenic livestock traits, such as increased growth rate, enhanced lean muscle mass, increased resistance to diseases, enhanced milk production have been achieved. Fish have been genetically engineered to grow faster and have increased muscle mass. Transgenic poultry, goats, swine, and cattle have been produced to generate large amounts of human proteins in their products (e.g., eggs, milk, and blood). The goal here is to use those products as human pharmaceuticals (e.g., antibodies, enzymes, and clotting factors).

The term "Knock-out" used to describe the Gene Knock-Out Technology refers to the inactivation of a specific gene in an animal. The main purpose of this technology is to create a possible source of replacement organs for humans. The process of transplanting cells, tissues, or organs from one species to another is known as "xenotransplantation." Among the different animals suitable for this kind of technology the pig has been found to be the most viable organ donor to humans. The main challenge facing the process of xenotransplantation is the lack of immunological compatibility between pig cells and human cells, which would result in rejection of the donated organ. The presence of markers on the cells of the pig makes it easy for the human immune system to recognize them as foreign and consequently reject them. GE is applied to knockout or inactivate the pig gene responsible for the protein that forms the marker associated with the pig cells. Another example of the "knockout" technology in animals is the inactivation of the "prion-related peptide" (PRP) gene that may produce animals resistant to some diseases linked to prions for example bovine spongiform encephalopathy (BSE), and Creutzfeldt-Jakob disease (CJD).

Somatic cell nuclear transfer (SCNT), alternatively known as "cloning," is another example of application of animal biotechnologies. It involves the use of somatic cell nuclear transfer to develop multiple copies of mammals, which are nearly identical copies of other animals, for example, transgenic animals, genetically superior animals, or animals that possess some other desirable characteristics. Some of the animals cloned using this technique include cattle, sheep, goats, pigs, horses, mules, cats, rats, and mice. Experience has shown that the degree of success for propagating animals through cloning is very low and is usually less than ten per cent. It is affected by multiple factors, for example, the animal species, source of the recipient ova, cell type of the donor nuclei, treatment of donor cells before nuclear transfer, and the technique followed for nuclear transfer.

The technique of producing infertile species is specific to aquatic organisms, for example fish and molluscs (aquatic invertebrates that include animals such as squid, octopuses, cuttlefish, snails, slugs, clams, oysters, and scallops). It has been developed to address one of the problems encountered in aquaculture production systems. This problem involves some species that are not indigenous to a certain area posing an ecological hazard to native species in case the foreign species escape confinement and enter the natural ecosystem. In addition to addressing the issue of confinement, sterility in fish allows for reproductive energy to be diverted toward somatic growth, resulting in higher growth rates for some triploid individuals. In practice, it has been a difficult task to achieve 100 per cent level of sterilization. This called for searching for alternative methods to fulfill the issue of reproductive confinement of fish.

As with any new technology, animal biotechnology is confronted with a number of challenges, faces a variety of uncertainties, and raises some concerns. The most important among these concerns are the issue of food safety, effects on human and animal health, possible environmental degradation, and most importantly animal welfare.

Another area where GMOs are used in agriculture is the production of animal feed. The feed of farm animals usually contains ingredients made from plants developed through GE. Additives and enzymes, for example Vitamin B12, biotin, amino acids, beta-carotene, which are sometimes incorporated in animal feed, are also produced using GE microorganisms. Different crops incorporated in the development of animal feed include soybean, maize, cottonseed, wheat, rye and oats, some of which are genetically engineered. The end products of animals fed GE ingredients, such as meat, milk and eggs, have been evaluated using advanced sensitive test methods to find out if there is any difference resulting from the type of feed (i.e., GE or non-GE). At present, it is not possible to tell if an animal was fed GM soy just by testing its resulting products. The only possible way to establish the presence or absence of GMOs in animal feed is to analyze the origin of the feed itself.

An important area where GMOs are used, and which sparked wide controversy, is the production of genetically modified foods. Various food categories have been produced through GE. Ghosh and Williams (2010) have cited the following general categories for foods produced through modern biotechnology (GE):

- Foods consisting of, or containing, living/viable organisms for example corn,
- Foods derived from, or containing, ingredients derived from GMOs for example corn meal containing proteins or oil from GM soy,
- Foods containing single ingredients or additives produced by GM microorganisms for example colors, vitamins, or essential amino acids,
- Foods containing ingredients processed by enzyme produced through GM microorganisms for example high fructose corn syrup produced from starch using the enzyme glucose isomerase or cheese produced using the enzyme chymosin.

Examples of GM crops used as food include apples, corn (maize), cotton seed (oil), papaya, peas, potato, rape seed or canola (oil), rice, soybean, squash, sugar cane, sweet corn, tomato, and honey (produced from flowers of GM crops).

The book published by Mahgoub (2016) discusses in depth the basics, applications, and controversy surrounding GM foods.

Some of the most exciting advances in genetically altered plants are for nonfood sources. Production of edible vaccinations is one such area. GE of plants has the potential to provide edible plant vaccines that could be used to immunize individuals against a wide variety of infectious diseases ranging from cholera to potentially AIDS. One such example is the development of transgenic potato plants that have been produced and tested successfully by utilizing a genetically engineered food to deliver a pharmaceutical immunization against diarrhea (Anon 2005).

### 1.5.2 Uses of GMOs in Medicine and the Pharmaceutical Industry

One of the first applications of GM was the creation a bacterial strain capable of producing human insulin. Insulin, the hormone lacking in people with diabetes, was previously isolated from pig pancreas. Recombinant insulin offers many advantages over pig insulin, including cost savings, fewer allergic reactions and putting an end to the practice of euthanizing pigs for their insulin (Wolfe 2013).

The pharmaceutical industry is another frontier for the use of GMOs. In 1986, human growth hormone was the first protein pharmaceutical made in plants, and in 1989, the first antibody was produced (Phillips 2008). Other examples of GMOs uses include pharmaceutical agents produced in sheep's milk and vaccines grown in chicken eggs (Wolfe 2013).

### 1.5.3 Uses of GMOs in Bioremediation

Bioremediation describes any process by which living organisms are used to clean up contaminated soil or water. Bioremediation generally uses microorganisms, small bacteria and yeasts, which ingest the contaminants in a given site and render them inert through the cells' own metabolic processes. Although certainly advantageous, bioremediation has had limited use because the organisms must be able to survive, and indeed thrive, in a contaminated environment in order to do their work. GM makes it possible to engineer bacteria that will be robust within a given environment, by inserting genes that will ensure their survival (Wolfe 2013).

## 1.6 REGULATION OF GMOs

### 1.6.1 Regulation-General Aspects

Regulation of GM crops and of GM foods is found to be a complex multidimensional issue that needs to be addressed carefully and from different angles. It has been an issue of concern to the public, policy makers, the food industry, as well as the wide pool of professionals such as food and agricultural scientists, economists, attorneys, legal scholars, bioethicists, and philosophers.

Since the advent of GE with its great potential, particularly in relation to GM foods, the need for a regulatory framework became evident. At international level, the two outstanding instruments are the Cartagena Protocol on Biosafety and the Codex Alimentarius. At country level, national laws that govern GMOs and GM foods are set. Governments of different countries around the globe have followed different strategies and taken various approaches with regard to GE and its applications to develop GMOs and products made from them particularly GM foods.

The development of a general regulatory framework on GE began in 1975 shortly after the first application of recombinant DNA (rDNA) new technology. The need for regulations resulted from the belief that this new technology can have some risks in addition to the identified benefits. Since the GE technology was then used to produce different types of foods, identified as GM or GE foods, it became necessary to regulate this category of foods as well. The main focus of the GM foods regulation has been safety assessment. The basic concepts for safety assessment of foods derived from GMOs have been developed through the collaborative work between the OECD and the United Nations' WHO and the FAO. An outcome of that collaboration came in the year 2003 when the Codex Alimentarius Commission (CAC) of the FAO/WHO produced the document "Principles and Guidelines on Foods Derived from Biotechnology" (Codex Alimentarius Commission 2003). The aim of that publication was to help countries establish, coordinate, and standardize regulations on GM foods to ensure consumer safety and at the same time harmonize and facilitate international trade. An additional related document updating the guidelines for import and export of food was released by CAC in 2005 (FAO Corporate Document Repository 2005).

Governments and the food industry have shared responsibilities in addressing the different issues and arising questions pertaining to GMOs and GM foods regulations for the benefit of the consumer. Some of the questions that face, and need clarification by, the regulators are: how prescriptive should the regulations be? Should there be any penalty or sanctions for non-compliance? What monitoring and enforcing procedures to follow? Are new regulations needed for gene technology or would already existing regulations suffice? To what extent can governments go in order to promote trade and commerce at regional and international levels? Would national governments be able to streamline and handle any conflict that might arise between international obligations and local needs? If so what modalities can be followed? (Mahgoub 2016).

A number of challenges face governments in the process of drafting regulatory framework for GM foods. Governments need to ensure consumer protection, as well as trust and confidence in what the government set as regulations. Consumers also need to be part of the decision-making process with regard to regulation development. Governments should have processes that will not impede development of the technology at all levels, for example, research and commercial levels. A reasonable balance between international regulatory systems and export and import trade and the national sovereignty of states needs to be observed by governments as well. The regulatory process is further complicated by the need for specific and different regulations for the different stages of the use of gene technology to produce foods, for example in the lab, and at the industrial and marketing levels.

Governments around the globe have considered GM regulation and labeling as an urgent priority and are working hard to set regulatory processes addressing GMOs and GM foods. Different governments have taken different approaches based on the specific political, social, and economic conditions prevailing around the region or in the country. In some cases, the GMO regulation varies within the same country. This depends on the intended use of the products of the GE for example for food or feed use. Differences in regulations among countries are clear and the most marked differences are occurring between the United States and Europe. Some countries ban or restrict GMOs and GM foods, while others permit them with varying degrees of regulation. In general, most governments have set "the protection of public health as affected by food consumption" as a first priority to be achieved through promoting and enforcing high standards of safety throughout the food chain.

The regulation of GE deals with the approaches taken by governments to assess and manage the benefits and the risks associated with the use of this technology and the development and release of GMOs. In some countries, for example, those in the EU, approval for cultivation of GM crops within those countries and approval for import and for processing of GM crops are treated differently. The EU has been stricter on cultivation of GM crops within its member states than on import and processing. The number of GM crops approved for cultivation is less than the number of GM crops approved for import and for processing. Many countries allow the import of GM food with authorization, but either do not allow its cultivation (Russia, Norway, Israel) or have provisions for cultivation, but no GM products are yet produced (Japan, South Korea). Most countries that do not allow for GMO cultivation do permit research (Law Library of Congress: LAW.gov 2015).

Being the world's leading producer of GM crops and the important role that the biotechnology industry plays in its economy, the United States has relatively favorable regulations toward the development of GM crops, as compared to other countries. GMOs are regulated in the United States under the Coordinated Framework for Regulation of Biotechnology, published in 1986, pursuant to previously existing statutory authority regulating conventional products, with a focus on the nature of the products rather than the process in which they are produced. Plant GMOs are regulated by the U.S. Department of Agriculture's Animal and Plant Health Inspection Service under the Plant Protection Act. GMOs in food, drugs, and biological products are regulated by the FDA under the Federal Food, Drug, and Cosmetic Act and the Public Health Service Act. GMO pesticides and microorganisms are regulated by the Environmental Protection Agency pursuant to the Federal Insecticide, Fungicide and Rodenticide Act and the Toxic Substances Control Act. The form of regulation varies depending on the type of GMO involved (Law Library of Congress: LAW.gov 2015).

### 1.6.2 Substantial Equivalence (SE)

A new concept, which has been developed and found to be helpful in the GM crops and GM foods regulatory process is "substantial equivalence" (SE). This is an internationally recognized standard that measures whether a biotech food or crop shares similar health and nutritional characteristics with its conventional counterpart (Council for Biotechnology Information 2001). It is considered as the starting point for the assessment of safety of GM foods, and it is widely used by national and international bodies dealing with GM foods, for example, FAO, WHO, OECD, USFDA, and by some countries such as United States (through the FDA), Canada (through the Canadian Food Inspection Agency), Japan (through Japan's Ministry of Health and Welfare), Lebanon, and Egypt. If the new crop or food is considered as substantially equivalent to an existing product, then further safety or nutritional concerns are considered insignificant. This product food would then be treated in a similar way to its natural counterpart to which it was compared.

Further insights on the meaning of SE are given by the FAO in this statement: "Substantial equivalence embodies the concept that if a new food or food component is found to be substantially equivalent to an existing food or food component, it can be treated in the same manner with respect to safety (i.e., the food or food component can be concluded to be as safe as the conventional food or food component)"(Codex Alimentarius Commission 2003).

To decide if a modified product is substantially equivalent, the product is tested by the manufacturer for unexpected changes in a limited set of components such as toxins, nutrients, or allergens that are present in the unmodified food. The manufacturer's data is then assessed by a regulatory agency, such as the U.S. FDA. That data, along with data on the GM itself and resulting proteins (or lack of protein), is submitted to regulators. If regulators determine that the submitted data show no significant difference between the modified and unmodified products, then the regulators will generally not require further food safety testing. However, if the product has no natural equivalent, or shows significant differences from the unmodified food, or for other reasons that regulators may have (for instance, if a gene produces a protein that had not been a food component before), the regulators may require that further safety testing be carried out (OECD 1993).

GM foods which are considered substantially equivalent are regarded to be as safe as their conventional counterparts. On the other hand, food products that are not substantially equivalent may still be safe on condition that they are subjected to a range of other tests to confirm their safety, before they can be marketed.

When applying the SE principle some aspects need to be taken into consideration. Such aspects include the composition and properties of the counterpart food as well as those of the novel food, the method used to alter the nature of the new food, and the way in which the new genetic material is expressed.

### 1.6.3 Labeling

Labeling of GM products, including GM foods, has been one of the main issues that concern regulators and authorities. Some of the debatable issues that lead to a lot of controversy come in the form of such questions as: Should GM products and GM foods be labeled or not? Should labeling be mandatory or voluntary? Who should be responsible for labeling? How would labeling affect consumers' choices?

In general, labeling of GM products can be mandatory up to a threshold GM content level (which varies between countries) or voluntary. There is a lot of controversy over this issue. People in the agribusiness industry believe that labeling should be voluntary and that the demands of the free market and consumer preferences would influence the labeling process. In case consumers prefer labeled foods over no-labeled ones, the industry would regulate itself or run the risk of losing consumers. On the other side of the controversy, stand the consumer interest groups who believe in mandatory labeling of GM foods stating that people have the right to know what they are eating. Whitman (2000) states that there are a number of questions that needs to be answered before regulating a mandatory nature for GM foods. One important question relates to the added cost of production incurred and the economic impact if labeling of GM foods becomes mandatory. This extra cost comes as a result of constructing two separate production lines at the industrial level as well as a result of practices at the farm level where farmers will try to keep GM crops separate from non-GM crops during planting, harvesting, and shipping. Testing and detailed record-keeping needs to be conducted at various stages of the food supply chain. Estimates of the cost of mandatory labeling vary from a few dollars per person per year to about ten per cent of a consumer's food bill (Gruère and Rao 2007). It is expected that the industry will shift the extra cost burden to the consumer in the form of higher food prices. The question here is: will consumers be ready to absorb the added cost of this initiative? Another question is about the acceptable limits of GM contamination (if any) in non-GM products. At what level can these limits be set? Who would be responsible to monitor food producing companies for compliance? What kind of penalty would be imposed? As with other issues related to GM technology there is a divided difference of opinion among different nations, for example the EU, has determined that 0.9 per cent is an acceptable level of cross contamination, Australia and New Zealand decided a threshold value of one per cent, while Japan has specified a five per cent threshold (Hansen 2001). Many consumer interest groups believe that only 0 per cent would be acceptable. On the other hand, some food producing companies such as Gerber baby foods and Frito Lay have pledged not to use any GM ingredients in manufacture of any of their products.

Another issue regulators need to take into consideration is how to verify the presence of GM components in different products. Auer (2003) discusses the methods used to detect GE components in crops and processed foods. Byrne et al. (2014) described two ways by which regulators can verify whether a food is, or is not, genetically engineered. The first one is content-based in which foods are tested for the physical presence of foreign DNA or protein. A current application of this type of procedure is the analysis and labeling of vitamin content of foods. The second one is process-based verification. It entails detailed record keeping of seed source, field location, harvest, transport, and storage. This is similar to the type of "identity preservation" system used to certify shade-grown coffee or organic foods. Details of this approach are explained by Sundstrom et al. (2002). Other issues that cause concern about GM foods labeling include the level of detectability of GM food cross contamination and public awareness about GM food labels. With regard to detecting GMO contamination, it has been found that current techniques are not able to detect minute quantities of contamination. This means that ensuring a 0 per cent level of contamination will not be possible. There is disagreement among scientists as to what level of contamination is practically possible. With regard to public awareness and to what extent would consumer understand the meaning of food label information, the question is who would be responsible to educate the public about GM food labels. Would it be of any benefit to label GM foods if consumers are not able to interpret the meaning of the information on the label? (Mahgoub 2016).

Many countries around the globe require GMO products and GM foods to be labeled; however, the United States and Canada do not. In Canada and in the United States, labeling of GM food is voluntary (Government of Canada 2012), while in Europe all food (including processed food or feed), which contains greater than 0.9 per cent of approved GMOs must be labelled (Davison 2010). While the United States does not require mandatory labeling of GM foods, other countries such as European countries, Japan, Australia, New Zealand, Brazil, China, and South Korea require labeling of products that contain GM ingredients. Currently, 64 countries around the world require labeling of genetically modified foods (Just Label it 2017). In January 2000, an international trade agreement for labeling GM foods was established with more than 130 countries signing the agreement. The policy states that exporters must be required to label all GM foods and that importing countries have the right to judge for themselves the potential risks and reject GM foods, if they so choose (Helmuth 2000).

The effects that GM labeling might have on local and international markets have been studied by many investigators. Golan and Kuchler (2011) investigated the possible role of GM labeling, whether mandatory or voluntary, on market outcomes. Their study focused on the role that mandatory GM labeling versus voluntary labeling has played in the split between those countries with small GM markets and those with large GM markets.

The study concluded that GM labeling has negligible effects on consumer choices or on GM differentiation costs, and therefore does not explain the split in GM market outcomes.

In the United States, a number of states have passed labeling laws, other states require that a coalition of regional government pass similar laws before labeling will be required (Takepart 2017). At the federal level there is no law in the United States requiring that GMO foods or foods with GMO ingredients be labeled to so indicate. Groups skeptical of biotechnology in some U.S. states have pushed for state-level laws mandating that GMO foods be labeled. Their rallying cry is that citizens have the right to know whether their food has been modified. The USFDA has regulatory authority to prevent false and misleading labeling of foods and drugs. With respect to GM foods, the FDA has stated in policy documents that if a GM food product is not materially different from its traditional counterpart, there is no need to label or change the name of the product, but name changes are appropriate when a food from a GM plant is so different from its traditional counterpart that the usual name no longer adequately describes the new food, or if there is a safety issue to which consumers should be alerted, such as the presence of allergens (FDA 1992).

## 1.7 PUBLIC AWARENESS ON GMOs

### 1.7.1 Public Awareness on GMO Products, with Special Reference to GM Foods

Recently consumer' opinions on GMO products have been in the spotlight and is greatly influencing governments policies related to GM technology in general and specifically to GM foods. The following discussion deals with GMO products in general with special reference to GM foods. Consumers' opinion and reaction toward different issues are considered as critical factors and powerful drivers that help to shape governmental policies in different parts of the world. It is extremely important for policy-makers, regulators as well as food producers and processors to understand the consumers' opinion because it very much influences the ultimate acceptance or rejection of GM foods in the marketplace. Governments usually design programs that aim at improving and maintaining its citizens' health. Part of these programs encompasses availing and dissemination of information related to health, which includes education, public information campaigns, and regulation of advertising and labeling (Aldrich 1999). Information on various issues related to GMO products, as well as on other sources of information, should be made available by the government, through its different departments, and should be made accessible to consumers.

A general societal anxiety over the GM tools is felt among consumers. This effect is caused by multiple factors such as consumer unfamiliarity with the technology, lack of reliable information, a steady stream of negative opinion in the news media, opposition by activist groups, growing mistrust of industry, and a general lack of awareness of how the food production system has evolved (Conko and Prakash 2004). Some of the reported factors that affect consumers' attitudes toward GM foods include socio-economic factors such as level of education, gender, and religious beliefs. Introduction of new information about GM technology would also affect consumers' attitudes and reaction toward GMOs. It is suggested that existence of negative new information on GM would increase negative attitudes toward the technology. At the same time, this negative attitude may be reversed with introduction of new positive information (Heiman and Zilberman 2011) and the existence of evidence of benefits from the use of GMOs. Some of the consumers' rights are the right to choose, the right to availability and access to credible information, and the right to participation in discussions and decisions of issues that affect their lives and well-being. Respect of consumers' rights has been a central issue and a focal area in the debate around GM technology and GM foods in different parts of the globe.

Generally consumers fall in different categories with regard to perception and attitude toward GMO products. Some have expressed their concerns about safety of GM foods and are hesitant to consume such modified foods, while others believe that this technology has benefits more than drawbacks and that it is safe to consume GM foods since there is no reported evidence of health risks. A third group has doubt and insecurity toward GM food, but at the same time acknowledges the benefits of biotechnology as an effective tool for sustainable food supply and availability.

A number of factors may affect consumers' perception and attitudes toward GM foods. Consumers use cognitive, affective, or behavioral responses to accept or reject GM foods (Frewer 2003). Many researchers concluded that acceptance or rejection of GM foods by consumers is likely to be associated with their risk/benefit beliefs about biotechnology (Mahgoub 2016). It is, therefore, logical to say that consumers who believe that GM food has benefits will be more willing to buy and consume GM food, while consumers who perceive GM food as a health risk, and risky to the environment, will be less willing to purchase GM food (Han and Harrison 2007). On the other hand, consumers' perceptions, attitudes, and responses toward GM foods are usually influenced by the type of information they receive about GM foods, for example positive statements, negative statements, both negative and positive, or no statements. Consumer purchasing behavior for GM foods is not necessarily similar to, or same as, their attitudes toward the GM technology or GM foods. In spite of the fact that consumer attitudes toward GM foods may be negative, there is a chance that these attitudes will not directly correlate with a negative purchasing behavior (Gaskell et al. 2003). This idea has been supported in a number of surveys conducted in the United Kingdom and reported by Halford and Shewry (2000).

The differences in attitudes toward GM observed between the United States and the EU consumers may be attributed to what is referred to as the "invisible flag." Coval and Moskowitz (1999) state that consumers generally prefer products and ideas originating from their own countries, described as "home bias." Many people have the perception that GM technologies are mainly linked to Monsanto, which is an American company, so some of the negative attitude by European consumers toward GM technology as a whole may be based on the perception that this is a technology that has been imposed on Europeans by a an American company.

The adoption of GM technology in countries other than the United States met a slow start. That resulted from a widespread resistance from consumers toward the technology and its various applications. Consumer objection to the technology was, to a large extent, fueled by various news against GM, which is expressed in the different media outlets (Knight et al. 2014). Due to the lack of global agreement on the issue of food labeling, consumers in different parts of the world have different perceptions and attitudes toward GM foods. Differences in "who to trust," when it comes to getting credible sources of information on GM technology, also exist between American consumers and other consumers around the world. Europeans are reported to place their trust in consumer and environmental groups, whereas Americans tend to trust scientific and academic resources more than consumer and environmental groups (Lang and Hallman 2005). The role of press in educating the public about technology issues has also been found to be different in Europe and the United States. The European press has covered the various biotechnology issues more extensively than press in the United States. This wide press coverage in Europe resulted in more public awareness, making European consumers to be both cognizant and wary of the GM technology (Durant et al. 1999; McInerney et al. 2004).

Supporters and critics of GM technology and GM foods try to convince consumers in what they say by presenting the benefits or drawbacks and risks of the technology, depending on what they want to portray about the technology. All this information is expected to be available to consumers to help them to decide for themselves on various issues related to GM technology. It is important and more ethical for both supporters and critics of GM foods to give all and honest information, and not only the points that support their cause, so that consumers get the whole true picture and make informed decisions.

One of the strongest opponents and critics of the application of GMO products in food production is the "NON-GMO Project." This project provides up-to-date information on GM foods and non-GM foods and sets standards for non-GMO verification. It aims to help consumers understand which products contain GMOs and the level of risk therein. The Non-GMO Project categorizes three levels of risk for GMOs inputs: high risk, low risk, and no risk. The Project designed this label "NON-GMO Project VERIFIED" to be shown on the package of food products that do not contain GM components. In order for a product to be "Non-GMO Project Verified," its inputs must comply with the standards set by the Non-GMO Project. The Project defined each risk level and cited some examples of genetically modified agricultural products (NON-GMO Project 2017). Detailed information about the project is available from its website: www.nongmoproject.org/gmo-facts/.

Consumer education about various aspects of GM foods is believed to be a useful strategy to address concerns around potential health risks and adverse effects on the environment and the ecosystem (Han and Harrison 2007). Educating consumers and raising their awareness on different GM food issues is not expected to bear fruits in the short-run. Consumers' knowledge and full understanding of GM foods would be a long process. In the meantime, it is expected that there will be an increasing demand for non-GM and organic foods. Nonetheless, effective management of safety verification and continuous public education on GM food may assure consumers of the safety of GM food in the long term, eventually leading to more acceptability of GM foods (Kim 2012).

### 1.7.2 Roles of Mass Media

It is believed that mass media have very strong influence in shaping people's views and perceptions of many aspects in human life. People tend to believe in what they read and view in different media sources, and become affected by the views expressed in them. That could be attributed to the easiness of access to information from media than from other professional or technical sources, or due to the easy-to-understand and comprehend language in which media reports are written or portrayed. Also, people find media sources at hand every day, or even every minute, while technical, scientific, or professional information is usually published less frequently than media reports. The power of media in disseminating messages of different types is widely used by different authorities and agencies to help them reach wider audiences.

Consumers usually get information about GM foods, or any other related issue, from various media channels such as newspapers, specialized magazines, periodicals, radio,

TV, or the internet. Views expressed in these media venues in most cases represent the author's, writer's, or presenter's views. In scientific and professional publications interpretation of research results may also be subjective and painted by the author's views and beliefs. All these media outlets present positive, negative, or balanced views and information about GM foods. This information has direct impact on the consumers' views, perceptions, and attitudes toward GM foods. Consumers need to be careful in evaluating information they receive from media to help them make the right decisions with regard to purchasing and consuming GM foods. Mass media reports on GM foods are widely controversial. Some reports support GM foods while others criticize it. At the same time, some balanced reports present both sides of the debate without any bias toward one side.

There are great expectations and hopes that mass media play a pivotal role in disseminating credible information and gain further consumer trust as a source of reliable reporting on various issues including biotechnology and GM foods.

Reports in the literature show that many studies, surveys, reviews, and polls have been, and continue to be, conducted among consumers on various issues surrounding GM products and GM foods in an effort to arrive at a conclusive, or at least a satisfactory answer to the pertinent question "is it safe to eat GM foods?" These studies have been conducted in different parts of the world, at different times, under different conditions, and with different goals. Results of such studies, surveys, and polls would carry more weight and be more meaningful if consumers are adequately informed and are knowledgeable on various issues surrounding GM technology and GM foods. Part of the responsibility to gain that knowledge falls on the consumers themselves. Consumers need to search for credible information from unbiased sources and understand it before expressing their views or making decisions on purchase or consumption of GM foods. Government authorities, food producers, and processors, as well as various media outlets have great responsibility in raising public awareness on issues related to GM foods. This has to be done in a way that does not mislead the consumers but help them to get the right information that would help them to decide for themselves to purchase or consume GM foods (Mahgoub 2016).

In an effort to raise public awareness on various issues related to GMOs, Trombitsky (2017) listed a number of effective tips (in his view) that might be helpful. The following tips are stated:

- Be scientific, not populist: do not give reasons to demonstrate your not scientific arguments and data; use simple but adequate language; use the EU arguing (i.e., there is no unique vision concerning danger of all GMOs): each GMO should be risk-evaluated; social-economic risk assessment should be equal on importance with other risk assessments—frequently here are main reasons do not permit GMO
- Work with media: media are the most efficient public awareness mechanism; be active and establish partnerships with mass-media; your position is strong: you are not against or in favor of GMOs, but fight for right to know of everybody; ask mass-media to consult with you and other specialists to avoid mistakes and incorrect evaluations of situation; criticize not-scientific articles or broadcasts appearing in mass media
- Work with stakeholders: people have to be motivated to participate—right identification of the groups; when possible—cooperate with the state and local authorities; take into consideration specific interests of groups; risks should be evaluated proportionally; stakeholders should also share their knowledge inside their group to multiply the effect of awareness

## 1.8 RECENT DEVELOPMENTS ON GMOs

Results of research and the various applications of GMOs in agriculture continue to be reported every day. Opposition of their utilization by critics has not hampered this activity. Yet, we still see the same trend of controversy in the reporting of information about developments by both sides: the proponents and the opponents. The problem is that each group highlights developments that support their views, and rarely report on failures, successes, or issues arising from their use. Supporters only report successes in application of GMOs, whereas critics only report failures and problems facing this technology. It is important that supporters and critics of the use of GMO technologies appreciate that consumers have the right to credible and correct information. The following sections give examples of developments reported by each group. The International Service for the Acquisition of Agri-biotech Applications (ISAAA- http://www.isaaa.org), a strong supporter of application GM technology in agriculture, publishes periodic reports on the successes of GM technology worldwide. On the other side, we find "GMWATCH" (www.gmwatch.org), a group strongly criticizing the applications of GM technology, and reporting on the problems and failures facing it.

Currently, GM crops are grown in every continent except Antarctica (Freedeman 2009). The ISAAA publishes annual reviews of the global status of biotech crops entitled "The Annual Global Review of Biotech Crops Commercialization or ISAAA Briefs." The "ISAAA Brief 52" is the 21st of the series which documents the latest information on the subject, global database on the adoption and distribution of biotech crops in 2016 as well as the accumulative data since 1996 (the first year of commercialization), country situations, trends in approval of biotech crops, and future prospects of the technology in the biotech crop growing countries and the world (ISAAA 2016).

According to the ISAAA 52 brief, a year after the second decade of commercialization of biotech/GM crops in 2016, 26 countries grew 185.1 million hectares of biotech crops representing an increase of 5.4 million hectares or 3 per cent from 179.7 million hectares in 2015. The observed increase in the total global area cultivated with biotech crops is reported to be about 110 folds (increasing from 1.7 million hectares in 1996 to 185.1 million hectares in 2016). As reflected in the figures in Table 1.1, there is a clear annual increase in the total global area planted with biotech crops. Out of those 26 countries growing biotech crops, 19 were developing and 7 were industrial countries. Developing countries grew 54 per cent (99.6 million hectares) of the global biotech crop area compared to 46 per cent (85.5 million hectares) for industrial countries (Table 1.2, Figure 1.1). Of the top five countries growing 91 per cent of biotech crops, three are developing countries (Brazil, Argentina, and India) and two are industrial (United States and Canada). The United States leads biotech crop planting in 2016 at 72.9 million hectares, followed by Brazil (49.1 million hectares), Argentina (23.8 million hectares), Canada (11.6 million hectares), and India (10.8 million hectares).

Trends of planting GM crops in different countries in the African continent change with time due to certain circumstances within those countries. By 2016, at least four countries had in the past placed a GM crop in the market—Burkina Faso, Egypt, South Africa, and Sudan. However, due to a temporary setback in Burkina Faso and Egypt, only South Africa and Sudan planted biotech crops at 2.8 million hectares (ISAAA 2016). On the other hand, some countries including Kenya, Malawi, and Nigeria are advancing from the stage of researching in GM crops toward granting environmental release approvals. Another group of African countries including Burkina Faso, Ethiopia, Ghana, Nigeria, Swaziland, and Uganda are moving toward considering commercial approval of

TABLE 1.1 Global Area of Biotech Crops, the First 21 Years, 1996–2016

| Year | Hectares (Million) | Acres (Million) |
|---|---|---|
| 1996 | 1.7 | 4.2 |
| 1997 | 11.0 | 27.2 |
| 1998 | 27.8 | 68.7 |
| 1999 | 39.9 | 98.6 |
| 2000 | 44.2 | 109.2 |
| 2001 | 52.6 | 130.0 |
| 2002 | 58.7 | 145.0 |
| 2003 | 67.7 | 167.3 |
| 2004 | 81.0 | 200.2 |
| 2005 | 90.0 | 222.4 |
| 2006 | 102.0 | 252.0 |
| 2007 | 114.3 | 282.4 |
| 2008 | 125.0 | 308.9 |
| 2009 | 134.0 | 331.1 |
| 2010 | 148.0 | 365.7 |
| 2011 | 160.0 | 395.4 |
| 2012 | 170.3 | 420.8 |
| 2013 | 175.2 | 432.9 |
| 2014 | 181.5 | 448.5 |
| 2015 | 179.7 | 444.0 |
| 2016 | 185.1 | 457.4 |
| Total | 2,149.7 | 5,312.0 |

*Note:* Global hectarage of biotech crops in 2016 increased to 185.1 million hectares compared with 179.7 million hectares in 2015, equivalent to 3 per cent or 5.4 million hectares.
*Source:* ISAAA, 2016 (with permission).

GM crops. These developments in the application of GM technology for crops in African countries represent a positive step toward wider spread of the technology, and further support for the GMOs advocates.

The main biotech crops to date are maize, soybean, cotton, canola, sugar beet, alfalfa, papaya, squash, potato brinjal/eggplant, and pineapple. From 1994 to 2016, a total of 40 countries have issued regulatory approvals to GM crops for consumption either as food and/or feed as well as for environmental release. From these countries, 3,768 approvals have been issued by regulatory authorities across 26 GM crops. Of these approvals, 1,777 are for food use (direct use or for processing), 1,238 are for feed use (direct use or for processing), and 753 are for environmental release or cultivation (ISAAA Brief 52–2016: Executive Summary). Maize still has the most number of approved events (218 in 29 countries), followed by cotton (58 events in 22 countries), potato (47 events in 11 countries), canola (38 events in 14 countries), and soybean (35 events in 28 countries. The top ten countries that granted food, feed, and cultivation/environment approvals are Japan, United States, Canada, Mexico, South Korea, Taiwan, Australia, New Zealand, EU, and Philippines (ISAAA Brief 52–2016: Executive Summary).

ISAAA (ISAAA Brief 52–2016: Executive Summary) projects that game-changing innovations will revolutionize the development of new biotech crops and traits. Three reasons justify this projection: first, the increasing adoption and appreciation by farmers of stacked traits; second, the advent of biotech crops and traits that not only cater to

TABLE 1.2 Global Area of Biotech Crops in 2015 and 2016: by Country (Million Hectares[b])

| | Country | 2015 | % | 2016 | % | +/- | % |
|---|---|---|---|---|---|---|---|
| 1 | United States[a] | 70.9 | 39 | 72.9 | 39 | 2.0 | 3 |
| 2 | Brazil[a] | 44.2 | 25 | 49.1 | 27 | 4.9 | 11 |
| 3 | Argentina[a] | 24.5 | 14 | 23.8 | 13 | −0.7 | −3 |
| 4 | Canada[a] | 11.0 | 6 | 11.6 | 6 | 0.6 | 5 |
| 5 | India[a] | 11.6 | 6 | 10.8 | 6 | −0.8 | −7 |
| 6 | Paraguay[a] | 3.6 | 2 | 3.6 | 2 | 0.4 | 0 |
| 7 | Pakistan[a] | 2.9 | 2 | 2.9 | 2 | −0.1 | −24 |
| 8 | China[a] | 3.7 | 2 | 2.8 | 2 | 0.1 | 17 |
| 9 | South Africa[a] | 2.3 | 1 | 2.7 | 1 | 0.2 | −7 |
| 10 | Uruguay[a] | 1.4 | 1 | 1.3 | 1 | 0.1 | 9 |
| 11 | Bolivia[a] | 1.1 | 1 | 1.2 | 1 | 0 | 29 |
| 12 | Australia[a] | 0.7 | <1 | 0.9 | <1 | 0.1 | 14 |
| 13 | Philippines[a] | 0.7 | <1 | 0.8 | <1 | 0.1 | 0 |
| 14 | Myanmar[a] | 0.3 | <1 | 0.3 | <1 | 0.1 | 0 |
| 15 | Spain[a] | 0.1 | <1 | 0.1 | <1 | <0.1 | 0 |
| 16 | Sudan[a] | 0.1 | <1 | 0.1 | <1 | <0.1 | 0 |
| 17 | Mexico[a] | 0.1 | <1 | 0.1 | <1 | <0.1 | <0.1 |
| 18 | Colombia[a] | 0.1 | <1 | 0.1 | <1 | <0.1 | <0.1 |
| 19 | Vietnam | <0.1 | <1 | <1 | <1 | <0.1 | <0.1 |
| 20 | Honduras | <0.1 | <1 | <1 | <1 | <0.1 | <0.1 |
| 21 | Chile | <0.1 | <1 | <1 | <1 | <0.1 | <0.1 |
| 22 | Portugal | <0.1 | <1 | <1 | <1 | <0.1 | <0.1 |
| 23 | Bangladesh | <0.1 | <1 | <1 | <1 | <0.1 | <0.1 |
| 24 | Costa Rica | <0.1 | <1 | <1 | <1 | <0.1 | <0.1 |
| 25 | Slovakia | <0.1 | <1 | <1 | <1 | <0.1 | <0.1 |
| 26 | Czech Republic | <0.1 | <1 | <1 | <1 | <0.1 | <0.1 |
| 27 | Burkina Faso | 0.5 | <1 | | | | |
| 28 | Romania | <0.1 | <1 | – | – | – | – |
| | Total | 179.7 | 100 | 185.1 | 100 | 5.4 | 3.0 |

[a] Biotech mega-countries growing 50,000 hectares or more.
[b] Rounded off to the nearest hundred thousand or more.
*Source:* ISAAA, 2016 (with permission).

farmers' agricultural needs but more so the preference and nutritional needs of consumers; and third, the heightened utilization of innovative tools of gene discovery and their subsequent use in crop improvement and varietal development.

In addition to the annual briefs, the ISAAA produce weekly updates on global developments in crop biotechnology under the title "Crop Biotech Update" (www.isaaa.org/kc/cropbiotechupdate).

On December 20, 2017, "Biotech Update" reported the following developments on the use of biotechnology and GMOs:

- "Society of toxicology: no verifiable evidence of potential for adverse health effects of GE crops"

The Society of Toxicology (SOT), a professional membership association of more than 8,200 scientists worldwide, has approved and released a new "Issue Statement" on food

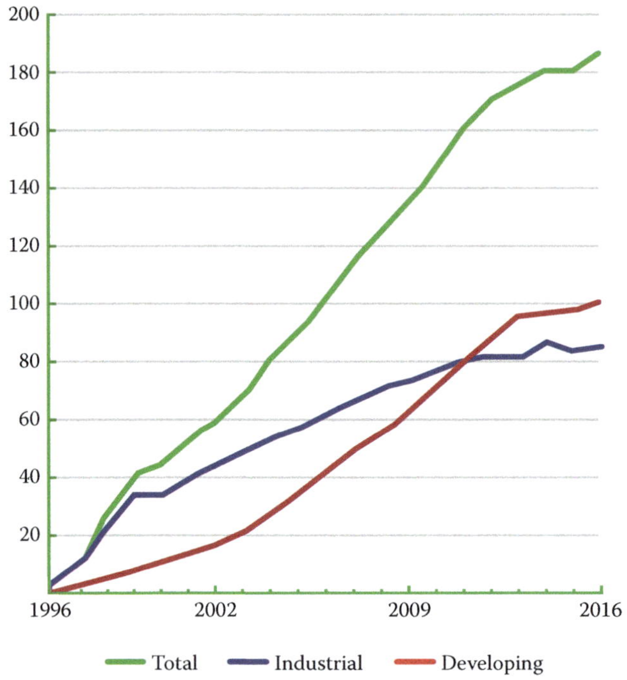


FIGURE 1.1 Global Area of Biotech Crops, 1996 to 2016: Industrial and Developing Countries (Million Hectares).

(*Source*: **ISAAA, 2016.**)

and feed safety related to GE crops. The Issue Statement has five key observations on safety, substantial equivalence, and labeling.

The Society affirms the safety of GE crops amid ongoing public debate about potential adverse impacts of GE crops on human or animal health, saying that each new event has been evaluated by regulatory authorities and all necessary regulatory approvals were secured before their commercial release. The Statement also mentioned that many GE events have achieved tremendous commercial success in the ensuing 20 years, and during that time, there has been no verifiable evidence of the potential for adverse health effects.

The following updates were reported on November 15, 2017, in the "Biotech Update" website:

- *"Biotech-improved golden potatoes contain higher levels of vitamins A and E."*

Scientists from Ohio State University and Italian National Agency for New Technologies have developed a "golden" potato with improved levels of vitamins A and E. The researchers used GE to boost provitamin A carotenoids and xanthophylls in potato, then studied the bioaccessibility of the nutrients in boiled wild type and golden (yellow-orange) tubers in a simulated digestive system. Results showed that a serving of golden potato can provide as much as 42 per cent of a child's recommended daily intake of vitamin A and 34 per cent of a child's recommended intake of vitamin E. They also found that women of reproductive age could get 15 per cent of their recommended vitamin A and 17 per cent of recommended vitamin E from that same 5.3-ounce (150-gram) serving. The result of their study is published in *PLOS One* journal.

The update of November 2, 2017, included the following report, among others:

- "Scientists develop late blight-resistant potato"

A research team at The Sainsbury Laboratory in Norwich Research Park, Norwich, United Kingdom, has successfully modified a popular potato variety (Maris Piper) to resist the devastating disease "late blight" by introducing a blight-resistant gene from a wild potato to the Maris Piper variety. This new blight-resistant gene introduced to the Maris Piper offers the promise of furthering its crop strength, and even the possibility of avoiding the use of chemical fungicides in its cultivation altogether.

On October 25, 2017, ISAAA reported the following news in its Biotech Updates:

- "Oxford scientists 'Supercharge' rice with maize gene; yields to increase by 50 per cent"

  To improve photosynthesis in rice plant, and increase its yield, scientists working on the Oxford University-led C4 Rice Project have, by introducing a single maize gene to the plant, moved toward "supercharging" rice to the level of more efficient crops. Scientists thought that if rice could be "switched" to use C4 photosynthesis (which is found to be more efficient than the C3 photosynthetic pathway naturally used by rice), its productivity will increase by 50 per cent.
- "Disease-resistant potato field tests show positive results in Uganda"

  Research on disease-resistant GM potato is underway in Uganda, according to the Director of Kachwekano Zonal Agriculture Research Institute. So far, three trials of Victoria potato variety have been conducted and the performance of the GM crop is good, no diseases were detected and the yield is high. It is expected that potatoes will be the first GMO crop to be commercialized in Uganda.

The following updates were reported on October 11, 2017, in the website:

- In relation to the potential role of GM on food security, a group of agricultural scientists comprising a team, from Rothamsted Research in the United Kingdom, Syngenta Crop Science and Symmetry Bioanalytics in the United States, reviewed how biotechnology developments over the past 35 years have shaped the efficiency of crop production. They concluded that GM of plants will reduce costs of production and increase productivity in farming, and will be essential to avert future food shortages.
- On the issue of the role of GM in enhancing the nutritional value of food crops, a study conducted by a group of scientists from Rutgers University, New Brunswick, New Jersey, USA discovered a way to enhance the nutritional value of corn. This could benefit millions of people around the world. The study involved inserting a bacterial gene that causes it to produce the key nutrient methionine.
- The potential role of GM technology on human health has been one of the debated issues. Researchers at the University of California, Riverside (UCR) tested a GM soybean oil used in restaurants, and found that while it induces less obesity and insulin resistance than conventional soybean oil, its effects on diabetes and fatty liver are similar to those of conventional soybean oil.

The update of October 4, 2017, included the following report, among others:

- A team of scientists from the Institute for Sustainable Agriculture in Cordoba, Spain, used GE to remove 90 per cent of the gliadins in wheat. They added genes that stop the production of the proteins. To prevent the wheat from making gliadins again, they knocked out 35 out of the 45 genes involved using CRISPR gene-editing. Though the resulting wheat cannot be used in baking sliced loaf breads because of less gluten content, it is found to be good enough for making baguettes and rolls.

On September 27, 2017, ISAAA reported the following news in its Biotech Updates:

- The National Biosafety Authority of Kenya has approved the field trial of Bt cotton (MON 15985 event). The Authority of the Republic of Kenya also published lists the approved GM applications in 2016–2017, including transgenic bananas for resistance to Banana Xanthomas Wilt (BXW) disease, and laboratory and greenhouse trials of modified sweet potato for weevil resistance.
- The Court of Justice of the European Union (CJEU) ruled that prejudices on GMOs are unfounded. This indicates more legal support to the use of GMO technology, in contrast to the general opposition by the EU states to the various applications of GMOs.

On September 13, 2017, Biotech Update reported the following developments on the use of biotechnology and GMOs:

- The non-aligned movement (NAM) scientists acknowledged the importance of biotechnology during the technical meeting on Science and Technology in Zimbabwe on August 22–24, 2017. Participants came from Cuba, Egypt, Gambia, India, Indonesia, Kenya, Malaysia, Mauritius, Myanmar, Nepal, Nigeria, South Africa, Sri Lanka, Sudan, Tanzania, Togo, Zambia, and Zimbabwe. A new resolution on biotechnology was adopted during the meeting. Member states of NAM were encouraged to invest more in scientific research to maximize the potential of biotechnology in driving economic progress.
- A group of the Chinese Academy of Agricultural Sciences (CAAS) researchers successfully incorporated a Bt gene into cabbage plants to improve resistance to the destructive pest, diamondback moth (*Plutella xylostella*).

GMWATCH publishes periodic reviews highlighting the negative aspects and failures of applying the GM technology to crop production, and how it might affect human health. Here are some of those reviews and articles reflecting their views on GM technology and GMOs and what the future might hold for them.

The following highlights are taken from the GMWatch Review 387, published on January 23, 2018 (GMWatch 2018).

- Thirty three thousand march in Berlin for better food and farming.

On 20 January, 33,000 people came together to demand a transformation of agriculture. Opposition to GMOs and dangerous pesticides, like glyphosate and the bee-killing neonicotinoids, were among the protest themes.

- Glyphosate and GM crops are harming no-till soils (Published in "No-Till Farmer Magazine")
- More pesticide runoff from no-till fields than ploughed fields
- Roundup causes changes in gut microbiome of rats

- Glyphosate herbicides contain toxic heavy metals, including arsenic
- Non-GMO yeast can reduce toxic acrylamide in potatoes and other foods
- GM among top ten food safety concerns posed by United States-United Kingdom

On October 11, 2017, GMWATCH published a report from Soil Association (2017) entitled "GM cotton's dramatic failure in India." The report was taken from the Soil Association website https://www.soilassociation.org/news/2017/october/gm-cotton-s-dramatic-failure-in-india/. It states that GM cotton grew to almost obliterate all other cotton production in India, and that the promised success of GM cotton rapidly turned to failure, with disastrous, even lethal, results for the poor farmers. The report indicated that alternative and more sustainable cotton production methods can replace GM cotton production. One proposed solution is to use the organic cotton production method, which uses non-GM seeds. The picture painted by the report shows that the promising good performance of GM cotton was short-lived, as the crop experienced severe pest attacks, causing a threefold increase in production costs due to the more expensive pesticide needed. The net result of that failure was mainly felt by the small-scale poor cotton growers, who represent most of India's cotton producers. Huge debts were incurred on those farmers due to this failure, the report states. The reported pest that caused the damage, and became immune to GM cotton, was the pink bollworm, the pest the plants were designed to resist. GMWATCH considers this failure as a big blow on the face of GM technology supporters, especially in crop production area.

Another article published by GMWATCH (GMWATCH 2017) on its website reports a case of plagiarism related to GM products of Monsanto. The article entitled "Glyphosate: expert finds BfR guilty of plagiarism from Monsanto" states that authors from the German authority BfR are guilty of "serious scientific misconduct" in copy-pasting a Monsanto report without giving citations or distinguishing between Monsanto's and their own assessments. A report by the Austrian NGO GLOBAL 2000 indicates that BfR had heavily plagiarized Monsanto's text, uncritically and without giving citations, leading to a situation where it was not possible to distinguish Monsanto's interpretation of the data from BfR's. This was regarded as a violation of guidance from the EU Commission, which states that comments and conclusions of national rapporteurs need to be clearly differentiated from the conclusions of the authors of any relevant studies and the industry applicant.

GMWATCH gives this as an example of the influence of Monsanto on other agencies and stakeholders to market its products and views. The findings in the report are said to add weight to the concern of NGOs and MEPs that Monsanto heavily influence the EU assessment of glyphosate. Both the European Food Safety Authority (EFSA) and the European Chemicals Agency (ECHA) concluded that glyphosate is not carcinogenic. Their conclusion does not agree with the view of the WHO's cancer agency International Agency for Research on Cancer (IARC), which classifies glyphosate as a probable human carcinogen and adds that evidence for its genotoxicity (ability to damage DNA) is strong.

## REFERENCES

Aldrich, L. 1999. *Consumer Use of Information: Implications for Food Policy*. Food and Rural Economics Division, Economic Research Service, U.S. Department of Agriculture. Agricultural Handbook No. 715.

Andrews, R. 2013. "All about" series. All about genetically modified foods. http://www.precisionnutrition.com/all-about-gm-foods. (accessed October 11, 2017).
Anon. 2005. Genetically modified foods: benefits of GM food. https://classes.soe.ucsc.edu/cmpe080e/Spring05/projects/gmo/benefits.htm (accessed September 25, 2017).
Auer, C.A. 2003. Tracking genes from seed to supermarket: techniques and trends. *Trends in Plant Science,* 8:591–597.
Australian Broadcasting Corporation (ABC) News. 2013. Scientists speak out against vandalism of genetically modified rice. http://www.abc.net.au/news/2013-09-20/scientists-speak-out-against-vandalism-of-gm-rice/4970626 (accessed August 26, 2017).
BBC News. 2012. GM wheat trial belongs in a laboratory. http://www.bbc.com/news/science-environment-17928172 (accessed August 26, 2017).
Bio. 2017. What is animal biotech? https://www.bio.org/articles/what-animal-biotechnology (accessed October 24, 2017).
Byrne, P., Pendell, D. and Graf, G. 2014. Labeling of genetically modified foods. 9.371 http://extension.colostate.edu/topic-areas/nutrition-food-safety-health/labeling-of-genetically-modified-foods-9-371/ (accessed October 25, 2017).
Codex Alimentarius Commission. 2003. Codex principles and guidelines on foods derived from biotechnology http://www.bfr.bund.de/cm/343/codex_principles_and_guidelines_on_foods_derived_from_biotechnology.pdf (accessed September 21, 2017).
Conko, G. and Prakash, C.S. 2004. Can GM crops play a role in developing countries? *AgBioWorld.* http://www.agbioworld.org/biotech-info/articles/agbio-articles/gm-crop-role.html (accessed October 26, 2017).
Coval, J.D., and Moskowitz, T.J. 1999. Home bias at home: Local equity preference in domestic portfolios. *Journal of Finance* 54:2045–2073.
CTV News Kitchener. 2013. March against Monsanto comes to King street in kitchener. CTV television network. http://kitchener.ctvnews.ca/march-against-monsanto-comes-to-king-street-in-kitchener-1.1296971 (accessed August 26, 2017).
Davison, J. 2010. GM plants: science, politics and EC regulations. *Plant Science,* 178(2):94–8.
Durant, J., Bauer, M., and Gaskell, G. 1999. *Biotechnology in the Public Sphere: A European Source Book.* Science Museum Press, London, UK.
EuropaBio. 2017. What is biotechnology? http://www.europabio.org/biotech-benefits/what-is-biotechnology (accessed October 22, 2017).
Experts. 2014. GMO answers. http://gmoanswers.com/experts (accessed August 26, 2017).
Fagan, J., Antoniou, M., and Robinson, C. 2014. *GMO Myths and Truths: An Evidence-Based Examination of the Claims Made for the Safety and Efficacy of Genetically Modified Crops and Foods.* Earth Open Source. 2nd edition, Version 1.0. http://responsibletechnology.org/GMO-Myths-and-Truths-edition2.pdf (accessed September 9, 2017).
Falck-Zepeda, J., Gruère, G., and Sithole-Niang, I. (Eds). 2013. *Genetically Modified Crops in Africa Economic and Policy Lessons from Countries South of the Sahara.* International Food Policy Research Institute, Washington, DC.
FAO Corporate Document Repository. 2005. Codex Alimentarius food import and export inspection and certification systems. http://www.fao.org/docrep/009/y6396e/Y6396E00.htm (accessed October 25, 2017).
FAO. 2005. Status of research and application of crop biotechnologies in developing countries (FAO-BioDeC). FAO Corporate Document Repository. http://www.fao.org/docrep/008/y5800e/Y5800E02.htm (accessed October 15, 2017).

FDA. 1992. Statement of policy: foods derived from new plant varieties, guidance to industry for foods derived from new plant varieties. VI, Labeling. FDA Federal Register, Volume 57. https://www.fda.gov/Food/GuidanceRegulation/GuidanceDocumentsRegulatoryInformation/Biotechnology/ucm096095.htm (accessed October 7, 2017).

Freedeman, J. 2009. *Genetically Modified Food: How Biotechnology is Changing What We Eat.* 1st Edition. The Rosen Publishing Group Inc., New York.

Frewer, L. 2003. Societal issues and public attitudes towards Genetically Modified foods. *Trends in Food Science and Technology,* 14:319–332.

Fusaro, D. 2013. European scientists ask for GMO research. *Food Processing.* http://www.foodprocessing.com/articles/2013/european-scientists-ask-for-gmo-research/ (accessed August 28, 2017).

Gaskell, G., Allum, N.C., and Stares, S.R. 2003. *Europeans and Biotechnology in 2002: Eurobarometer 58.0.* European Commission, Brussels.

Gaskell, G., Stares, S., Allansdottir, A., et al. 2010. Europeans and biotechnology in 2010: winds of change? A report to the European Commission's Directorate-General for Research. https://ec.europa.eu/research/swafs/pdf/pub_archive/europeans-biotechnology-in-2010_en.pdf (accessed October 24, 2017).

Ghosh, D. K. and Williams, P. 2010. Global food biotechnology regulations and urgency for harmonization. Chapter 29, in Bagchi, D., Lau F.C. and Ghosh, D. K. (Eds.) *Biotechnology in Functional Foods and Nutraceuticals.* CRC Press. Boca Raton, FL, pp 531–541.

GMWatch. 2017. Glyphosate: expert finds BfR guilty of plagiarism from Monsanto http://www.gmwatch.org/en/news/latest-news/17898-glyphosate-expert-finds-bfr-guilty-of-plagiarism-from-monsanto-demolishes-excuses (accessed October 12, 2017).

GMWatch. 2018. GMWatch review 387, January 23, 2018. https://gmwatch.us6.list-manage.com/track/click?u=29cbc7e6c21e0a8fd2a82aeb8&id=90906ea823&e=7995e6f1a4.

Golan, E., and Kuchler, F. 2011. Chapter 11 The effect of GM labeling regime on market outcomes, in Carter, C.A., Moschini, G., and Sheldon, I. (Eds.) *Genetically Modified Food and Global Welfare (Frontiers of Economics and Globalization,* Volume 10), Emerald Group Publishing Limited, pp. 263–281.

Government of Canada. 2012. The regulation of genetically modified food. https://www.canada.ca/en/health-canada/services/science-research/reports-publications/biotechnology/regulation-genetically-modified-foods.html (accessed June 22, 2017).

Gruère, G.P., and Rao, S.R. 2007. A review of international labeling policies of genetically modified food to evaluate India's propose rule. *AgBioForum,* 10(1):51–64. http://www.agbioforum.org/v10n1/index.htm (accessed October 25, 2017).

Halford, N. and Shewry, P. 2000. Genetically modified crops: methodology, benefits, regulation and public concerns. *British Medical Bulletin* 56:62–73.

Han, J.H., and Harrison, R.W. 2007. Factors influencing urban consumers' acceptance of Genetically Modified foods. *Review of Agricultural Economics* 29(4):700–719.

Hansen, M. 2001. Genetically engineered food: Make sure it's safe and label it, in Nelson, G.C. (Ed.) *Genetically Modified Organisms in Agriculture.* Academic Press, San Diego. pp. 239–255.

Harmon, A. 2013. A race to save the orange by altering its DNA. *The New York Times.* http://www.nytimes.com/2013/07/28/science/a-race-to-save-the-orange-by-altering-its-dna.html?pagewanted=all&_r=1& (accessed October 20, 2017).

Health and Safety Executive. 2017. What are GMOs? http://www.hse.gov.uk/biosafety/gmo/whatare.htm (accessed March 27, 2017).

Heiman, A. and Zilberman, D. 2011. The effects of farming on consumers' choice of GM foods. *Agbioforum.org* 14, article 9.

Helmuth, L. 2000. Biotechnology. Both sides claim victory in trade pact. *Science*, 287(5454):782–783.

Hilbeck, A., Binimelis, R., Defarge, N. et al. 2015. No scientific consensus on GMO safety. *Environmental Sciences Europe* 27 article 4, 1–6.

Husby, J. 2007. Definitions of GMO/LMO and modern biotechnology. Chapter 23 in: *Biosafety First*. Traavik, T. and Lim, L.C. (Eds.), Tapir Academic Publishers. http://genok.no/wp-content/uploads/2013/04/Chapter-23.pdf (accessed April 22, 2017).

ISAAA Brief 52–2016: Executive Summary. http://www.isaaa.org/resources/publications/briefs/52/executivesummary/default.asp.

ISAAA. 2016. *Global Status of Commercialized Biotech/GM Crops: 2016*. ISAAA Brief No. 52. ISAAA, Ithaca, NY.

Just Label it. 2017. Labeling around the world. http://www.justlabelit.org/right-to-know-center/labeling-around-the-world/ (accessed October 25, 2017).

Kiguli, L.N. 2000. The utilisation of Azolla filiculoides Lam. as a biofertiliser under dryland conditions. Master thesis, University of Rhodes, South Africa.

Kim, R.B. 2012. Consumer attitude of risk and benefits toward genetically modified (GM) foods in South Korea: implications for food policy. *Inzinerine Ekonomika-Engineering Economics* 23(2):189–199.

Knight, J.G., Mather, D.W., and Holdsworth, D.K. 2014. Consumer benefits and acceptance of genetically modified food. http://otago.ourarchive.ac.nz/bitstream/handle/10523/1605/ConsumerbenefitsGMOs.pdf (accessed September 14, 2017).

Kopicki, A. 2013. Strong support for labeling modified foods. *The New York Times*. http://www.nytimes.com/2013/07/28/science/strong-support-for-labeling-modified-foods.html?_r=1& (accessed October 26, 2017).

Lang, J. T., and Hallman, W.K. 2005. Who does the public trust? The case of genetically modified food in the United States. *Risk Analysis* 25(5):1241–52.

Law Library of Congress: LAW.gov. 2015. Restrictions on genetically modified organisms: United States. http://www.loc.gov/law/help/restrictions-on-gmos/usa.php (accessed October 4, 2017).

Mahgoub, S.E.O. 2016. *Genetically Modified Foods: Basics, Applications, and Controversy*. CRC Press, Taylor & Francis Group, Boca Raton, FL.

Martínez, V.D. 2011. The colors of biotechnology. BiotechSpain. http://biotechspain.com/en/article.cfm?iid=colores_biotecnologia (accessed May 16, 2017).

McInerney, C., Bird, N., and Nucci, M. 2004. The flow of scientific knowledge from lab to the lay public: the case of genetically modified food. *Science Communication* 26:75–106.

National Academies of Sciences, Engineering, and Medicine. 2016. *Genetically Engineered Crops: Experiences and Prospects*. The National Academies Press, Washington, DC. Available from: http://www.nap.edu/23395 (accessed August 16, 2017).

National Research Council of the National Academies. 2008. *Global Challenges and Directions for Agricultural Biotechnology: Workshop Report*. The National Academies Press, Washington, DC. http://www.nap.edu/catalog/12216.html (accessed August 16, 2017).

Naveen. 2012. Genetic engineering vs biotechnology. Difference between.com. http://www.differencebetween.com/difference-between-genetic-engineering-and-vs-biotechnology/ (accessed September 11, 2017).

NC State Extension: Ag Bio Tech. 2017. What is the difference between genetically modified organisms and genetically engineered organisms. https://agbiotech.ces.ncsu.edu/q1-what-is-the-difference-between-genetically-modified-organisms-and-genetically-engineered-organisms-we-seem-to-use-the-terms-interchangeably/ (accessed September 11, 2017).

NON-GMO Project. 2017. GMO facts. https://www.nongmoproject.org/gmo-facts/. (accessed October 11, 2017).

Novella, S. 2014. The GMO controversy. Neurologica blog http://theness.com/neurologicablog/index.php/the-gmo-controversy/ (accessed September 12, 2017).

OECD. 1993. *Safety Evaluation of Foods Derived by Modern Biotechnology: Concepts and Principles*. Chapter 2, pp 13–16. Organisation for Economic Co-operation and Development, Paris, France. http://www.oecd.org/science/biotrack/41036698.pdf (accessed September 21, 2017).

Penn State College of Agricultural Sciences. 2015. The science of GMOs. What Are GMOs? http://agsci.psu.edu/magazine/articles/2015/spring-summer/the-science-of-gmos (accessed January 20, 2017).

Pew Initiative on Food and Biotechnology. 2007. Application of biotechnology for functional foods. http://www.pewtrusts.org/~/media/legacy/uploadedfiles/wwwpewtrustsorg/reports/food_and_biotechnology/pifbfunctionalfoodspdf.pdf (accessed October 24, 2017).

Phillips, T. 2008. Genetically modified organisms (GMOs): Transgenic crops and recombinant DNA technology. *Nature Education* 1(1):213. Available from: Scitable by Nature Education: a collaborative space learning for science http://www.nature.com/scitable/topicpage/Genetically-Modified-Organisms-GMOs-Transgenic-Crops-and-732 (accessed September 22, 2017).

Pollack, A. 2013. Seeking support, biotech food companies pledge transparency. *The New York Times*. http://www.nytimes.com/2013/07/29/business/seeking-support-biotech-food-companies-pledge-transparency.html (accessed October 24, 2017).

Powell, C. 2015. How to make a GMO. Harvard University, The Graduate School of Arts and Sciences Blog, Special Edition on GMOs. http://sitn.hms.harvard.edu/flash/2015/how-to-make-a-gmo/ (accessed March 27, 2017).

Quick, D. 2013. Seeds at root of protest march. *The Post and Courier*. http://www.postandcourier.com/archives/seeds-at-root-of-protest-march/article_7ac72306-db2b-5d18-a8e2-08f15e38512b.html (accessed October 24, 2017).

Science Daily. 2013. Fighting GM crop vandalism with a government-protected research site. http://www.sciencedaily.com/releases/2013/02/130228124134.htm (accessed October 26, 2017).

Sense About Science. 2012. Don't destroy research Q & A.: plant scientists answer your questions. http://archive.senseaboutscience.org/pages/rothamsted-appeal.html (accessed October 25, 2017).

Shrestha, R. 2010. The Importance of biotechnology in today's time. Aakhayan. A Chapter Scripting Life. http://raunakms.wordpress.com/2010/06/04/the-importance-of-biotechnology-in-todays-time/ (accessed October 10, 2017).

Sleenhoff, S. and Osseweijer, P. 2013. Consumer choice linking consumer intentions to actual purchase of GM labeled food products. *GM Crops and Food: Biotechnology in Agriculture and the Food Chain*, 4(3):166–171.

Soil Association. 2017. GM cotton's dramatic failure in India. https://www.soilassociation.org/news/2017/october/gm-cotton-s-dramatic-failure-in-india/ (accessed October 12, 2017).

Sundstrom, F.J., Williams, J., VanDeynze, A. and Bradford, K.J. 2002. Identity preservation of agricultural commodities. *Agricultural Biotechnology in California Series* Pub 8077. http://anrcatalog.ucdavis.edu/pdf/8077.pdf (accessed October 23, 2017).
Takepart. 2017. What are GMOs? http://www.takepart.com/flashcards/what-are-gmos (accessed March 26, 2017).
The Illinois Farm Bureau. 2017. Let's talk about: Biotechnology and GMOs https://www.ilfb.org/media/2397646/lets-talk-about-biotechnology-and-gmos.pdf (accessed September 12, 2017).
Trombitsky, I. 2017. Public Awareness on GMO issues: Practical outcomes (PPT). Eco-TIRAS, Moldova. http://www.unece.org/fileadmin//DAM//env/pp/gmo/Pres_Trombitsky-Nagoya-GMO (accessed October 10, 2017).
UNCTAD Secretariat. 2002 (1). UNCTAD/ITE/TEB/10. United Nations Conference on Trade and Development. KEY ISSUES IN BIOTECHNOLOGY. United Nations New York and Geneva, 2002. https://studylib.net/doc/10430005/key-issues-in-biotechnology--unctad-ite-teb-10-united-nat... (accessed September 11, 2017).
UNCTAD Secretariat. 2002 (2). Genetically modified crops and food biotechnology and health pp: 8–10 In: UNCTAD/ITE/TEB/10. United Nations Conference on Trade and Development. Key issues in biotechnology. United Nations New York and Geneva, 2002. https://studylib.net/doc/10430005/key-issues-in-biotechnology--unctad-ite-teb-10-united-nat... (accessed September 11, 2017).
von Mogel, K. H. 2013. GMO crops vandalized in Oregon. Biology Fortified. http://www.biofortified.org/2013/06/gmo-crops-vandalized-in-oregon/ (accessed October 26, 2017).
Whitman, D.B. 2000. Genetically modified foods: harmful or helpful? CSA discovery guides. https://biomed.brown.edu/arise/resources/docs/GM%20foods%20review.pdf (accessed October 25, 2017).
WHO. 2014. Food safety. Frequently asked questions on genetically modified foods. http://www.who.int/foodsafety/areas_work/food-technology/faq-genetically-modified-food/en/ (accessed January 20, 2017).
Wolfe, M. 2013. What are the uses of GMOs? Livestrong.com. http://www.livestrong.com/article/213053-pros-cons-of-gmo-foods/ (accessed September 22, 2017).
Yahoo News. A.P. 2013. Millions march against Monsanto in over 400 cities. http://news.yahoo.com/millions-march-against-monsanto-over-400-cities-222259976.html (accessed October 24, 2017).

## SUGGESTED REFERENCES

Biotech and Pharmaceutical Industries. *The Balance*. What exactly is a GMO? https://www.thebalance.com/biotech-4074047 (accessed February 15, 2017).
GMO Awareness. GMO facts. https://gmoawareness.org/gmo-facts/.
Haas, R. 2015. Food for thought: The difference between GMO and GE foods. http://www.opb.org/news/blog/newsblog/food-for-thought-the-difference-between-gmo-and-ge-foods/ (accessed May 11, 2017).
Illinois Farm Bureau. 2016. Biotechnology and GMOs. https://www.ilfb.org/resources/consumer-resources/hidden-biotechnology-and-gmos.aspx (accessed June 22, 2017).
Living non. GMO: a lifestyle site created by the Non-GMO project http://livingnongmo.org/learn/gmo-faq/?gclid=CISpmu-nndACFZWFaQodTjEANA.
Non-GMO Project. GMO facts. http://www.nongmoproject.org/gmo-facts/.

Penn State College of Agricultural Sciences. 2015. How GMOs are made—simplified. The science of GMOs http://agsci.psu.edu/magazine/articles/2015/spring-summer/the-science-of-gmos (accessed April 10, 2017).
Phillips, T. 2017. What are genetically modified organisms or GMOs? *The Balance* https://www.thebalance.com/what-are-gmos-375532 (accessed February 15, 2017).
The facts about GMOs. https://factsaboutgmos.org/.

# SECTION 2

# Sampling

CHAPTER 2

# Guidelines for Sample Preparation Procedures in GMO Analysis

*European Commission*
Joint Research Centre, Institute for Health and Consumer Protection

CONTENTS

## 2.1 INTRODUCTION

The ad hoc working group on sample preparation procedures was established on the basis of a mandate adopted at the 19th ENGL steering committee meeting held on October 6, 2010. The working group has been chaired by Gilbert Berben, Walloon Agricultural Research Centre (CRA-W), Gembloux, Belgium. The other members of the working group have been Diana Charels, Joint Research Centre (JRC), Institute of Health and Consumer Protection (IHCP), Ispra, Italy; Tina Demšar, National Institute of Biology (NIB), Ljubljana, Slovenia; Rupert Hochegger, Austrian Agency for Health and Food Safety (AGES), Vienna, Austria; Elena Nardini, Joint Research Centre (JRC), Institute of Health and Consumer Protection (IHCP), Ispra, Italy; Roberta Onori, Istituto Superiore di Sanità (ISS), Rome, Italy; Manuela Schulze, Rötgesbüttel, Germany; Patrick Philipp, Service Commun des Laboratoires, Strasbourg, France; and Thomas Weber, Joint Research Centre (JRC), Institute of Health and Consumer Protection (IHCP), Ispra, Italy.

The mandate of the working group was the following:

- Evaluation of the reference documents (ISO norms, CEN standards, legislative provisions) at national, European, and international levels related to sample preparation issues, both in general and focused on GM product analysis.
- Characterization of the most relevant scientific publications associated with sample preparation issues.

The text of the mandate also stressed particular issues to consider within the working group.

Within the cited reference documents and publications, the following issues will be covered:

- Evaluation of the correlation between particle size and DNA extraction yield for GMO crops.
- Comparison and evaluation of pros and cons derived from the use of different grinding devices.
- Evaluation of cross-contamination problems.
- Comparison between slurry technique and dry milling.
- Evaluation of practicability in terms of time of grinding operations, safety of operators, and working areas environmental issues.
- Evaluation of the weight of each of the above considered issues in order to analyze their contribution and identify the best sample preparation procedure.
- Set up of ad hoc standard operating procedures.

Finally, the mandate also gave some indications about the expected outcome:

> All this information should represent the basis to building up an operative guideline for laboratory technicians and to identifying correct pathways for a reliable analysis.

This document is the result of the ENGL working group on sample preparation procedures. However, it was based on other existing documents and mainly on an ISO document that existed as a draft when the working group started its mandate:

> '*Animal feeding stuffs—Guidelines for sample preparation*' as *document* ISO 6498 jointly prepared by Technical Committee ISO/TC 34, *Food products*, Subcommittee SC 10 and Technical Committee CEN/TC 327, *Animal feeding stuffs* (ISO/FDIS 6498:2011 (E)) It gave rise to the standard ISO 6498:2012 which specifically states that its *guidelines are overruled by special instructions and regulations for sample preparation demanded by specific analysis methods.*

Since GMO analysis using DNA-based techniques has special requirements related to cross-contamination risks, a specific document was still deemed necessary and the present report kept the format of a standard. The rules or guidelines described in it may probably be applied to any other DNA-based analysis covering the same range of matrices as those considered here for GMOs (food, feed, and seeds).

The guidelines were elaborated with the perspective that the test portion would be submitted to a DNA extraction step in view of a polymerase chain reaction (PCR) analysis. However, most of the principles outlined here should remain valid even if the final target analyte does not consist of DNA but of proteins (or polypeptides).

## 2.2 SCOPE

This document aims at providing guidelines for a correct sample preparation during GMO analysis on food, feed, seed, plants, and propagating material samples. For seed sample preparation, the reader is also referred to the ISTA rules (ISTA, 2013).

## 2.3 PRINCIPLE

The sample preparation guidelines describe the procedure for handling a laboratory sample upon its arrival in the laboratory to obtain homogeneous and representative test portions avoiding cross contamination.

In general, the whole laboratory sample is homogenized to obtain a test sample for the analysis. Sometimes, mass reduction (subsampling) has to be done. The procedure followed has to be documented.

All the sample preparation steps should be done under conditions avoiding cross contaminations and minimizing degradation of the target analyte (DNA or proteins) in the test portion.

Storage of the samples prior to and during the sample preparation as well as after the process should be performed under adequate conditions (e.g., at room temperature, refrigerated, frozen), depending on the sample.

## 2.4 DEFINITIONS

The following section provides an overview of definitions generally taken from GMO European legislation and standards (ISO and CEN).

### 2.4.1 General Definitions

#### *2.4.1.1 Lot*

A "lot" is a distinct and specified quantity of material dispatched or received at one time and covered by a particular contract or shipping document (Commission Recommendation 787/2004. European Commission (2004)).

#### *2.4.1.2 Grab Sampling*

Any "lump" or material from the lot, taken in a single operation (Minkkinen and Esbensen, 2009). Adapted at laboratory level in the context of sample preparation, it means that this material is taken from the laboratory sample or from the test sample. The focus of grab sampling is exclusively on getting the final subsample mass in one go (based on Petersen et al., 2005). Or in other words: "Catch whatever you can in the cheapest possible way!" (Lischer, 2001a).

### 2.4.2 Definitions Concerning the "Sample"

Since the model taken for this text is based on the standard for sample preparation relating to animal feeding stuffs, the working group recommends to use the definitions listed in ISO 6498:2012 with a small adaptation of the definition regarding the "reserve sample":

#### *2.4.2.1 Laboratory Sample*

Sample as prepared (from the lot) for sending to the laboratory and intended for inspection or testing (ISO/FDIS 6498:2011).

#### *2.4.2.2 Reserve Sample*

Leftover material from the test samples where test portions (or from the laboratory sample if both are the same) are taken away from and where no further particle size reduction is done (adapted from ISO/FDIS 6498:2011).

#### *2.4.2.3 Test Portion*

Quantity of material drawn from the test sample (or from the laboratory sample if both are the same) (ISO/FDIS 6498:2011).

Note: The definition for "test portion" provided by ISO 24266:2006 adds aspects that are not considered here: sample, as prepared for testing or analysis, the whole quantity being used for analyte extraction at one time.

#### *2.4.2.4 Test Sample*

(Sub-) sample prepared from the laboratory sample and from which test portions will be taken (ISO/FDIS 6498:2011).

Note: Mind that the definition provided here corresponds to what is called the "analytical sample" in Commission Recommendation 787/2004 (European Commission, 2004), while the concept of test sample in this recommendation is set equal to the notion of test portion as defined in ISO 24276:2006 and CEN TS 15568:2007.

#### *2.4.2.5 Other Definitions Related to the Sample*

Other definitions of the concept of "sample" and closely related issues according to various standards and regulatory texts are detailed in Appendix A.

### 2.4.3 Definitions Concerning the "Sample Preparation Procedure"

#### *2.4.3.1 Coarse Grinding (or Pre-grinding)*

A first grinding step of the whole sample to be carried out before mass reduction when the laboratory sample contains large lumps or if its mean particle size exceeds about 6 mm (ISO/FDIS 6498:2011).

#### *2.4.3.2 Comminution*

Any process (see a nonexhaustive list of possibilities in Section 2.9.3.1) that enables reduction of the average particle size of a solid material and thereby reduces its constitutional heterogeneity.

#### *2.4.3.3 Constitutional (Compositional) Heterogeneity*

Definition of the concept can be found under Section 2.5.1.1.

#### *2.4.3.4 Distributional Heterogeneity*

Definition of the concept can be found under Section 2.5.1.2.

#### *2.4.3.5 Fragment—Particle*

The smallest physically separable unit that is not affected by the subsampling process (based on Petersen et al., 2005). Comminution will affect the mean size of the fragments or particles.

#### *2.4.3.6 Homogeneity*

Degree to which a property or a constituent is uniformly distributed throughout a quantity of material (ISO/FDIS 6498:2011).

Note: Homogeneity may be considered to have been achieved in a practical sense when the sampling error of the processed portion is negligible compared to the total error of the measurement system. Since homogeneity depends on the size of the units under consideration, a mixture of two materials may not be homogeneous at the molecular or atomic level, but homogeneous at the particulate level. However, a uniform visual appearance does not ensure compositional homogeneity (ISO/FDIS 6498:2011). Heterogeneity has a larger impact on errors when the concentration of the property or the constituent to measure is low in the sample.

#### *2.4.3.7 Increment*

An increment in this context will be considered as a portion of material extracted from the laboratory sample when a subsampling process is required (adapted from Minkkinen and Esbensen, 2009).

#### *2.4.3.8 Incrementing (Composite Sampling)*

Collection of many random increments from the laboratory sample to make up the subsample. More generally, incrementing can be considered as the combination of a number of random increments to obtain a subsample before further processing or further analysis (based on ISO/FDIS 6498:2011).

Note: To meet the fundamental sampling principle, all increments must have the same probability of ending up in the sample.

#### *2.4.3.9 Mass Reduction*

Part of the sample preparation procedure to reduce the mass of a laboratory sample through subsampling (ISO/FDIS 6498:2011).

Note: After mass reduction, all subsamples should have the same properties as the original laboratory sample (ISO/FDIS 6498:2011).

#### *2.4.3.10 Mixing–blending-Homogenization*

Any process that enables a reduction of the grouping and segregation effects and thereby reduces the distributional heterogeneity of a sample.

Note: Comminution processes like grinding may not only contribute to particle size reduction but can also homogenize the sample.

#### *2.4.3.11 Particle Size Reduction*

Part of the sample preparation procedure done by chopping, crushing, cutting, blending (homogenizing), milling (grinding), and pulverizing to obtain a homogenous test sample for further analysis (based on ISO/FDIS 6498:2011).

Note: In general, the particle size reduction follows the mass reduction step of the sample preparation procedure with different sieve-size options to ensure integrity of the test sample(s) (ISO/FDIS 6498:2011).

## 2.5 GENERAL CONSIDERATIONS RELATED TO THE THEORY OF SAMPLING

Sample preparation steps have been shown to contribute to the largest error component in an analytical determination. This kind of error, which is generally overlooked, is in essence a sampling error, and therefore, it is generally much larger than the errors arising from subsequent analytical procedures. To fully comprehend the reasons of some actions to be undertaken in sample preparation, it is important to understand possible error sources and the means to reduce them.

### 2.5.1 Errors Linked to Characteristics of the Material under Analysis

Errors deriving from sample heterogeneity (i.e., properties of the material under analysis) contribute to the total subsampling error in two ways: through constitutional heterogeneity and through distributional heterogeneity. One should also bear in mind that the level of the analyte to be measured has a decisive influence on the possible error size. It must therefore be considered as a rule of thumb that the lower the content of the target analyte, the higher the measurement uncertainty on this parameter.

#### *2.5.1.1 Constitutional Heterogeneity*

When a great overall composition-based difference exists between the individual smallest inseparable fragments of a sample exists, the constitutional heterogeneity is large (Figure 2.1). The total contribution to heterogeneity is never zero, however, as that would be the case of all fragments being strictly identical. Mixing and blending does not change constitutional heterogeneity.

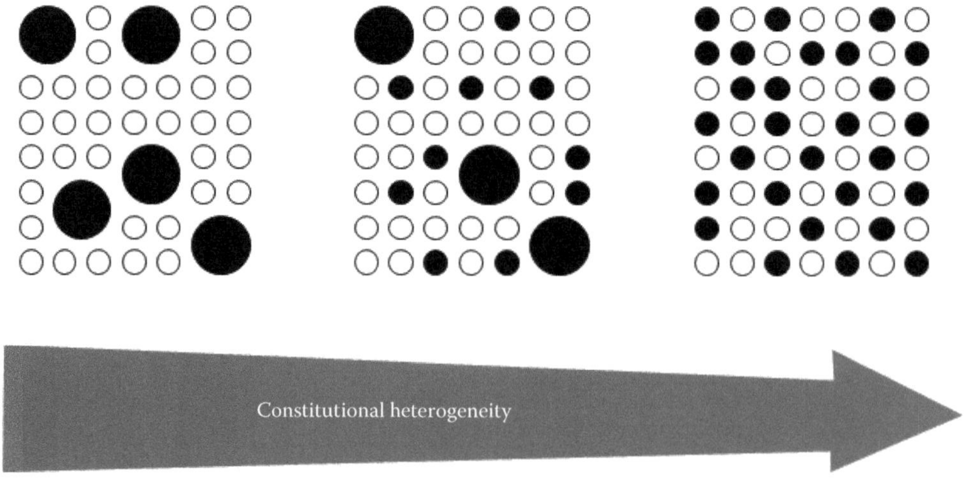


FIGURE 2.1 Illustration of a decreasing constitutional heterogeneity.

The only way to alter the constitutional heterogeneity of any given material is by comminution (crushing/cutting) or by other methods changing the physical properties of a sample. The reduction of the average particle size is the dominating factor in reducing constitutional heterogeneity. The other possibility to limit the constitutional heterogeneity is to consider a sufficient mass of test portion that can reflect the properties of the sample. In most cases, this is not an option because in GMO detection, the test portion size should generally remain small to be compatible with extraction procedures.

#### *2.5.1.2 Distributional Heterogeneity*

The grouping and segregation error is linked to the distributional heterogeneity. This heterogeneity reflects the nonrandom distribution of particles in the sample. It results mainly from the gravitational forces on particles of different densities, sizes, and shapes that cause grouping and segregation of all particles. Particles with large differences in size and/or density tend to segregate or stratify heavily, with the smallest and/or densest particles at the bottom of the sample.

"Mixing and blending" are techniques that can reduce the grouping and segregation error.

Distributional heterogeneity can best be illustrated by a laboratory sample consisting of black and white spheres. If all the black spheres are located at the bottom of the sample and the white spheres are more to the top, the system displays a very high distributional heterogeneity. If, on the other hand, the spheres have been mixed well (i.e., homogenized), the system's distributional heterogeneity would be significantly reduced (Figure 2.2).

Mixing is not an appropriate technique for many materials because it may, for some materials and under certain circumstances, increase segregation instead of reducing the grouping and segregation error. Segregation will always occur because of the force of gravity. Many materials will always display an innate propensity for segregation, even immediately after mixing, for example, highly density-fractionated materials and suspensions. Such systems require constant monitoring and treatment, but once this feature has been duly recognized, it can always be dealt with.

"Incrementing" is another technique that helps to reduce the distributional heterogeneity.

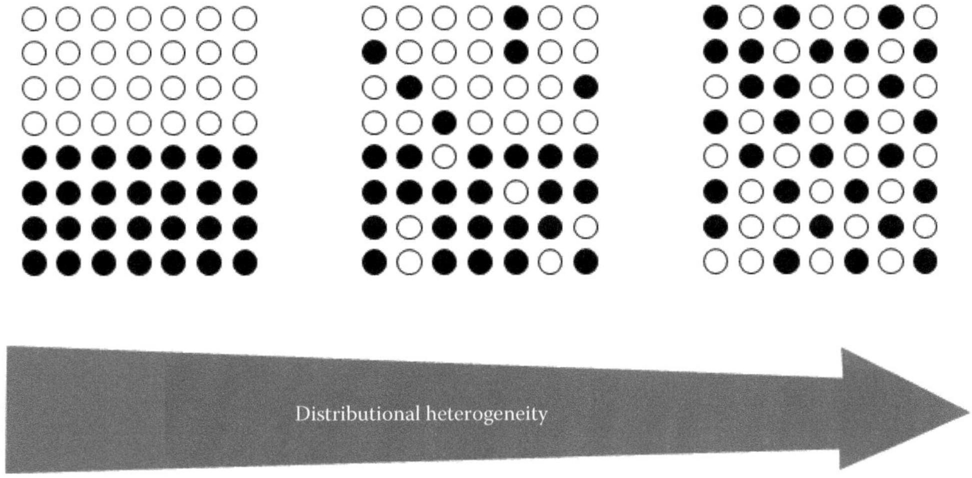


FIGURE 2.2 Illustration of a decreasing distributional heterogeneity.

### 2.5.2 Errors linked to the Subsampling Process

The way in which subsampling is achieved is also a source of possible errors. Any subsampling process produces its own sampling errors. Incorrect sampling errors (ISE) are to be avoided at any cost. These errors are the root cause of all sampling bias. Elimination of ISE, therefore, has absolute priority in all practical subsampling steps. These errors can be subdivided in three main types (Esbensen and Julius, 2010): increment delineation errors, increment extraction errors, and increment preparation errors.

#### *2.5.2.1 Increment Delineation Errors*

Errors linked to a delineation of the increment introduce a bias whereby the distributional heterogeneity of the increment systematically increases or decreases toward the mean distributional heterogeneity of the sample.

In correctly delineated increments, any part of the subsample or laboratory sample is represented in identical proportions. For three-dimensional samples, it is important to subsample also at the very bottom layer (to avoid the so-called "Brazil nut effect" linked to gravity). For material spread in a long pile, a complete cross-sectional slice avoids the increment delineation error. This concept can be illustrated by the use of shovels which are not square-edged (see Figure 2.3). In the illustrated examples, the correct delineation of the increment is shown in B and D, where all materials in between the vertical lines are sampled. The extraction is done incorrectly in A and C because of the extraction tools (e.g., round-edged shovel) used, which results in an incomplete sampling of the material in between the vertical lines (see 2.5.2.2).

#### *2.5.2.2 Increment Extraction Errors*

This error arises when fragments inside the delineated increment do not end up in the composite subsample (due to bouncing or dusting or due to the use of inappropriate sampling tools) or if fragments outside the delineated increment migrate into the composite subsample. Only fragments with their center of gravity inside the several delineated increments should become part of the composite subsample (as illustrated in Figure 2.4).

#### *2.5.2.3 Increment Preparation Errors*

This error arises when the sample is altered during its handling (e.g., contamination).

### 2.5.3 Subsampling Operations

There are only four subsampling operations to reduce the subsampling errors (Esbensen and Paasch-Mortensen, 2010):

- Composite subsampling (or incrementing),
- Comminution (particle size reduction),
- Mixing/blending,
- Representative mass reduction.

The first three aim to limit errors linked to the characteristics of the matrix under analysis. The last operation is linked to how subsampling itself has to be carried out in order to avoid ISE.

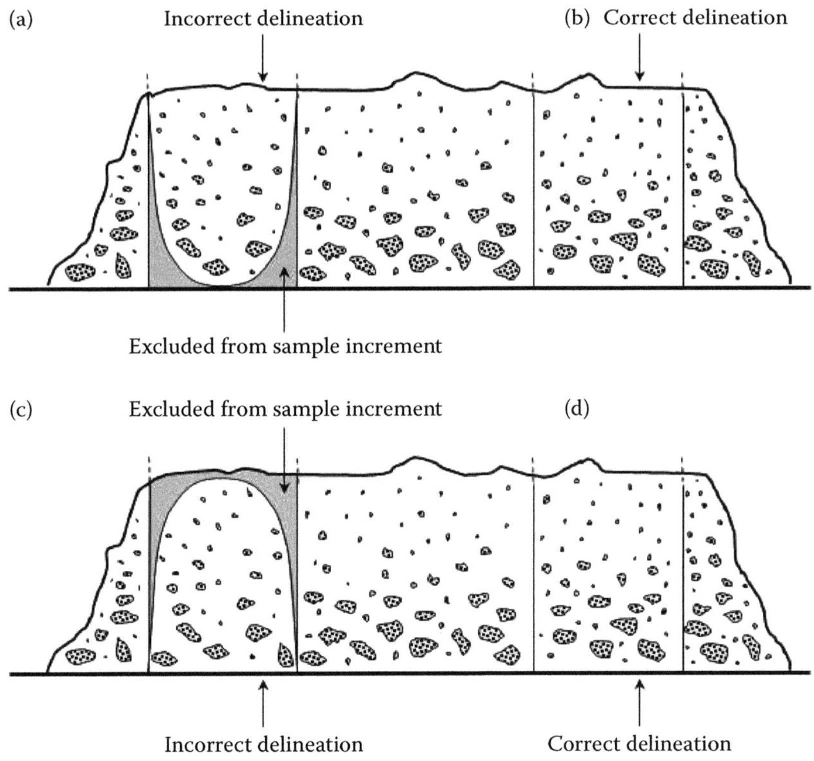


FIGURE 2.3 Use of inappropriate extraction tools can result in an incorrect delineation of the increment that will lead to over-representation (C) or under-representation (A) of some fractions present in the sample. (Adapted from Myers, 2004.)

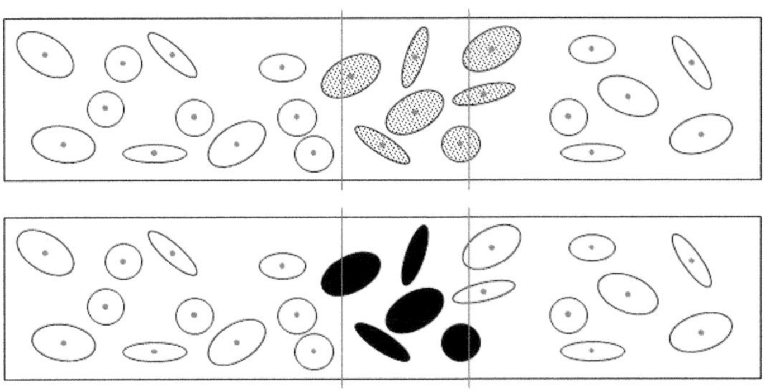

FIGURE 2.4 Sample extraction—only those fragments with their center of gravity (red dot) within the delineated increment should be extracted. The upper part of the figure shows all fragments which are in the increment or at least overlap it, while the lower part illustrates which fragments (in black) have to be extracted. (Adapted from Esbensen and Paasch-Mortensen, 2010.)

Representative mass reduction is a way to perform correct subsampling and avoid ISE.

## 2.6 EQUIPMENT

In the following section, examples of equipment that may be needed in sample preparation are given. The selection of the equipment depends on the specific needs of the laboratory.

### 2.6.1 Cleaning Tools

a. "Brushes" for cleaning grinders, etc.
b. "Compressed air blower" for cleaning
c. "Vacuum cleaner"
d. "Ultrasound bath" (e.g., useful for cleaning sieves)

### 2.6.2 Sampling Tools

Spoons, spatulas, and shovels.

To avoid the increment delineation errors, it is advised that spoons, spatulas, and shovels should be square-edged (e.g., Figure 2.5).

### 2.6.3 Sample Preparation

1. Balance
2. Seed Counting Device (Optional)

### 2.6.4 Drying Systems

1. Lyophilization (or Freeze-drying) System
2. Drying Ovens or Incubators

### 2.6.5 Equipment for Particle Size Reduction and Mixing

1. Mass Reduction Devices: Riffle Splitters
2. Grinders

For practical examples of grinders used in GMO laboratories, see Appendix B.

1. Dust Extractor
2. Mortar and Pestle or More Automatic Disruption Devices (e.g., TissueLyser)
3. Overhead Mixer, Tumbling Mixer, and Other Types of Mixers (e.g., Rotating Mixer, etc.)
4. Plastic Bags (see Section 2.9.3.4.2)

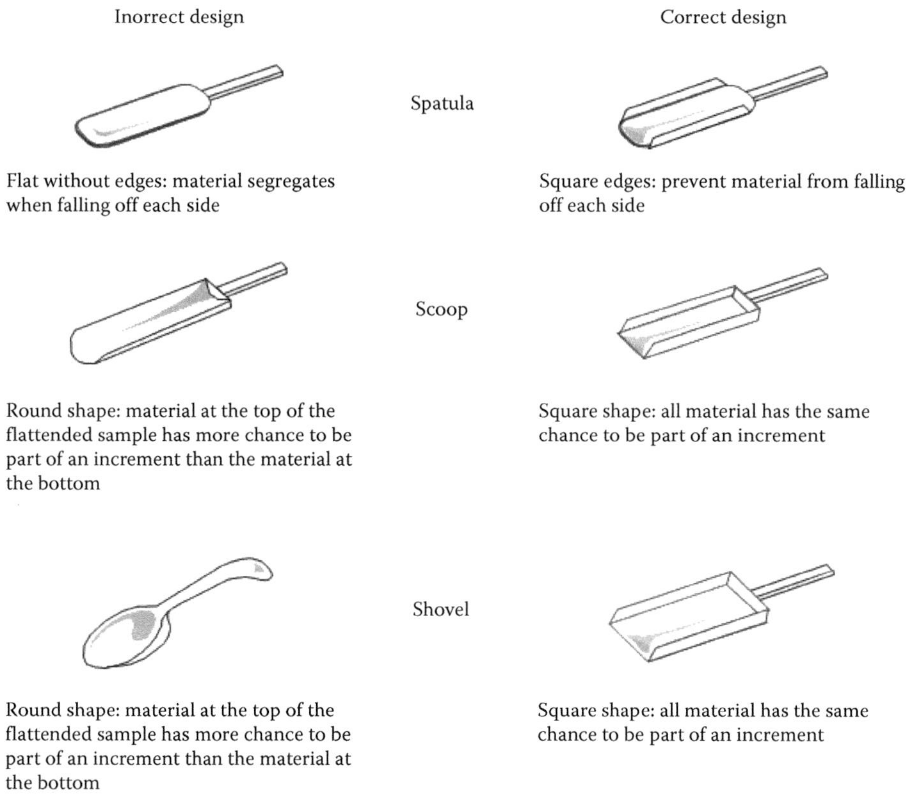


FIGURE 2.5 Some recommendations related to appropriate design of spatulas, scoops, and shovels used in sampling. (Adapted from Myers, 2004.)

### 2.6.6 Equipment for the Storage of Samples

1. Wide Mouth Plastic Bottles with Screw Cap
2. Plastic Bags

Eventually with seals (and seal number), if it is to be used in relation with the implementation of EU Regulation 691/2013.

1. Refrigerator
2. Freezer

## 2.7 ENVIRONMENT AND ROOMS

### 2.7.1 Rooms

According to ISO Standard 24276 (2006), grinding of samples should be carried out in a room or working area dedicated to that purpose. Special attention should be paid to follow the forward flow in order to avoid contamination.

### 2.7.2 Cleaning and Decontaminating Reagents

All equipment (e.g., mills, grinders, blending devices, sampling tools, balances, laboratory benches, etc.) used in the sample preparation procedure must be carefully cleaned upon completing and, if deemed necessary, during sample preparation. Vacuum cleaning alone is not sufficient, a wet cleaning is necessary to eliminate contaminating particles.

Apart from washing solutions such as detergents, it is possible, when necessary, to eliminate or degrade DNA with the following reagents:

- Bleach (e.g., 5–10 v/v per cent, i.e., a 10–20 fold dilution of commercial bleach at 12° Chl—in Gay-Lussac chlorometric degrees—or 3.61–3.65 per cent of active chlorine),
- Hydrochloric acid 1N,
- Hydrogen peroxide solution at 3 per cent (US Patent 20070289605 A1, 2007) as well as solutions of several cationic compounds (US Patent US 7687027 B2, 2010),
- Ready-to-use DNA removal products (e.g., ELIMINase® of Decon Labs, King of Prussia, Pennsylvania, USA; DNA-ERASE™ of MPBiomedicals, Solon, Ohio, USA).

## 2.8 SAFETY PRECAUTIONS

Appropriate personnel protective equipment (e.g., lab coat) should be worn as required in the laboratory. In an extremely noisy environment (85–90 dB or more), ear protectors (earmuffs or ear plugs) are necessary to prevent ear damage. For noisy equipment, noise reduction enclosures may also be considered.

The mills for crushing, cutting, and grinding have sharp blades. One should never put hands or fingers past the edges of the introduction chamber during operation of the equipment nor open the mills until they have completely stopped. It is advised to regularly check that safety interlocks on all equipment are operating properly.

If available, the dust ventilation system has to be operated during dust generation procedures. For instance, a vacuum cleaner can be used to minimize dust in the hood area and the working area. One should also be careful when handling (but especially grinding) seeds treated with phyto-pharmaceutical products by wearing appropriate respiratory protective equipment because the dust may be contaminated with these chemicals.

## 2.9 PROCEDURE

After registration and check of the laboratory sample (see Section 2.9.1), a first optional step may consist of a representative mass reduction of this laboratory sample (see 2.9.2).

In a next step, the particles in the test samples are reduced to adequate sizes to minimize the subsampling error arising when the test portion is taken from the test sample (see Section 2.9.3).

For samples with a high moisture content, partial drying prior to grinding could be necessary (see Section 2.9.4). For liquid samples and some fatty and/or sticky samples (e.g., oil, oilseeds, pet foods, fluid lecithin), special sample preparation procedures are useful/necessary (see Section 2.9.5).

Storage of the samples before and during sample preparation, as well as after the analysis, should be performed under adequate conditions, be it at room temperature, refrigerated, or frozen (see Section 2.9.7).

For particulate material, a flow chart of the several steps with a decision tree can be found in Appendix C.

### 2.9.1 Laboratory Sample Check

Firstly, the laboratory sample will be registered and uniquely identified (e.g., with a unique code number).

Before starting the proper sample preparation procedure, some laboratory sample checks have to be carried out.

#### *2.9.1.1 Check of Laboratory Sample Constitution*

Upon arrival in the laboratory, the sample should be free from any sign of damage and should be cooled or frozen if prescribed by the shipment conditions. Furthermore, all information concerning the sample should be available and complete.

Deficiencies (e.g., missing important information about the type of sample, an open laboratory sample container, the sampling protocol does not correspond to the sample received) should be documented and eliminated whenever possible.

In case of suspected cross contaminations between samples, these laboratory samples are not appropriate for analysis. The customer should be informed about the deficiencies in the samples provided.

Another point to consider during laboratory sample check at its reception is the sample size. Table 2.1 provides a list of recommended laboratory sample sizes.

The received laboratory sample size should be stated in the analysis report. It should be stated when the sample size is below the recommended minimal sample intake.

Just as an indication, Table 2.2 provides information on what is the average mass of 1,000 kernels of cropped plants that might have an interest with relation to GMO detection.

TABLE 2.1 Recommended Laboratory Sample Sizes According to the Type of Matrix

| Products | Recommended Laboratory Sample Size |
|---|---|
| Seeds | Mass equivalent of 3,000 kernels (see table below for mass equivalent of 1,000 kernels) |
| Commodity grains | Mass equivalent of 10,000 grains (see table below for mass equivalent of 1,000 kernels) |
| First transformation products (semolina, flour, grits, oilcake etc.) | From 100 g to 1 kg |
| Liquids | 500 ml |
| Doughy and viscous products | 500 g |
| End products (e.g., packed rice noodles) | From 100 g to 1 kg |

*Source:* Adapted from AFNOR, 2006.

*Note:* The numbers provided are indicative. In special cases, other quantities might be required. Some legislative texts specify other values for the laboratory sample size (e.g., for rice as a commodity at least 960 g are required according to Commission Decision 287/2013).

TABLE 2.2 Data Concerning the Mean Mass of 1,000 kernels for Different Plant Species

| Plant species | Mean mass of 1,000 kernels (in g) |
|---|---|
| Barley | 37 |
| Linseed | 6 |
| Millet | 23 |
| Oat | 32 |
| Maize | 285 |
| Rapeseed | 4 |
| Rice | 27 |
| Rye | 30 |
| Soybean | 200 |
| Sugar beet | 11 |
| Sunflower | 100 |
| Tomato | 4 |
| Wheat | 37 |

*Source:* Data derived from AFNOR (2006), Belitz et al. (2009), the Canadian Grain Commission (2013), and Hübner et al. (2001).

Note: be careful that for some species, especially maize, these average values are just an indication and it is better to really establish the mass of a sufficient number of kernels to determine the mass equivalence of 1,000 kernels for that specific variety than to rely on these average values.

Appendix D provides a very useful way to determine what minimal sample size to be taken into consideration when it consists of kernels and that one wants to check that presence of a GMO is below a certain level with a given probability. The outcome should not necessarily be analyzed at once, you might do it in subsamples as long as you know in which amount of seeds one transgenic seed can still be detected with your complete method (going up to the PCR results).

There are of course limitations to the use of that statistical approach. It is not usable for potatoes, neither for some fresh fruits (e.g., papaya). This is, however, briefly considered in the conclusion.

#### *2.9.1.2 Maximum Mass of the Laboratory Sample*

Apart from minimal size requirements of the laboratory sample, it is also advisable to fix a maximum size. This will enable avoiding the mass reduction step on a large quantity of laboratory samples. Maximum numbers should not be fixed in a single unit for all samples but should be adapted to the kind of matrix analyzed.

### 2.9.2 Mass Reduction

When a laboratory sample needs to be ground (for examples of matrices that do not need to be ground, see Appendix E), it is recommended to use the whole laboratory sample in as far as possible. The mass reduction process used has to be documented when only a part of the laboratory sample is used. Several subsampling procedures for mass reduction are outlined below (see 2.9.2.2). However, in some cases, a pre-grinding step has to be carried out before any mass reduction (see 2.9.2.1).

#### *2.9.2.1 Coarse Grinding (or Pre-grinding)*

When a "dry laboratory sample" is composed of lumps or its particle sizes are above 6 mm, the whole laboratory sample should be pre-ground (e.g., using a cutting mill, or chopped to particle sizes in the range of 4–6 mm) before mass reduction/subsampling.

#### *2.9.2.2 Subsampling Procedures*

From a mere statistical viewpoint, mass reduction with the use of dedicated devices such as rotational dividers or riffle splitters is generally recommended because the resulting sampling errors are reduced (Petersen et al., 2004). The problem with most of these devices in the case of GMO detection is the risk of cross contamination. That is why the approaches which are generally considered to be more simplistic and less efficient are those most frequently applied. All these techniques include incrementing.

Unfortunately, it is common practice to take only a limited number of increments. When a small number of increments is selected, there can be very large subsampling errors due to sample heterogeneity. The number of increments has to be determined in view of the size of the error deemed acceptable and not according to the ease of handling. As a rule of thumb, it is recommended to take ten increments when there is no prior knowledge about the sample heterogeneity.

*2.9.2.2.1 Fractional (Alternate) Shoveling* It is a very simple splitting technique with the following advantages:

- No costly equipment involved (e.g., riffle splitters);
- Minimal clean up and decontamination requirements;
- Can be implemented in the lab or field;
- Any number of splits can be generated;
- Very low sample splitting error.

The laboratory sample is split into the desired number of samples by collecting increments from the laboratory sample. Increments that should be of identical sizes are alternately placed in containers or piles to create split subsamples.

When a sample is to be split into two equal subsamples, one split would contain the odd increments and the other subsample would contain the even increments (= alternate shoveling). Fractional shoveling implies at least three splits.

When a sample is to be split into three subsamples, the first split would contain increments 1, 4, 7, the second split would contain increments 2, 5, 8, and the third split would contain increments 3, 6, 9, etc. (see Figure 2.6).

The same pattern as the one described above has to be followed when a large number of split subsamples are considered.

The following formula can be used to calculate the mass increment:

$$m_{(\text{increment})} = m_{(\text{lab sample})} \Big/ \left[ n_{(\text{subsamples})} \times N_{(\text{increments})} \right] \quad (2.1)$$

where m = mass and n and N = number

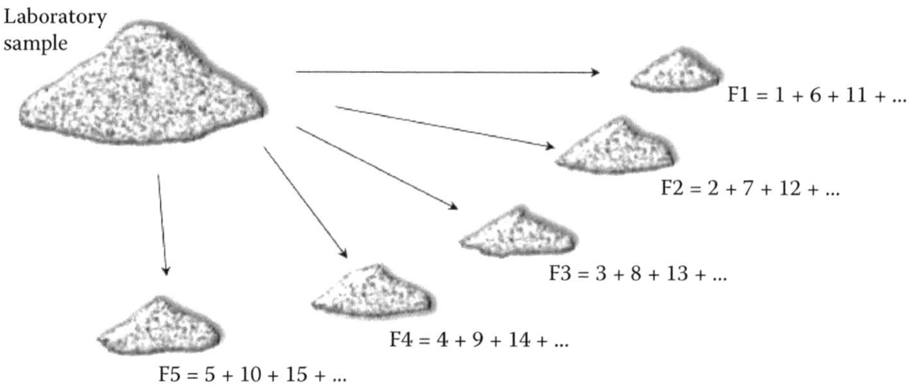


FIGURE 2.6 Illustration of fractional shoveling from a laboratory sample into five subsamples (F1–F5). (Adapted from Gerlach et al., 2002.)

The following precautions must be considered:

- All increments must have approximately the same size;
- Each subsample must have an identical number of increments;
- Split subsamples must be randomly selected;
- All material must be used.

Note: Toward the end of the splitting process there can be a small amount of very small particles called fines; it is advisable to reduce the increment size so that the fines are equally apportioned among the splits; when this is not done, it is possible that all fines will end up in only one of the subsamples.

*2.9.2.2.2 The Spoon Method* The spoon method (based on Petersen et al., 2004) can be used when a relatively low sampling ratio is needed (reduction by less than a factor of 10). The method is somewhat related to bed blending. The laboratory sample is spread out in an even layer. To do so, the laboratory sample has to be poured out as a thin layer (<2 cm) in an S-shape movement in one direction (Figure 2.7A). This is subsequently repeated in the traverse direction (i.e., perpendicular to the first one—see Figure 2.7A). If needed, the procedure is repeated until the laboratory sample is poured into the tray but the thickness of the entire layer or bed should reach at least 3–4 cm. After the spreading step, the spoon method simply consists in extracting randomly spread increments (Figure 2.7B) using a spatula and a square-edged shovel ensuring that for each of these increments the bottom of the tray is reached. The combination of the several increments will lead to a subsample. The method can be greatly user-dependent but with the aforementioned guidelines, the user-dependency should be reduced.

*2.9.2.2.3 The Long pile Method (*)* In this method, the sample is poured out of the bag and spread on flat surface in a long pile (Figure 2.8A). The pile should have a length of at least 20 times its width and the height should not exceed the width of the pile. Several cross

* Based on a discussion with K. Esbensen during a training course on sampling given at CRA-W (Gembloux, Belgium) in March 2012.

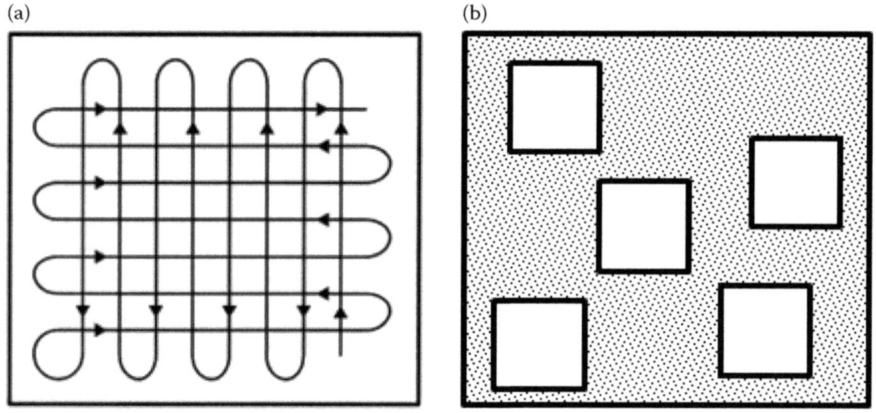


FIGURE 2.7 Mass reduction with the spoon method. (A) The "S-shaped" pattern used for spreading the laboratory sample in a tray when performing mass reduction by the spoon method. (Adapted from Petersen et al., 2004.) (B) Random spread location of the extracted increments.

sections are then taken out of the pile (Figure 2.8B and C) and all the cross sections put together (Figure 2.8D) lead to a mass reduction of the original sample.

The best is to take a sufficient number of not too large sections. The several cross sections are not distributed with the same distance in between each of them (as ideally this should be at random). If nothing is known about heterogeneity, it is advised to take at least ten cross sections. Like the spoon method, this technique is advised when a low sampling ratio (less than a factor of 10) is needed. Basically, the technique tries to mimic on a static sample what happens with a sample in motion where cross sections are taken at a given place. Here, the sample is static, and the cross sections are dispersed along the pile.

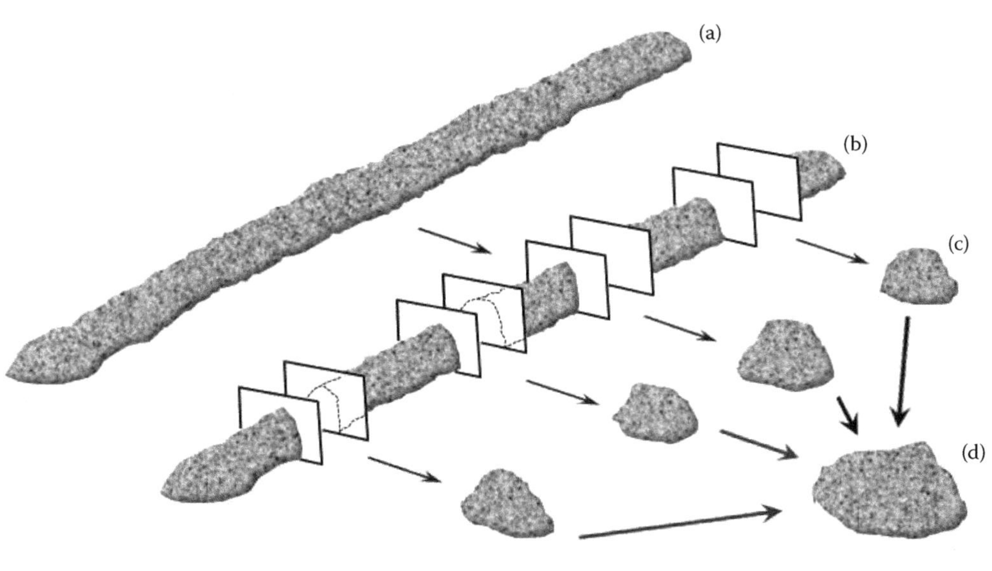


FIGURE 2.8 Schematic representation of mass reduction by the long pile method.

*2.9.2.2.4 Other Mass Reduction Techniques* A separate section is added for other mass reduction techniques that are not favored by the working group as they might have some disadvantages. However, if they are used while correctly understanding the limits of the technique and the results are still satisfying, there is no reason not to use them.

The techniques are briefly outlined here:

"Coning and quartering": This is an old technique that according to literature (but never on matrices for GMO analysis) has a poor performance (Mullins and Hutchison, 1982; Gerlach et al., 2002). Basically, it does comply with the fundamental rules required to avoid ISE. So, other than the warning that it might have a low performance (i.e., it would deliver subsamples on which there is a too large variation; essentially because incrementing is low), which means in other words that parameters measured on such subsamples would have a greater measurement uncertainty, the technique has the big advantage to be very simple and cleaning is easy to carry out. More detailed explanation on coning and quartering can be found, for instance, in the ISTA guidelines (2013).

"Techniques with more elaborate devices": There is wealth of much more elaborate devices, some being automatic (revolving splitters, rotational dividers, etc.) and some not (riffle splitters).

The very big disadvantage of such devices is the risk of contamination as once used it is difficult to get rid of the material that was put in it. Cleaning is, therefore, generally rather difficult to carry out or is time-consuming and therefore not cost-efficient. There is one exception that should however be mentioned among these devices, which is the riffle splitters. No one in the working group had experience with such devices. It was only when the working group was ending that at least one of the labs had to consider such a device to implement regulation 691/2013. More detailed information on splitters can be found in the ISTA guidelines (2013) as well as in Petersen et al. (2004). Appendix F gives an example of what could be a paper-cone riffle splitter that might be a suitable device but that does not exist commercially.

### 2.9.3 Particle Size Reduction

Some samples might not require any grinding (for a list of examples, see Appendix E).

#### *2.9.3.1 General Methods*

Comminution, the generic term for particle reduction can be achieved through several processes (list based on ISO 6498:2011):

- Chopping: a material is mechanically cut into smaller parts;
- Crushing: applying pressure to particles to fragment them into smaller particles, especially for samples with large and hard lumps;
- Cutting: cutting mills reduce soft to medium-hard and fibrous materials using rotating and stationary cutting knives;
- Blending (homogenizing): materials that are generally semi-solid (i.e., with a certain water content) are mixed with rotating knives which break fragments in

smaller particles and blend the entire sample to a macroscopically more uniform texture (at least in appearance) and consistency (e.g., "Waring blenders");
- Milling/grinding: reduces solid particles by a combination of cutting, shearing, and pressure;
- Pulverizing: describes the action of various mills, which further reduce small-sized material (<10 mm) to an average particle size usually below 75 μm.

#### *2.9.3.2 Requirements Regarding the Choice of Size Reduction Equipment*

The requirements for suitable size reduction methods differ widely and depend on the sample material. To keep track of possible cross contamination between successive samples processed by grinding equipment, a logbook should mention the order in which samples have been handled on a specific device.

Considerations for selecting a size reduction equipment for a specific application include the following aspects (list based on ISO 6498:2011):

- What are the physical (e.g., hardness) and chemical properties (e.g., composition, very fatty or not) of the material? Is the size reduction process affected by heat generation, moisture change, or chemical reactions?;
- Maximum allowed initial particle size (e.g., chunks, powder, etc.);
- Final desired particle size range (mm, μm);
- Quantity of material to be ground and number of laboratory samples to be processed daily or weekly (taking into account also the time for cleaning the grinder);
- Importance of sample loss due to adherence to the grinding surface;
- It is essential that all parts of the device in contact with the sample be washed completely using decontamination solutions (only vacuum cleaning will not be sufficient);
- The choice of a grinding device should also take account of the possibility to periodically check the grinding efficiency (see examples in Appendix B).

Other general considerations for grinding are:

- Devices with integrated sieves will give some control of the particle size independently of the kind of matrix processed;
- When successive grinding steps have to be applied with sieves of decreasing mesh sizes, a factor of 4 between successive mesh sizes should be used as a rule of thumb: for example, a first grinding with a sieve at mesh size of 2 mm followed by a subsequent grinding with a sieve at the mesh size of 0.5 mm;
- Especially for fatty samples, it may be difficult to make use of sieves of a mesh size of 0.5 mm as this might generate a heating of the sample, which could be detrimental for the DNA content. In such cases, it is advisable to avoid grinding at a mesh size of 0.5 mm but to replace it by a second grinding at a mesh size of 2 mm. As illustrated in Table 2.3, on two kind of rice products, repeated grinding with the same mesh size sieve may lead to results comparable to a first grinding at the mesh size of 2 mm followed by a second one at the mesh size of 0.5 mm;
- Mind that particle size may have an influence on DNA yield during extraction (e.g., Moreano et al., 2005);
- Wet milling is not appropriate for GMO analysis. According to Corbisier et al. (2005), DNA degradation occurred after exposure of ground seed powder to

TABLE 2.3 Percentage of Recovery of Ground Rice Products According to the Granulometry

| Sample | Grinding (Retsch ZM200) (mm sieve) | Percentage of Recovery According to the Granulometry | | | |
|---|---|---|---|---|---|
| | | > 0.5 mm | [0.5–0.25] mm | <0.25 mm | ≤ 0.5 mm |
| Rice kernels 1 | 1 × 2 | 17.5 | 38.6 | 43.8 | 82.4 |
| | 2 × 2 | 3.4 | 30.0 | 66.4 | 96.3 |
| | 3 × 2 | 0.6 | 17.3 | 81.9 | 99.2 |
| | 1 × 2 + 1 × 0.5 | 0.2 | 10.1 | 89.7 | 99.7 |
| Rice kernels 2 | 1 × 2 | 19.6 | 40.8 | 39.5 | 80.3 |
| | 2 × 2 | 4.2 | 33.7 | 62.2 | 95.8 |
| | 3 × 2 | 0.8 | 19.5 | 79.9 | 99.3 |
| | 1 × 2 + 1 × 0.5 | 0.3 | 11.5 | 88.2 | 99.7 |
| Rice noodles 1 | 1 × 2 | 20.4 | 43.4 | 36.4 | 79.8 |
| | 2 × 2 | 3.1 | 33.0 | 64.0 | 96.9 |
| | 3 × 2 | 1.3 | 26.7 | 72.0 | 98.7 |
| | 1 × 2 + 1 × 0.5 | 0.1 | 16.4 | 83.4 | 99.8 |
| Rice noodles 2 | 1 × 2 | 21.2 | 43.1 | 35.7 | 78.8 |
| | 2 × 2 | 4.8 | 37.3 | 58.0 | 95.3 |
| | 3 × 2 | 1.3 | 28.0 | 70.8 | 98.8 |
| | 1 × 2 + 1 × 0.5 | 0.3 | 21.3 | 78.6 | 99.9 |

*Source:* Data from Janssen, 2013.

*Note:* Grinding was performed on a ultracentifugal mill with sieves at a given mesh size. A single passage or several passages through the 2 mm mesh size sieve is compared to a passage with the 2 mm mesh size sieve followed by another passage through the 0.5 mm mesh size sieve.

water. DNA degradation is proportional to the vigor of the mixing process. It can be assumed that in the slurry the DNA is enzymatically degraded by endonucleases released by the cells.

Note: There is no industry standard for classifying particle size reduction equipment. A comprehensive summary of several types of grinders is provided in ISO 6498:2012.

#### *2.9.3.3 Maintaining Integrity of the Laboratory Sample*

To minimize the loss of integrity of DNA molecules of the sample, heating during the grinding process must be limited (e.g., when grinding some fatty matrices like linseed with a 0.5 mm mesh size sieve).

#### *2.9.3.4 Mixing Techniques*

*2.9.3.4.1 General Considerations on Mixing Techniques* Mixing is used by many laboratories in an attempt to "homogenize" the sample. Once the sample is "homogenized," any increment or grab from the sample is then deemed representative of the sample without any further considerations. This assumption, however, does not hold true for particulate matter. Appendix E gives a list of matrices that are considered as homogenous and therefore do not need any mixing technique before taking the test portion.

While mixing may be possible in some cases, it might actually promote segregation in other cases. This is especially true for material with diverging particle sizes and densities.

One type of mixing technique, which is strongly discouraged, is putting a spatula in the top of a sample container and stirring it a few times vertically.

A second unacceptable technique for dry, ground material is shaking a sample container when the jar is full or almost completely filled. The material at the bottom of the container is not properly mixed in and the stirring might have actually promoted segregation, thus enlarging the mass reduction error. It is recommended to leave at least one third of open space in the jar.

There are many other mixing techniques available that are superior to stirring (e.g., drum mixer, stirring vane mixer, V-shaped double cylinder mixer, overhead mixer, tumbler mixer). One practical technique carried out in a laboratory of one of the Working Group members is outlined hereafter.

*2.9.3.4.2 The Plastic Bag Technique* The ground material is put in a plastic bag that can be closed (sealed, zipper). Leave approximately one half of open space in the bag. Homogenization occurs through 20 successive reversals of the bag (Figure 2.9).

Although it may depend on the nature of the material, for commonly treated samples, the following bag sizes can be considered:

- for 1 kg of ground sample: a plastic bag of 30 cm by 40 cm,
- for 2 kg of ground sample: a plastic bag of 37 cm by 50 cm.

### 2.9.4 Partial Drying

For some semi-solid matrices with less than 85 per cent dry matter (e.g., forages, fresh bread, but not for liquids), it is necessary to partially dry them prior to fine grinding.

Partial drying can be done using either a forced-air oven or a microwave oven. The aim is to dry the sample while keeping its temperature below 55–60°C to minimally affect its chemical composition. Drying at higher temperatures (i.e., above 60°C) might cause chemical changes which could affect the DNA content of the sample. Following drying, the subsample is ground.

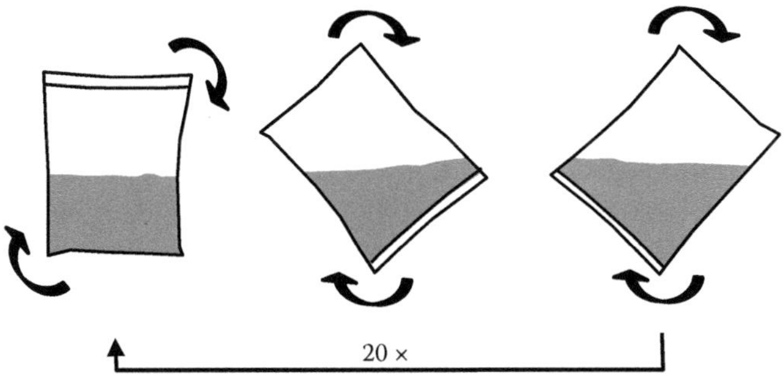


FIGURE 2.9 Homogenization by mixing with the plastic bag technique.

### 2.9.5 Special Sample Preparation Procedures

#### *2.9.5.1 Gelatine, Molasses, and Samples with High Fat Content*

For samples composed of high contents of fat, gelatine, and/or molasses, some special sample preparation procedures help in obtaining a representative subsample and finely ground test samples:

- Cool the entire laboratory sample in a freezer overnight and process the sample in a frozen or chilled state;
- Use dry ice during grinding to keep the sample cold enough to prevent clumping or melting;
- Use blending type mills, operated in intervals of 30 s.

#### *2.9.5.2 Viscous Samples*

For viscous samples such as fluid lecithin and honey, heating the sample at 40–60°C improves the homogeneity of the sample and helps obtaining a representative subsample.

#### *2.9.5.3 Liquid Samples*

Liquid samples are generally considered as homogeneous (Ministero della Salute, 2012) and do not require prior homogenization. However, there may be exceptions like for oil where DNA is present in solid particles that may be in suspension in the liquid. In such a case, it seems preferable to use a method described by Costa et al. (2010), where the laboratory sample is submitted to a centrifugation of 30 minutes at ~ 18,000 g. The supernatant is discarded and DNA extraction is performed on the pellet.

#### *2.9.5.4 Plant Tissues*

For plant tissues, two possibilities can be considered:

- A technique which generally works well on fresh tissues is to freeze the material in the presence of liquid nitrogen using a mortar and pestle or eventual other disruption devices to crush the material;
- An alternative to the liquid nitrogen technique consists of freeze-drying the material (which might take more than one day) and subsequently grinding the dried material.

### 2.9.6 Test Portion

#### *2.9.6.1 Homogenization of the Test Sample (or Analytical Sample) Prior to Test Portion Uptake*

Most solid samples will first be ground before taking the test portion from the homogenized test sample or analytical sample. It is, however, possible to store the homogenized material for a while before the test portion uptake. When proceeding in such a way to include a resting period for the homogenized test sample, it is advisable to homogenize this sample by agitation of the jar in which it was kept (hence requiring at least one third of available volume) before the uptake of the test portion. Special equipment (e.g., overhead mixer) can be used for this purpose.

#### 2.9.6.2 Minimum Mass of Test Portion

To properly represent a laboratory sample, the test portion (i.e., the final subsample submitted to the further analytical process) must contain an adequate mass in accordance with the fundamental subsampling error (FSE) and maximum particle size ("minimum mass"). The test portion mass should increase by a factor of 8 when the particle size doubles to maintain the same representativeness of the laboratory sample (Table 2.4). This is because the test portion size is proportional to the power 3 of the particle size. It clearly shows that if the maximum particle size exceeds 3 mm, this will lead to an excessive fundamental sampling error when taking into account that the maximum test portion size for DNA extraction is of 5 g (Terry et al., 2002). As most generally the test portion size does not even exceed 2 g, it is advised to be below 2 mm as a maximum size of particles.

Because of technical limitations and reagent costs, the sample intake for DNA extraction is relatively small. This implies that special care must be devoted to obtain a sufficiently small size of particles to be integrated in the test portion; otherwise, errors linked to constitutional heterogeneity of the material will become too high.

Other tables (Table 2.5A and B) concerning the test portion size are based on data from Berben and Janssen (2008) that are derived from Lischer (2001b). They indicate the minimal test portion required to detect a certain threshold amount of GMO in a given context of sampling error. It should be mentioned that the figures are theoretical. Moreover, in practice, it is difficult to estimate the size as well as the weight of a particle (Janssen et al., 2010).

Table 2.6 gathers experimental data collected during the Co-Extra project (Janssen et al., 2010). Samples consisting of soybean with known amounts of genetically modified soybean kernels were tested at different test portion sizes. The DNA extraction method used was checked to provide enough DNA within a PCR even with the smallest test portion to make detection at the lowest level possible, but due to a random distribution of ground material (constitutional heterogeneity), the outcome is that the relative standard deviation on the measured content at 0.1 per cent for most of the test portion sizes considered is above 25 per cent. This result has a consequence for quantification of low-level presence event quantification. The test portion size considered on the tested sample should be large enough because otherwise the measurement uncertainty is unacceptable with respect to EU Regulation No 619/2011.

#### 2.9.6.3 Test Portion Uptake

The test portion uptake is generally done using so-called grab sampling. Since care has been taken to prepare a rather homogeneous test sample, grab sampling at the level of sample preparation is generally deemed acceptable. As the test portion size is generally determined by weighing, care should be taken to perform this according to good weighing practices. Use of antistatic devices may sometimes be helpful with finely ground material to avoid weighing errors but also to limit contamination of the balance.

### 2.9.7 Storage and Disposal

Once a representative test sample has been prepared from the laboratory sample, it is essential to maintain its integrity throughout the analytical and post-analytical phases

TABLE 2.4 Theoretical Calculations of the Minimum Mass of the Test Portion: Expected Relative Standard Deviation (RSD) Linked to the Maximum Particle Size (Assumed Density of 1 g/cm³

| **FSE (expected RSD)→** **Maximum particle size** ↓ | 25% | 20% | 10% | 5% | 2% | 1% |
|---|---|---|---|---|---|---|
| 0.5 mm | 0.02 g | 0.03 g | 0.13 g | 0.5 g | 3 g | 12.5 g |
| 0.75 mm | 0.07 g | 0.1 g | 0.42 g | 1.7 g | 10.5 g | 42 g |
| 1 mm | 0.16 g | 0.25 g | 1 g | 4 g | 25 g | 100 g |
| 2 mm | 1.28 g | 2 g | 8 g | 32 g | 200 g | 800 g |
| 3 mm | 4.3 g | 6.7 g | 27 g | 108 g | 672 g | 2,688 g |
| 4 mm | 10.2 g | 16 g | 64 g | 256 g | 1,600 g | 6,400 g |

*Source:* Data adapted from ISO/FDIS 6498:2011. The grey cells are those compatible with common sample intakes for DNA extraction (maximum 5 g).

*Note:* For materials with densities other than 1 g/cm³, this table can be modified by multiplying the minimum mass with a corrective factor corresponding to the density of the material expressed in g/cm³.

TABLE 2.5 Minimum test portion in mg to reach a sampling reproducibility (at a 95 per cent probability level) of 20 per cent **A**) if grouping and segregation error and also analytical error are assumed as negligible, **B**) if grouping and segregation error is considered equivalent to the fundamental error and if the analytical error is set at 5 per cent

| **Mean mass of Particles** | **Critical GMO content** | | | |
|---|---|---|---|---|
| | 0.1% | 0.5% | 0.9% | 1.0% |
| A | | | | |
| 5 µg | 500 mg | 100 mg | 55 mg | 50 mg |
| 10 µg | 999 mg | 199 mg | 110 mg | 99 mg |
| 20 µg | 1,998 mg | 398 mg | 220 mg | 198 mg |
| B | | | | |
| 5 µg | 499.5 mg | 265 mg | 147 mg | 132 mg |
| 10 µg | 2,664 mg | 531 mg | 293 mg | 264 mg |
| 20 µg | 5,328 mg | 1,061 mg | 586 mg | 528 mg |

*Source:* From Berben and Janssen, 2008 based on data from Lischer, 2001b.

(i.e., including all analytical processes and reporting of data) until the ultimate disposal of any leftover material.

A proper storage may include cooling (i.e., refrigeration or freezing), controlled humidity conditions to protect samples from moisture gain or loss, protection from UV light, etc. The aim of these storage conditions is to prevent the breakdown of organic compounds by an excess of harmful microorganisms.

The proper storage conditions will depend on the various types of matrices to be analyzed. One should bear in mind that the storage of the laboratory sample and of

TABLE 2.6 Experimental Data Collected During the Co-Extra Project on Test Portion Size for Detection of Genetically Modified Soybean in Soybean Kernels

| | GMO% | | | | | | |
|---|---|---|---|---|---|---|---|
| **Test Portion Size** | **0.1%** | **0.3%** | **0.6%** | **0.9%** | **1.2%** | **1.5%** | **1.8%** |
| 50 mg | ! | Y | Y | Y | Y | Y | Y |
| 100 mg | ! | Y | Y | Y | Y | Y | Y |
| 200 mg | ! | Y | Y | Y | Y | Y | Y |
| 400 mg | ! | Y | Y | Y | Y | Y | Y |
| 800 mg | Y | Y | Y | Y | Y | Y | Y |

*Source:* Janssen et al., 2010.
*Note:* An exclamation point indicates for what combination of test portion size and GMO content the relative standard deviation on the measured content exceeded 25 per cent.

the reserve sample can be completely different. For example, fresh papayas can be kept some days at room temperature or in a refrigerator, whereas the reserve sample that has to be kept for some months will have to be frozen.

Storage and disposal policy should be established and documented by the laboratory.

When the matrix consists of living GMOs (grains, kernels, seeds) care should be taken to avoid their dissemination into the environment upon elimination of this material (e.g., the whole sample should be ground).

## 2.10 PERFORMANCE TESTS (QUALITY CONTROL)

Performance tests are described to estimate the sample preparation error, the latter depending on the procedure, the material, the analytes, and the analyst.

Performance tests can be used to evaluate new equipment by comparing results obtained with the new and the previous equipment.

Some performance test procedures are given below. These procedures have to be adapted to meet the laboratory needs.

### 2.10.1 Performance Test for Particle Size Reduction (Grinding)

#### *2.10.1.1 Grinding Quality*

When using centrifugal grinders with sieves at defined mesh sizes several regular performance tests (e.g., on an annual basis) can be designed:

- It is generally considered that for a given mesh size of a sieve in a centrifugal grinder, the ground product should consist of at least 80 per cent of particles below half of the mesh size;
- Due to repetitive use, the mesh size of a sieve in a centrifugal mill increases with time. Its proper functioning is confirmed when at least 95 per cent of the material ground is below the nominal mesh size of the sieve.

For performing these tests, the ground material has to be analyzed using calibrated sieves. Not every matrix is suitable for that purpose. Ground soybeans give rise to a fatty and sticky material, which is very difficult to analyze with calibrated sieves. A good matrix for these performance tests is, for example, wheat or rice. It is recommended to store a wheat lot intended for performance tests in order to have comparable figures over several years. For instance, it will become evident that the proportion of particles exceeding the nominal mesh size of the sieve will progressively increase due to repetitive use of the sieve.

#### *2.10.1.2 Carry-over*

*2.10.1.2.1 Negative Sample Test* A way to check the prerequisites of the cleaning process of a mill and its correct execution by different operators consists in analyzing a negative sample following a positive sample with preferably a rather high content of genetically modified material (>5 per cent). Alternatively, the test can be done on different species (e.g., soybean and maize). The cleaning process will of course have been carried out in between samples.

The major difficulty with this technique, however, for genetically modified material is that one can never be completely sure of the real negative character of the so-called negative sample (for more details linked to how to check this, see Appendix D). The laboratory has to decide about the frequency of the test and the acceptance criteria.

*2.10.1.2.2 IKI Carryover Test* This is another example of a carryover test that is fully described in ISO 6498:2012 and which is probably of less interest with respect to the scope of this guideline. It consists to check if starch particles could contaminate another sample by coloring the starch with a lugol solution (IKI for iodine- potassium iodide solution). The ISO 6498:2012 standard accepts 0.25 per cent (m/m) of contamination, which for GMO analysis is not acceptable.

### 2.10.2 Performance Test for Mixing

Grinding is often a source of segregation, because particles which are more difficult to grind may not pass the sieve as quickly as the softer particles. Improper mixing will only emphasize this problem.

The mixing container should never be more than two-thirds full and preferably only half full. An example of a performance test for mixing is given hereafter.

#### *2.10.2.1 Unmixed Layers Method*

One fourth of the container volume of the normal storage container is filled with ground wheat or a similar light-colored material. One-fourth volume of a ground colored mineral mix is added on top (taking into consideration realistic densities of test material, which are routinely analyzed). The content of the container is mixed. The time needed to mix the contents until they are visually blended is recorded. This unmixed layers method can be used to test any mixing method in the lab.

### 2.10.3 Environmental Control

ISO 24276 (2006) considers the possibility of using environmental controls.

The other controls prescribed for the PCR analysis by ISO 24276 do not cover the sample preparation step. The environmental control is a possible mean to regularly check the cleanliness of the air in the grinding room or any other workspace linked to sample preparation considered to be critical for the environmental control described in ISO 24276 (2006).

### 2.10.4 Representativeness of the Test Portion

As the test portion used in GMO analysis is always small, it is essential to check that its size combined with the grinding technique used ensures a sufficient representativity of the sample within the test portion. A way to do this is to check on kernels (GM—non-GM or different species) if a level somewhat above the limit of detection can be reliably detected during replicate analyses on the ground material: for example, analyze six test portions and all should deliver a positive result. Similarly, for quantitative analysis when a level somewhat above the limit of quantification is analyzed, the results of a replicate analysis on the test portion should deliver a relative standard deviation that does not exceed 25 per cent. If the performance level is not reached, it means that either the test portion should be increased or the mean particle size of the yielded ground material should be smaller.

### 2.10.5 Overall Performance Test on Sample Preparation Steps through a Replication Experiment

A way to evaluate the variability of the entire sample preparation procedure can be done through a replication experiment as suggested for sampling strategies by Esbensen and Julius (2010). The interest of this approach is that it also points out per step from where the largest variability is coming. An example is outlined in Appendix G.

## 2.11 IDENTIFIED GAPS AND CONCLUSIONS

The present document set up a global framework for the several actions involved in sample preparation during GMO analyses. To that aim, it could benefit from an already existing structure laid down in a standard intended for feed samples. It was adapted to a specific use for GMO analysis, but with an enlargement of the matrices considered as next to feed, seeds, food, and environmental samples were also to be taken on board. The existing text is useful for most of the common samples a laboratory could get, but it is impossible to be complete and consider all cases that might need a special handling. That is also why a reminder of the fundamental principles of sampling and the errors associated with it are crucial as it allows; considering if for a given special matrix, the procedure intended to be followed will not generate ISE.

This document that is the deliverable of the working group is meeting the general expectations of the mandate set by the ENGL steering committee. However, it still is more a catalog of possibilities that can be considered with some highlights on possible caveats or errors that should be avoided than a real list of fully documented standard operation procedures that are directly usable by a technician. Intended readerships are more the laboratory responsibles than the technicians. In that sense, the deliverable was unable to meet some of the more specific aims of the mandate but this is due to the fact that the so set aim was simply too ambitious. Another example is giving some weight to several steps in the final measurement uncertainty. Doing this was simply impossible because it will largely vary between the several types of matrices under analysis. However, a procedure is detailed in Appendix G on how to perform this if one would like to have an idea about it on a defined matrix.

Because of the fact that is was built on a model of an existing standard, it might eventually be suggested to serve as model for setting up a real standard with that same purpose of sample preparation in the field of GMO analysis. This means that it certainly requires to be regularly updated which then could be a possibility to add progressively more detailed standard operational procedures. Some of the documents it contains might need a larger discussion. For instance, the document of Appendix E concerning the list of homogenous material or of material that does not require grinding is coming from the Italian authorities. It might require some enlargement or even revision of some of the existing items that it is listing.

One of the essential aims of the document especially through some of the data provided is to attract the attention of the reader on the fact that sample preparation is probably the step that at laboratory level will account for most of the measurement uncertainty on the result that is delivered. An easy example for that is to be found in Table 2.4 on test portion size in relation to main particle size of the sample. It clearly shows that if the mean size of the particle is not below 4 mm (and we know some laboratories do not grind with sieves below 4 mm), this would require to perform the analysis on a test portion with a much larger size than what is commonly considered, just to keep the uncertainty within an acceptable range. So if this text would just open the eyes of some persons in the sense that some of the procedures they use generate too large measurement uncertainties, it would already be a large success.

Among the gaps that could be identified in setting up these guidelines is the fact that at several occasions, ten replicates have to be considered but without a real scientific underpinning of this figure. For sure, there is a difference between already homogenous samples and more heterogeneous ones, and the figure of ten is probably a kind of compromise. Nevertheless, it is not even sure that on really widely heterogeneous samples, this figure of ten is really sufficient. The only way to check this would be to perform more practical research on this kind of topic but this was not part of the mandate. We just kept our action to available data.

Another difficulty that was met is that statistical considerations sometimes arrive to figures that are scientifically right but nevertheless unrealistic for practical application. An example for this is that for seeds or kernels, either 3,000 or 10,000 kernels are generally advised as an ideal sample size for the laboratory sample. Extending this to potato would of course be an error. Although already challenging, it would certainly be possible to gather the required number of tubers but going on in a cost-efficient way to analyze this laboratory sample remains for time being a quite impossible task. That is why, in such a situation, one must try to circumvent the problem by alternative approaches. In the very special cases of potatoes, which are in some way clones, it seems that an expert easily finds out in the field which plant is different from the others. That is why for potato it is apparently much more practical to work on leaf material collected from the field and focusing on plants that are morphologically different from others than to work on the commercialized products. Of course, such a way of thinking has then to be integrated into control plans of the authorities.

As outlined in the introduction, we considered sample preparation here as all operations between the laboratory sample and the test portion. It should be stressed that subsampling as such may still exist afterward (e.g., during the DNA extraction step if only part of the material is considered to go through the process). Moreover, most of the principles outlined in the guideline remain valid before reaching the laboratory sample. Therefore, the sections on mass reduction and on homogenization or coarse grinding of this guideline may also be of interest to those who have to make final samples from aggregate samples as requested by EU Regulation 691/2013 European Commission (2013b), that entered into force for feed analysis since the January 1, 2014. Nevertheless, it was not the aim of the working group to focus on that as it is outside the mandate. As a consequence, someone wanting to use this guideline for that purpose may not find an answer to all his questions.

Finally, we also hope that this document may help to better harmonize the practice in sample preparation as a survey carried out during the Co-Extra project showed that there was a very large variety of actions among labs (Berben et al., 2010).

## BIBLIOGRAPHIC REFERENCES

AFNOR (2006), Implementation guide for standards NF EN ISO 24276, NF EN ISO 21569, NF EN ISO 21570 and NF EN ISO 21571—Nucleic acid based methods of analysis for the detection of genetically modified organisms and derived products (in French), Document GA V03–042, 24 pp., AFNOR, France.

Belitz, H.D., Grosch, W., Schieberle, P. (2009), *Food Chemistry*, 4th revised and extended edition. Springer-Verlag, Berlin-Heidelberg, ISBN 978-3-540-69933-0.

Berben, G., Janssen, E. (2008), Subsampling (or secondary sampling) approaches, Chapter 10 in CO- EXTRA Deliverable 4.3, "Existing sampling plans and needs for the development of novel sampling approaches for genetically modified organisms (GMO) evaluation" (Miraglia, M. ed.), pp. 49–60.

Berben, G., Janssen, E., Onori, R. (2010), Report on the results of the questionnaire on sample preparation, Co-Extra project, Deliverable D4.6.

Canadian Grain Commission (2013), Sampling and testing protocol for Canadian flaxseed exported to the European Union, Available at: www.grainscanada.gc.ca/gmflax-lingm/stpf-peevl-eng.htm (consulted on 20 February 2014).

CEN TS 15568 (2007), Methods of analysis for the detection of genetically modified organisms and derived products—Sampling strategies.

Corbisier, P., Trapmann, S., Gancberg, D., Hannes, L., Van Iwaarden, P., Berben, G., Schimmel, H., Emons, H. (2005), Quantitative determination of roundup ready soybean (Glycine max) extracted from highly processed flour. *Analytical and Bioanalytical Chemistry* 383 (2), 282–290.

Costa, J., Mafra, I., Amaral, J.S., Oliveira, M.B.P.P. (2010), Monitoring genetically modified soybean oil extraction and refining processes by polymerase chain reaction techniques. *Food Research International* 43, 301–306.

European Commission (2004), Commission Recommendation No 2004/787/EC of 4 October 2004 on technical guidance for sampling and detection of genetically modified organisms and material produced from genetically modified organisms as or in products in the context of Regulation (EC) No 1830/2003. *Official Journal of the European Union* 348, 18–26.
European Commission (2009), Regulation (EC) No 152/2009 of 27 January 2009 laying down the methods of sampling and analysis for the official control of feed. *Official Journal of the European Union* 54, 1–130.
European Commission (2011), Regulation (EU) No 619/2011 of 24 June 2011 laying down the methods of sampling and analysis for the official control of feed as regards presence of genetically modified material for which an authorisation procedure is pending or the authorisation of which has expired. *Official Journal of the European Union* 166, 9–15.
European Commission (2013a), Commission Implementing Decision 2013/287/EU of 13 June 2013 amending Implementing Decision 2011/884/EU on emergency measures regarding unauthorised genetically modified rice in rice products originating from China. *Official Journal of the European Union* 162, 10–14.
European Commission (2013b), Regulation (EU) No 691/2013 of 19 July 2013 amending Regulation (EC) No 152/2009 as regards methods of sampling and analysis. *Official Journal of the European Union* 197, 1–12.
Esbensen, K.H., Julius L.P. (2010), Representative sampling, data quality, validation—a necessary trinity in chemometrics. *Comprehensive Chemometrics* 4, 1–20.
Esbensen, K.H., Paasch-Mortensen, P. (2010), Process sampling: Theory of sampling—the missing link in process analytical technologies (PAT). In *Process Analytical Technology: Spectroscopic Tools and Implementation Strategies for the Chemical and Pharmaceutical Industries* (ed. Bakeev, K.), Second edition, John Wiley and sons, pp. 37–80.
Gerlach, R.W., Dobb D.E., Raab, G.A., Nocerino J.N. (2002), Gy sampling theory in environmental studies. 1. Assessing soil splitting protocols. *Journal of Chemometrics* 16, 321–328.
Hübner, P., Waiblinger, H.-U., Pietsch, K., Brodmann, P. (2001), Validation of PCR methods for quantitation of genetically modified plants in food. *Journal of AOAC International* 84 (6), 1855–1864.
ISO 24276 (2006)/Amd 1:2013, Foodstuffs—Methods of analysis for the detection of genetically modified organisms and derived products—General requirements and definitions.
ISO 3534-1 (2006), Statistics—Vocabulary and symbols—Part 1: General statistical terms and terms used in probability.
ISO 6498 (2011), Draft version ISO/FDIS 6498:2011(E) of CEN/TC 327 and ISO/FDIS 6498 "Animal feeding stuffs—Guidelines for sample preparation."
ISO 6498 (2012), Animal feeding stuffs—Guidelines for sample preparation.
ISO 7002 (1986), Agricultural food products—Layout for a standard method of sampling from a lot.
ISTA (2013), *International Rules for Seed Testing*, International Seed Testing Association, Bassersdorf, Switzerland, ISBN 978-3-906549-68-2.

Janssen, E., Planchon, V., Oger, R., Berben, G. (2010), Assessing the validity of procedures deriving test portion from laboratory sample. In Deliverable D4.9. Survey, analysis and development of cost efficient sampling plans, Co-Extra project.

Janssen, E. (2013), DNA extraction from fresh papayas and rice products. NRL-GMO practical workshop "sample preparation—DNA extraction from different matrices," Brussels, 6 June 2013. Available on: https://intralab.favv-afsca.be/labo/formations/presentations/_documents/2-NRL-GMOworkshop_06062013_E.Jansens.pdf (consulted on 18 November 2013).

Lischer, P. (2001a), Sampling procedures to determine the proportion of genetically modified organisms in raw materials. Part I: Correct sampling, good sampling practices. *Mitteilungen aus Lebensmitteluntersuchung und Hygiene* 92, 290–304.

Lischer, P. (2001b), Sampling procedures to determine the proportion of genetically modified organisms in raw materials. Part II: Sampling from batches of grain. *Mitteilungen aus Lebensmitteluntersuchung und Hygiene* 92, 305–311.

Ministero della Salute (2012), Piano nazionale di controlo ufficiale sulla presenza di organismi geneticamente modificati negli alimenti, 36 pp., available from www.salute.gov.it/imgs/C_17_pubblicazioni_1666_allegato.pdf (consulted on 15 May 2013).

Minkkinen, P.O., Esbensen, K.H. (2009), Grab vs. composite sampling of particulate materials with significant spatial heterogeneity—A simulation study of "correct sampling errors." *Analytica Chimica Acta* 653 (1), 59–70.

Moreano, F., Busch, U., Engel K.-H. (2005), Distortion of genetically modified organism quantification in processed foods: Influence of particle size compositions and heat-induced DNA degradation. *Journal of Agricultural and Food Chemistry* 53, 9971–9979.

Mullins, C.E., Hutchison, B.J. (1982), The variability introduced by various subsampling techniques. *Journal of Soil Science* 33 (3), 547–561.

Myers, J. (2004), Representative subsampling at the laboratory: New guidance from USEPA, Powerpoint presentation of Washington Group International available on Internet at http://www.dtic.mil/ndia/2004Chemistry/Myers_AFCEE_PresJCM.pdf (consulted on 2 January 2007).

Petersen, L., Dahl, C.K., Esbensen, K.H. (2004), Representative mass reduction in sampling—a critical survey of techniques and hardware. *Chemometrics and Intelligent Laboratory Systems* 74, 95–114.

Petersen, L., Minkkinen, P., Esbensen, K. H. (2005), Representative sampling for reliable data analysis: Theory of Sampling. *Chemometrics and Intelligent Laboratory System* 77, 261–277.

Terry, C.F., Harris, N., Parkes, N. (2002), Detection of genetically modified crops and their derivatives: Critical steps in sample preparation and extraction. *Journal of AOAC International* 85 (3), 768–774.

US Patent 20070289605 A1 (2007), Use of dilute hydrogen peroxide to remove DNA contamination, (Available online: www.google.com/patents/US20070289605, consulted on 29 October 2013).

US Patent US 7687027 B2 (2010), Leaning compositions, methods and materials for reducing nucleic acid contamination, (Available online: www.google.com/patents/US7687027?hl=fr&cl=en, consulted on 29 October 2013).

# APPENDIX A: DEFINITIONS RELATED TO THE CONCEPT OF "SAMPLE" ACCORDING TO STANDARDS AND EUROPEAN LEGISLATION

The comparisons between definitions are summarized in Table A.1.

TABLE A.1 Comparison of Several Definitions

| | **Laboratory Sample** | | | **Test portion—(Test Sample[a])** |
|---|---|---|---|---|
| CEN/TS 15568:2007 (E) ISO 24276:2006 | Sample as prepared for sending to the laboratory and intended for inspection or testing [ISO 7002:1986] | | | Sample, as prepared for testing or analysis, the whole quantity being used for analysis or testing at one time [ISO 3534 1:2006] |
| Regulation (EU) No 691/2013 | A sample intended for the laboratory (as received by the laboratory) and can be the final, reduced or aggregate sample. | | | |
| | **Laboratory sample** | **Counter sample** | **Analytical sample** | **Test sample** |
| Recommendation 2004/787/EC | Quantity of product taken from the bulk sample intended for laboratory inspection and testing | Sample retained for a specific period of time for enforcement or referee purposes | Homogenized laboratory sample, consisting either of the whole laboratory sample or a representative portion thereof. | According to: CEN/TS 15568:2007 and ISO 24276:2006 |
| | Final sample | | | Test portion—(Test sample) |
| Regulation (EU) No 152/2009 Regulation (EU) No 619/2011 Regulation (EU) No 691/2013 | A part of the reduced sample or of the homogenized aggregate sample. | | | According to CEN/TS 15568:2007 and ISO 24276:2006 |

# APPENDIX B: EXAMPLES OF GRINDERS USED BY LABORATORIES INVOLVED IN GMO DETECTION

TABLE B.1 Grinders Used in GMO Detection (Based on a Small Enquiry Among the Laboratories Participating to the Working Group—Based on Five Replies)

| **Brand (of the grinder)** | **Retsch** | **Retsch** | **Vorwerk** | **IKA** | **IKA** | **Maxi Grinder** | **Waring** |
|---|---|---|---|---|---|---|---|
| **Type** | **ZM200** | **Grindomix GM200** | **Thermomix 21** | **A11 basic** | **M20** | **Solo** | **Blender, 1, 2 and 4 l capacities** |
| Maximal capacity that can be ground at once (in grams unless other unit used) | Up to 300 ml with standard cassette (4,500 ml with cyclone) | Up to 700 ml | 2,000 (depending on mass and volume) | 250 (depending on mass and volume) | 500 (depending on mass and volume) | 2,000 (depending on mass and volume) | From 200 to 2,000 according to the capacity |
| Number of laboratories using this equipment | 5 (7)[a] | 3 | 1 | 1 | 1 | 1 | 1 |
| Is there any integrated system for "size control of particles"? | Yes (due to sieve) | No | No | No | No | No | No |
| "Easiness of cleaning" —When a sample is ground. How long does it take to have all cleaned and ready for the next sample? | Difficult 15–60 minutes (depending of the mesh-size, material used); Time reduction when using extra containers/sieves and rotors | Medium 10 minutes Time reduction when using extra blades and bowls | Simple 1–5 minutes (pot, lid, blade) Time reduction when using extra pots/ blades and dishwasher | Simple 3–5 minutes | Medium 5–10 minutes | Simple 3–5 minutes Time reduction when using extra containers/ blades and dishwasher | Medium 10 minutes |

(*Continued*)

TABLE B.1 (Continued) Grinders Used in GMO Detection (Based on a Small Enquiry Among the Laboratories Participating to the Working Group—Based on Five Replies)

| **Brand (of the grinder)** | **Retsch** | **Retsch** | **Vorwerk** | **IKA** | **IKA** | **Maxi Grinder** | **Waring** |
|---|---|---|---|---|---|---|---|
| **Type** | **ZM200** | **Grindomix GM200** | **Thermomix 21** | **A11 basic** | **M20** | **Solo** | **Blender, 1, 2 and 4 l capacities** |
| Are there "matrices that do not fit"? | Oily and fatty material (e.g., linseed), depending on the mesh-size (difficult with sieves below 1 mm); particles of sample should not exceed 10 mm.); not suitable for very hard material as well as pasty material | Not suitable for very hard material | Soft/elastic material (e.g., fresh leaves) | Soft/elastic material (e.g., fresh leaves) | Soft/elastic material (e.g., fresh leaves) | Soft/elastic material (e.g., fresh leaves) | Matrices with high content of fat are difficult to grind; the grinding speed must be decreased |
| Additional remarks (if any) | Additional mixing step necessary when using cyclone; can reach a final fineness of <40 µm<br>Use of an ultrasonic cleaner helps to wash the sieves<br>Successive grindings through a sieve at the same mesh size result in a higher yield of small material | Can generally reach a final fineness of <300 µm | Minimum quantity/volume of material necessary | Fit for small quantities | / | Challenging handling, minimum quantity/volume of material necessary | In order to facilitate the work, several blades and bowls are needed |

[a] 7 is because there are also two ZM100 versions which is an older version of the ZM200 grinder.

## APPENDIX C: FLOW CHART OF THE SUCCESSIVE STEPS OF THE SAMPLE PREPARATION PROCEDURE FOR PARTICULATE MATERIAL

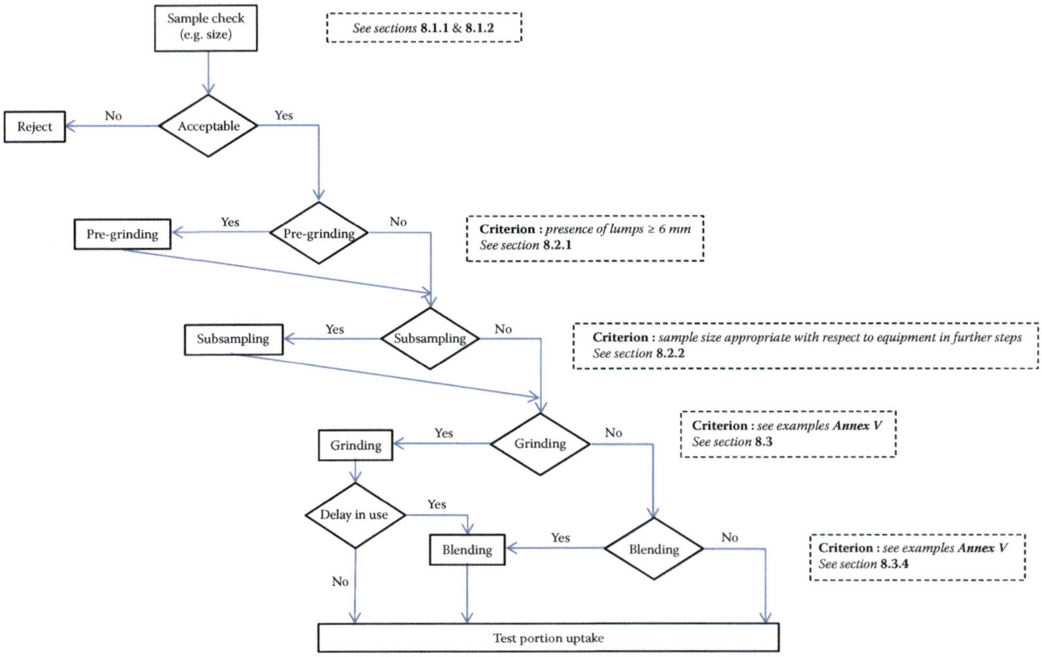


## APPENDIX D: MATHEMATICAL FORMULA THAT MIGHT BE VERY HELPFUL IN GMO DETECTION FOR DETERMINATION OF THE LABORATORY SAMPLE SIZE WHEN TESTING KERNELS

When a lot of kernels is analyzed, it is impossible to state that it does not contain any transgenic kernel because this can only be stated if all kernels have been analyzed. However, what can be provided is a probability level that the lot does not exceed a certain content of transgenic kernels.

When a lot is spiked at a certain level with transgenic kernels into a lot of negative kernels, a certain amount of transgenic kernels will be added to what is considered as an amount of negative material. This negative material should have been checked to not exceed a level of transgenic material that is 20 times less the amount of the spiking level and this at a probability of 95 per cent. To determine this, the following formula is of great help:

$$\alpha = (1-p)^N$$

Where:

$\alpha$ is the complement of the probability level, i.e., if $\alpha = 0.05$, this corresponds to a probability level of 95 per cent (in fact $1-\alpha$).

$p$ is the amount of transgenic material not to be exceeded in the negative lot and expressed as a ratio.

$N$ is the number of kernels to be analyzed.

So, if one wants to spike a maize lot at 0.1 per cent of transgenic maize, the lot of non-transgenic maize should first be analyzed in order to check that it does not already exceed a concentration of 0.1%/20 = 0.005% of that maize in what is the negative material. To check this, one should analyze N kernels:

$$N = \frac{\text{Log } \alpha}{\log(1-p)}$$

This will deliver that approximately 60,000 kernels (in fact exactly 59,913 kernels) should be analyzed to check that they are all negative.

Other examples of application of the formula:

If one wants to check that a lot contains less than 0.01 per cent of transgenic linseed in a linseed batch at a probability of 95 per cent, the numbers of kernels to be analyzed is around 30,000 (the exact outcome of the formula is 29,956).

The formula might also be of interest for operators to know what amount of kernels to check if for instance one fears that a soybean or a maize lot might be contaminated by linseed and to check if decontamination was done correctly. Let us consider that the background contamination level of linseed is 0.005 per cent. What is then the number of contaminating linseeds that should not be exceeded in the laboratory sample of maize or soybean in order to avoid its detection in 99 per cent of cases? The formula provides the answer that is 918 kernels, so close to 1,000 kernels, which in weight will be close to 6 g according to Table 2.2.

## APPENDIX E: LIST OF FOOD MATRICES THAT DO NOT NEED HOMOGENIZATION OR GRINDING

The list provided in Table E.1 is based on an official Italian document (Ministero della Salute, 2012), which makes a classification between food products that are considered as homogeneous and those that are not. Moreover, within the non-homogeneous products, it also makes the distinction between the ones needing grinding and those that do not. Mind that for this classification, what is aimed to look at is important because energy bars for instance are ranked in homogeneous products (but only when looking for genetically modified soybean or maize not for something else). Moreover, it is not because a product is homogeneous that there is no need for a comminution step. Bread is considered as homogeneous but to perform the extraction comminution is required.

TABLE E.1 List of Food Matrices that Do not Need Homogenization or Grinding

| Main Food type | Product that Can Be Considered as Homogeneous (which does not mean that comminution is not necessary, it might be required for the DNA extraction step) | Product that Cannot be Considered as Homogeneous: Product Requiring Only Homogenization | Product that Cannot be Considered as Homogeneous: Product Requiring Homogenization and Grinding |
|---|---|---|---|
| Cereal corn and rice products and bakery products | Noodles, dumplings, etc. of corn and rice | Maize and rice flour or mixes | Maize kernels, maize for popcorn, sweet maize, rice kernels |
| | | | Corn flakes, muesli, pop corn |
| | | Bread, cakes, pastry biscuits | |
| Edible vegetables and derived products | | | Canned sweet corn and soybeans, even presented in mixed salads with baby corn |
| Roots and tubers | | Potato starch, potato flour and flakes of potato | Potato, cooked potatoes |
| Oil seeds | | Soybean flour | Soybean kernels, linseeds, canola seeds, cotton seeds |
| Fruit | Papaya juice | | Papaya (if coming from one same fruit, it is genetically homogenous—however, avoid taking the seeds) |
| Vegetable drinks and products derived from vegetable milk | Soy milk and drink, soy cheese, béchamel, soy yoghurt, tofu, soy fluid | | |
| Baby food | Soy milk vegetable baby food | | |
| Miscellaneous edible preparations | Ice creams and sorbets, desserts, puddings, creams, custards, products coming from extrusion processes (tortilla chips), energy bars (for this latter ones, only if detection is addressing genetically modified soybean or maize) | | |
| Meat imitates | Textured soy protein products | | |

*Source:* Derived from Ministero della Salute, 2012.

## APPENDIX F: THE PAPER-CONE RIFFLE SPLITTER (FOR INFORMATION ONLY)

A device presented by Gerlach et al. (2002), called paper cone riffle splitter (see Figure F.1) might be compatible with sample preparation for GMO detection because the risk of cross contamination could be avoided by replacing the filter for each sample. However, this device does not seem to be commercially available. Moreover, in the configuration illustrated in Figure F.1, there is also a problem of loss of sample to be solved. This device is cited here just because it integrates improvements that would make its use feasible for GMO detection, but in practice, the device does not seem to be available.

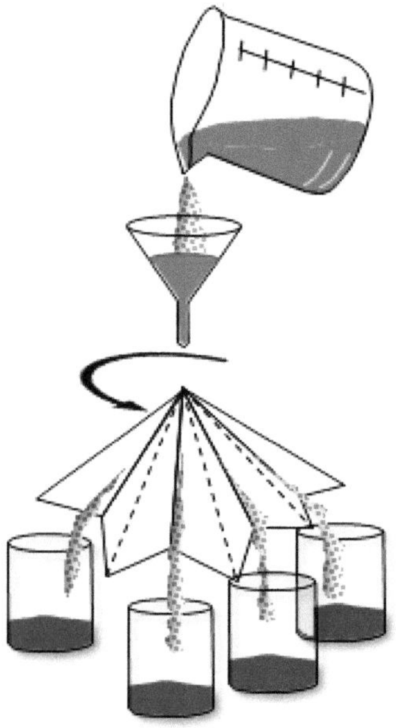

FIGURE F.1 The paper cone riffle splitter. (Adapted from Gerlach et al., 2002.)

## APPENDIX G: REPLICATION EXPERIMENT

To perform this replication experiment, at least 10 replicates are to be considered and this should be carried out as indicated in Table G.1. In this table, three levels have been considered but it is possible to extend it to a fourth or a fifth level if required. It is then possible to calculate the total relative subsampling variation but also the contribution of each step to the whole variability. The three steps considered in Table G.1 could for instance be:

A. a mass reduction step + the grinding of the resulting subsample
B. the uptake of the test portion + the DNA extraction
C. the PCR analysis

Step A should be done in 10 replicates and the total analysis with steps B and C should be performed on each of the replicates (from A100 to A10 00). This will lead to ten results

TABLE G.1 The Replicate Analysis to Distinguish the Source of Variability of Three Successive Steps (A, B and C).

1) from level A to C

A: A1.0.0 A2.0.0 A3.0.0 A4.0.0 A5.0.0 A6.0.0 A7.0.0 A8.0.0 A9.0.0 A10.0.0
B: B1.1.0 B2.0.0 B3.0.0 B4.0.0 B5.0.0 B6.0.0 B7.0.0 B8.0.0 B9.0.0 B10.0.0
C: C1.1.1 C2.0.0 C3.0.0 C4.0.0 C5.0.0 C6.0.0 C7.0.0 C8.0.0 C9.0.0 C10.0.0 ⇨ $RSV_1$.

$RSV_1$ provides the global subsampling variability from step A to C

2) from level B to C

B: B1.1.0 B1.2.0 B1.3.0 B1.4.0 B1.5.0 B1.6.0 B1.7.0 B1.8.0 B1.9.0 B1.10.0
C: C1.1.1 C1.2.0 C1.3.0 C1.4.0 C1.5.0 C1.6.0 C1.7.0 C1.8.0 C1.9.0 C1.10.0 ⇨ $RSV_2$

$RSV_2$ provides the subsampling variability from step B to C

3) level C

C: C1.1.1 C1.1.2 C1.1.3 C1.1.4 C1.1.5 C1.1.6 C1.1.7 C1.1.8 C1.1.9 C1.1.10 ⇨ $RSV_3$

$RSV_3$ provides the variability of level C

To calculate the specific contribution of variability of level B:

$$RSV_B = \sqrt{(RSV_2)^2 - (RSV_3)^2}$$

To calculate the specific contribution of variability of level A:

$$RSV_A = \sqrt{(RSV_1)^2 - (RSV_2)^2} = \sqrt{(RSV_1)^2 - (RSV_B)^2 - (RSV_3)^2}$$

(C111, C200 to C10 00) from which the relative standard deviation (corresponding to $RSV_1$ in Table G.1) can be calculated.

Step B will also be submitted to a special replicate analysis on the material of step A100. This will also generate ten results (C111, C120 to C1 10 0) from which the relative standard deviation (corresponding to $RSV_2$ in Table G.1) can be calculated.

Step C will then lastly also be submitted to a separate replicate analysis but limited to the material generated by step B110.

For sampling, the whole variability expressed in terms of relative standard variation should not exceed 33 per cent. As we are here, in fact at subsampling level, it should even be less, and therefore, a figure of 25 per cent seems appropriate as value that should not be exceeded. However, it is not at all impossible that in some cases the variability cannot be below that figure.

# SECTION 3

# GMO Testing Methods

# CHAPTER 3

# Immunoassays (Protein-Based Methods)

*Rajesh Kumar and Vishal Srivashtav*
Banaras Hindu University

*Abhilasha Tripathi*
Sanjay Gandhi Postgraduate Institute of Medical Sciences

CONTENTS



The specific detection of a novel protein synthesized by inserted transgene constitutes an expression-based approach for the identification of genetically modified (GM) crops. Protein-based detection is primarily based on immunoassays, i.e., specific binding between a protein and an antibody. There are many different immunoassay formats, and the choice of format is dependent on the target proteins and application. The immunoassay includes dipstick strip assay, enzyme-linked immunosorbent assay (ELISA), immuno-polymerase chain reaction (PCR), Western blot, and dot immuno-binding assay. ELISA and dipstick are most commonly used test formats for the screening of transgenic proteins in plants. The dipstick is designed for qualitative yes/no testing, whereas ELISA can be used as either a qualitative or a quantitative assay. The Western blot is primarily a qualitative analytical method and particularly useful in the characterization of transgenic protein.

## 3.1 KEY COMPONENTS OF IMMUNOASSAY

The key components of immunoassay are an antibody, antigen, sensitivity, and specificity. The availability of specific antibodies against transgenic proteins with the desired affinity is the most important factor for developing these immunoassays. Monoclonal, polyclonal, or recombinant single chain variable fragment (scFv) antibodies can be employed for developing the immunoassays. Polyclonal antibodies are relatively easy to prepare in a relatively short time (e.g., 2–3 months); however, monoclonal antibodies require greater time (e.g., 5–6 months) and skill to produce and are comparatively more expensive to develop than polyclonal antibodies. The recombinant scFv antibody is developed by antibody engineering technology such as phage antibodies displayed technology, which makes it possible to generate monoclonal scFvs with desired binding affinity and specificities (Golchin and Aitken 2008, Garet et al. 2010).

The extraction of transgenic proteins from plant leaf tissues with high efficiency and consistency is a critical step for accurately determining the amount of such protein in a GM sample. The extraction efficiency depends on the tissue sample, buffer, and buffer-tissue ratios (Shan et al. 2007). The sensitivity and specificity of detection are also sometimes limited by the interference by the biological matrix. The presence of a large variety and quantity of phenolics and quinones may adversely affect the extraction of protein, binding of antibody–antigen, and enzyme activities (Loomis 1974, Gegenheimer 1990). To minimize matrix effects, polymers such as polyvinylpyrrolidone (PVP) may be usually added to the extracting media as a phenol adsorbent or quinone scavenger (Shan et al. 2007). PVP is effective against binding those phenolic compounds that form strong hydrogen-bonded complexes.

The specificity and sensitivity are important characteristics of the immunoassay, which depends on the quality of antibody and should be analyzed properly before developing protein-based test kit. An antibody binds only to the antigenic determinant site that elicits its production. This specificity of antibodies enables the development of test methods without any cross-reaction to nontarget proteins. Cross-reactivity can result in false-positive signal or overestimation of amount of transgenic protein; therefore, it should be minimized. The sensitivity of immunoassay depends on the strength of specific binding (affinity) between antibody and protein. High affinity of the bond may lead to high sensitivity (lower limit of detection; LOD) of the test method. The sensitivity of an immunoassay is determined not only by the affinity of the antibody for the protein but also by other factors such as transgenic protein expression level, protein extraction efficiency, and the size of the GM sample taken for analysis.

## 3.2 ENZYME-LINKED IMMUNOSORBENT ASSAY

ELISA, also known as an enzyme immunoassay (EIA), is a biochemical technique mainly used in immunological detection for the presence of antigens in a sample. ELISA is distinguished from other antibody-based assays because the separation of specific and nonspecific interactions occur via serial binding to a solid surface, usually a polystyrene multi-well plate, and also quantitative results can be achieved. ELISA can be performed in two ways: sandwich and competitive format. Sandwich type of ELISA has frequently been followed for the screening of GM samples. This involves a combination of two types of antibodies specific to transgenic protein: first, capture antibody (i.e., immobilized directly onto well surface) and second, detection antibody (i.e., linked to the enzyme). Further, it can be classified as the direct and indirect type based on attachment of enzyme label either to detection antibody or to secondary antibody. In the direct type, the enzyme is directly linked to detection antibody, whereas in indirect type, enzyme is linked to the secondary antibody, which is against primary transgenic specific antibody (Figure 3.1).

The stepwise procedure for direct sandwich ELISA has been given in the flow chart (Figure 3.2), and the simple plate layout has been depicted in Figure 3.3a. Performing a sandwich ELISA involves the first step of immobilization of transgenic specific first antibody (capture antibody) to a multi-well solid plate. Then, the sample solution with known and unknown amounts of transgenic protein or sample to be detected is added to respective wells. If the transgenic protein is present in the sample to be tested, it will bind to the capture antibody. When performing direct type, a transgenic specific second antibody tagged with an enzyme (detection antibody) is added in the next step to each well. In indirect type, transgenic specific second antibody without enzyme-tagged (primary antibody) is added to each well, and in the next step, secondary antibody (specific to primary antibody) tagged with an HRP enzyme (horseradish peroxidase) is added to well. Between each step, the plate is typically washed with a mild detergent solution to remove any proteins or antibodies that are nonspecifically bound. Then, the substrate TMB (3,3′,5,5′-tetramethylbenzidine) for the enzyme is added, which induces a color change in the solution that can be read through visual inspection or by an optical plate reader. The degree of color change is directly proportional to the amount of transgenic protein present in the well (Figure 3.3b). This method produces a qualitative result if read through visual inspection. However, a quantitative result of unknown samples to be tested can be obtained if the necessary transgenic protein standards are included in

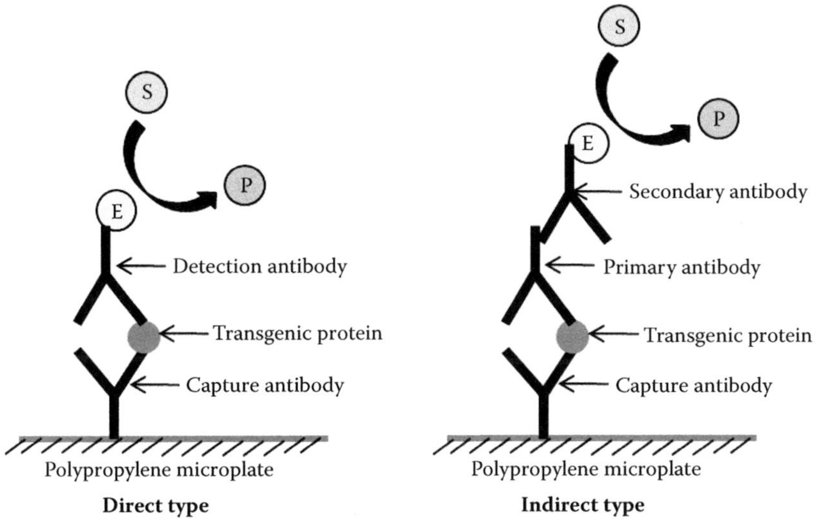


FIGURE 3.1 Schematic representation of direct and indirect sandwich ELISA. E, enzyme HRP. S, substrate (TMB). P, product (produce color).

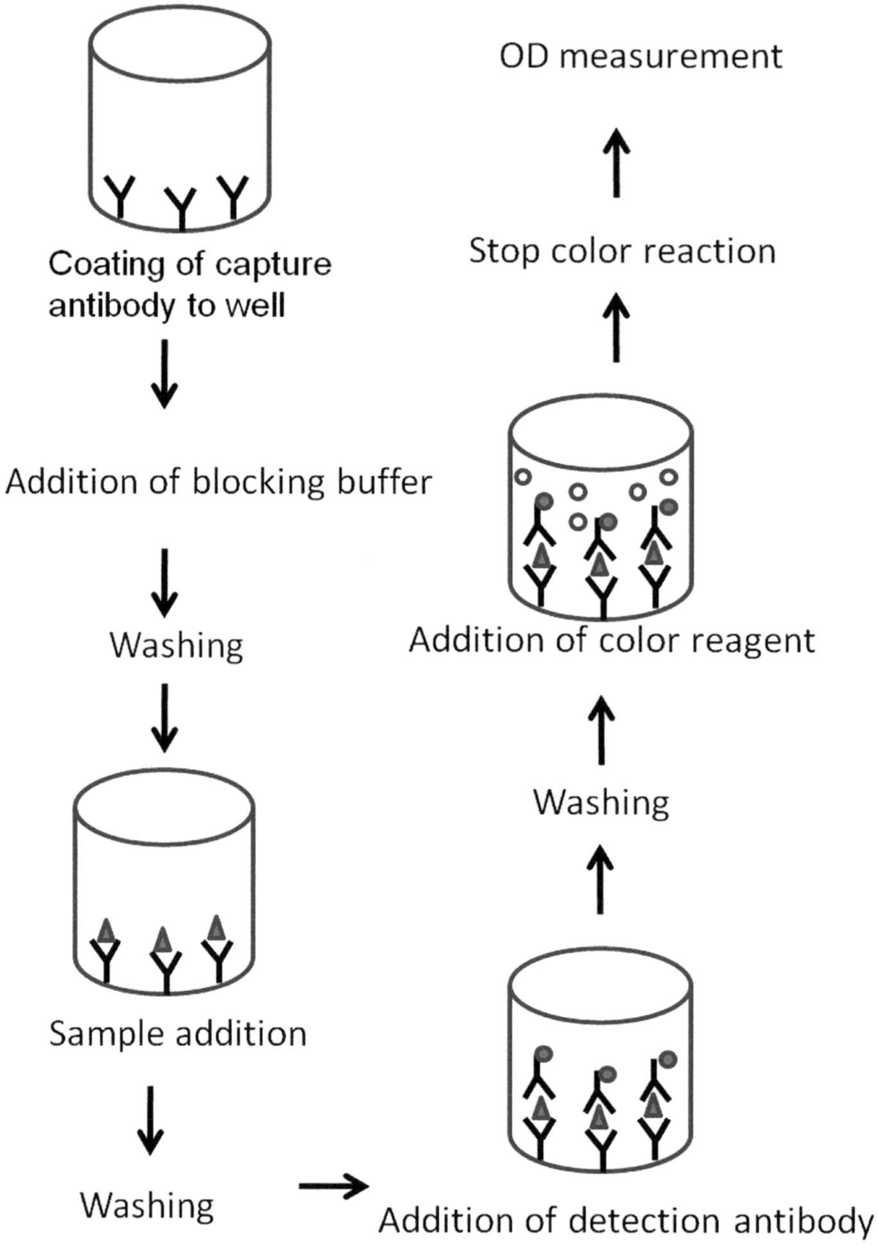


FIGURE 3.2 Flow chart for procedure of direct sandwich ELISA. The well is coated with the primary antibody against the target transgenic protein. The sample is added and upon presence, the analyte binds to the antibody and forms an antibody-protein complex. Only the specific protein is bound. After incubation, the test well is washed several times to remove unbound protein. The secondary antibody (detecting antibody) is added that recognizes the protein-antibody complex. It is coupled to an enzyme for the detection procedure. After incubation, unbound antibody is washed away. The substrate for enzyme is added. The enzyme coupled to the secondary antibody converts the substrate into a colored end product that can be measured photometrically.

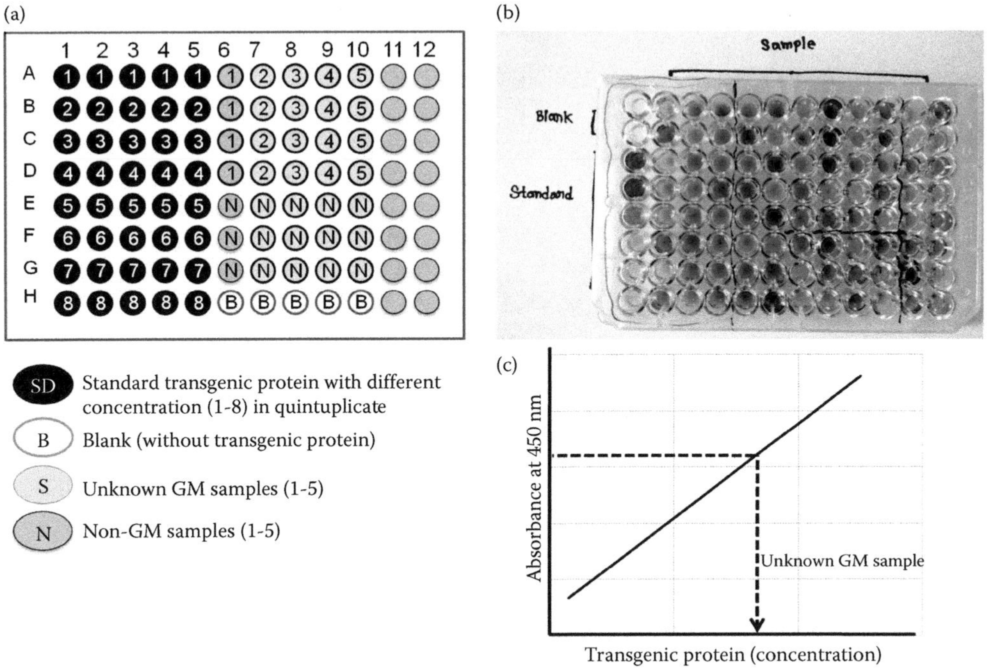


FIGURE 3.3 (a) A 96-well plate layout for ELISA with standard protein (SD), blank wells (B), and unknown GM samples (S). (b) A typical plate showing color development after indirect sandwich ELISA (plate layout not same). Lighter color indicates lower concentration, and the darker color indicates higher concentration of transgenic protein. (c) Schematic representation for standard curve for transgenic protein with sandwich ELISA and measurement of transgenic protein unknown samples.

the assay and an optical plate reader is used to evaluate the intensity of the color reaction resulting from antibody recognition of the target protein in the sample (Figure 3.3c).

In the competitive type of ELISA, only one transgenic specific antibody is used, which is linked with an enzyme HRP in the direct type. First, standard transgenic protein is immobilized onto the well surface, and then the unknown GM sample solution and the enzyme-linked specific antibody are added to the well sequentially. Free protein in liquid phase competes with the immobilized protein for binding to the enzyme-linked specific antibody. With a greater concentration of protein in the sample, the lower amount of labeled antibodies bind to the immobilized protein; hence, lower color will be developed. Competitive ELISA is further classified as the direct and indirect type and performed as in case of sandwich ELISA (Figure 3.4). The competitive type ELISA is less followed to develop kits for screening of GM crops.

The ELISA test is faster and less expensive than PCR-based methods and can be set up in any laboratory. The test provides high-throughput screening results with rapid and consistent manner. Use of highly purified and specific antibodies gives the best result without any cross-reaction to other closely related transgenic proteins. The ELISA test has some advantages over dipstick test; for example, quantitative and more sensitive results can be obtained. The commercial specific ELISA kits available for GMO testing are providing the screening results in hours up to approximately 0.04 per cent GMO content

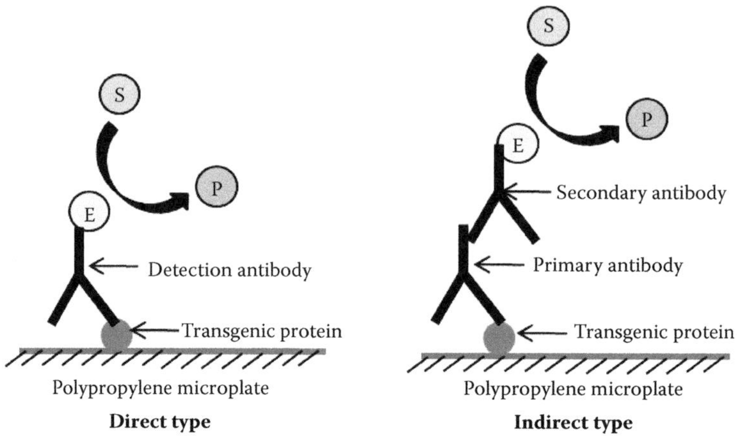


FIGURE 3.4 Schematic representation of direct and indirect competitive ELISA. E, enzyme HRP. S, substrate (TMB). P, product (produce color).

in the sample (Biogenetic Services Inc.), whereas the sensitivity in terms of amount of protein level in the sample has been reported up to pg/ml by ELISA kits (EnviroLogix).

However, ELISA has some drawbacks; for example, the antibodies may cross-react with closely related proteins Cry1Ab and Cry1Ac (Shan et al. 2007). Further, if the protein structure is altered or the antibody binding sites are damaged, there can be reduced antibody–antigen binding, which may affect the accuracy of the analysis (Clapper and Kurman 2011). Further, ELISAs are also not readily conducive for quantitative analysis of multiple transgenic proteins in a single reaction.

## 3.3 ELISA TESTS FOR GM CROPS

The ELISA technique has been widely applied for evaluating, at the experimental stage, the expression level of the novel protein synthesized by the inserted transgene. The technique has been utilized for the detection and quantification of different transgenic proteins (Table 3.1) in various GM samples such as 5-enol pyruvyl shikimate-3-phosphate synthase (EPSPS), *Bacillus thuringiensis* (Bt) proteins (Cry1Ab, Cry1Ac, Cry1B, Cry1Ie, Cry2Ab, Cry3Bb1, Cry4, Vip3) herbicide-tolerant phosphinothricin acetyltransferase (PAT) protein.

Various in-house ELISA tests have been reported for quantitative analysis of Cry1Ab transgenic protein in different samples. Walschus et al. (2002) developed a monoclonal antibody-based sandwich ELISA for detection of Cry1Ab with LODs of 0.10 per cent for Bt-11 maize and 0.23 per cent for MON810 maize. Similarly, Roda et al. (2006) reported polyclonal and monoclonal antibodies-based sandwich ELISA test for Cry1Ab expressed in MON810 maize with LOD of 0.1 per cent sample. Ermolli et al. (2006) developed a monoclonal antibody-based sandwich ELISA for Cry1Ab in Bt-11 maize with LOD of 0.0056 per cent sample. Fantozzi et al. (2007) reported ELISA for quantification of the Cry1Ab present in MON810 and Bt11 GM maize lines with LOD and LOQ (limit of quantification) of 0.018 and 0.054 per cent, respectively. Paul et al. (2008) developed highly specific and sensitive sandwich ELISA with LOD of 0.4 ng/ml for Cry1Ab protein in Bt-maize. Kumar (2012a) developed polyclonal antibody-based sandwich ELISA for Cry1Ab with LOD of 1 ng/ml of pure protein. Dong et al. (2017a) established a sandwich ELISA utilizing monoclonal

TABLE 3.1 Summary of Some In-House Developed ELISA for the Detection of Transgenic Proteins in GM Sample

| S. No. | Transgenic Proteins | Type of ELISA | Matrices | Sensitivity (LOD) | Reference |
|---|---|---|---|---|---|
| 1 | Cry1 toxins | Sandwich ELISA | Pure proteins | 15 ng/ml | Dong et al. (2016) |
| 2 | Cry1Aa | Sandwich ELISA | Soil | 4 µg/l | Helassa et al. (2011) |
| 3 | Cry1Ab | Sandwich ELISA | Spiked leaf and rice | 0.008 µg/ml | Zhang et al. (2014) |
| 4 | Cry1Ab | Sandwich ELISA | Bt-Maize | 0.10 per cent sample | Walschus et al. (2002) |
| 5 | Cry1Ab | Sandwich ELISA | Maize | 0.4 ng/ml | Paul et al. (2008) |
| 6 | Cry1Ab | Sandwich ELISA | Maize | 0.4 ng/ml | Guertler et al. (2009) |
| 7 | Cry1Ab | Sandwich ELISA | Soil | 0.4 ng/g | Gruber et al. (2012) |
| 8 | Cry1Ab | Sandwich ELISA | Water | 2.1 ng/l | Strain et al. (2014) |
| 9 | Cry1Ab | Sandwich ELISA | Pure protein | 1 ng/ml | Kumar (2012a) |
| 10 | Cry1Ab | Sandwich ELISA | Bt-11 maize | 0.0056 per cent | Ermolli et al. (2006) |
| 11 | Cry1Ab | Sandwich ELISA | Bt maize | 3–5 pg/ml, 0.1 per cent | Roda et al. (2006) |
| 12 | Cry1Ab | Sandwich ELISA | Spiked rice leaf and flour | 0.47 ± 0.11 ng/ml | Dong et al. (2017a) |
| 13 | Cry1Ac | Sandwich ELISA | Cotton Seed | 0.075 µg/g | Shan et al. (2007) |
| 14 | Cry1Ac | Sandwich ELISA | Cotton leaves | 5 ng/ml | Wang et al. (2007) |
| 15 | Cry1B | Indirect competitive ELISA | Rice leaves | Not reported | Zhang et al. (2012) |
| 16 | Cry1C | Indirect competitive ELISA | Spiked rice | Not available | Wang et al. (2012) |
| 17 | Cry1Ie | Sandwich ELISA | Maize plant | 0.27–0.51 ng/ml | Zhang et al. (2016) |
| 18 | Cry1F | Indirect competitive ELISA | Spiked rice, wheat, corn | 0.18 ng/ml | Xu et al. (2017) |
| 19 | Cry2Ab | Sandwich ELISA | Cotton seed | 1 pg/g | Kamle et al. (2011) |
| 20 | Cry4 | Sandwich ELISA | Water | 2 ng/ml pure protein, 170–900 ng/ml in samples | Fejes et al. (2012) |

*(Continued)*

TABLE 3.1 (*Continued*) Summary of Some In-House Developed ELISA for the Detection of Transgenic Proteins in GM Sample

| S. No. | Transgenic Proteins | Type of ELISA | Matrices | Sensitivity (LOD) | Reference |
|---|---|---|---|---|---|
| 21 | Vip3Aa9 | Sandwich ELISA | Pure protein | 10 ng/ml | Kumar (2011) |
| 22 | Cry1Ab, Cry1Ac, Cry1B, Cry1C, and Cry1F | Indirect competitive ELISA | Wheat | 0.029–0.074 mg/ml | Xu et al. (2016) |
| 23 | Dm-AMP1 and Rs-AFP2 | Indirect competitive ELISA | Rice leaf | Not available | Jha and Chattoo (2009) |
| 24 | CP4-EPSPS | Sandwich ELISA | Soybean | 0.35 per cent | Lipp et al. (2000) |
| 25 | CP4-EPSPS | Sandwich ELISA | Soybean | 0.25–1.4 per cent | Rogan et al. (1999) |
| 26 | PAT | Indirect competitive ELISA and sandwich ELISA | Pepper | 0.01 μg/ml | Shim et al. (2007) |
| 27 | AAD-1 and AAD-12 | Sandwich ELISA | Maize | Not reported | Wright et al. (2010) |

antibody for highly specific detection of Cry1Ab with LOD of 0.47 ± 0.11 ng/ml and LOQ of 2.43 ± 0.19 ng/ml samples and having no cross-reaction with Cry1Ac. Zhang et al. (2014) established a new sandwich ELISA for detection of Cry1Ab protein using recombinant scFv antibody with LOD of 0.008 μg/ml but having cross-reactivity to the Cry1Ac toxin.

The ELISA tests have also been developed for other Cry toxins. Head et al. (2002) developed ELISA plates for detection of Bt cotton Cry1Ac protein in the soil matrix with LOD of 3.68 ng/g. Shan et al. (2007) reported a monoclonal antibody-based sandwich ELISA for Cry1Ac protein in GM cotton with LOD of 100 ng/g. Wang et al. (2007) developed polyclonal antibody-based sandwich ELISA for the detection of Cry1Ac protein in GM cotton tissue with LOD of 5 ng/ml. Zhang et al. (2012) developed an indirect competitive ELISA for Cry1B toxin using recombinant single-chain variable fragment antibody (scFv) with a linear range of detection for standards approximately 0.19–1.1 μg/ml showing cross-reactivity with Cry1Ab, Cry1Ac, and Cry1C toxins. Wang et al. (2012) developed indirect competitive ELISA for Cry1C toxin using scFv antibody with determination range from 0.023 μg/ml to 4.35 μg/ml. Xu et al. (2017) developed indirect competitive ELISA for Cry1F toxin using monoclonal scFv antibody with LOD of 0.18 ng/ml and detected Cry1F toxin spiked in rice, wheat, corn, and soil samples with good accuracy, stability, and repeatability.

Dong et al. (2016) developed a polyclonal and monoclonal antibody-based sandwich ELISA with broad recognition of seven major Cry1 toxins (Cry1Aa, Cry1Ab, Cry1Ac, Cry1B, Cry1C, Cry1E, and Cry1F) with LOD and LOQ of 15 and 30 ng/ml for each Cry1 toxin, respectively. Further, Dong et al. (2017b) developed sandwich ELISA using specific monoclonal antibodies that can specifically detect the seven Cry1 toxins with the LOD and LOQ of 6.37–11.35 ng/ml and 17.36–24.48 ng/ml, respectively, without showing cross-reactivity to Cry2A and Vip3. Xu et al. (2016) developed an indirect competitive ELISA for Cry1Ab, Cry1Ac, Cry1B, Cry1C, and Cry1F toxins, respectively, using broad-specificity phage domain antibody with detection limit 0.029–0.074 μg/ml for those Bt Cry toxins. Kamle et al. (2011) developed sandwich type ELISA for Cry2Ab protein in transgenic cottonseed with monoclonal antibody and reported LOD of 1 pg/g concentration of the test sample with LOQ of 4 pg/g.

ELISA tests have been developed for detection of transgenic proteins other than Cry toxin. Kumar (2011) developed polyclonal antibody-based sandwich ELISA for Vip3A protein with LOD of 10 ng/ml of pure protein. Shim et al. (2007) developed polyclonal antibody ELISA for detection of phosphinothricin-N-acetyltransferase (PAT) encoded by the Bialaphos resistance (bar) gene in GM pepper with LOD of 0.01 μg/ml for a sandwich and 0.01 μg/ml for competitive ELISA. Jha and Chattoo (2009) developed polyclonal antibody indirect competitive ELISA to check the expression level of Dm-AMP1 and Rs-AFP2 in the leaf of GM rice plants. Rogan et al. (1999) developed monoclonal and polyclonal antibody-based sandwich ELISA to check the level of CP4-EPSPS in soybean. Lipp et al. (2000) developed a direct sandwich ELISA to check the level of CP4-EPSPS in soybean with LOD of 0.35 per cent sample. Further, Ermolli et al. (2006) developed a qualitative multiplex assay to assess the presence of two GM proteins Cry1Ab and the CP4-EPSPS simultaneously. Mire et al. (2010) developed a multiplexed sandwich assay for quantification of transgenic proteins in GM crops using the Luminex® FLEXMAP 3D® System.

Currently, several manufacturers such as Agdia, (Elkhart, IN), EnviroLogix, Inc. (Portland, ME), Amar Immunodiagnostics (Hyderabad, AP, India), Romer Labs (Austria), Abraxis, Inc. (Warminster, PA), Biogenetic Services, Inc. (Aurora, SD), and DesiGen diagnostics (Maharashtra, India) produce ELISA test kits for the detection and quantification of several transgenic proteins such as Cry proteins, Vip3A, PAT, EPSPS, CspB, DMO, HPPD, etc., in GM crops (Table 3.2).

TABLE 3.2 Commercially Available Protein Based Kits for Testing of GM Crops

| Company | Test Format | Test Kit for Transgenic Proteins |
|---|---|---|
| Agdia Inc., United States | Sandwich ELISA kit | Cry 1Ab, Cry1Ac, Cry1F, Cry2A, Cry2Ab, Cry3A, Cry34Ab1, Cry3Bb1, eCry3.1Ab, Vip3A, CP4-EPSPS, CspB |
| | Dipstick (Immunostrips) | AAD-12, Cry1Ab, Cry1Ac, Cry1F, Cry2A, Cry2Ab2, Cry34Ab1, Cry3Bb1, eCry3.1Ab, Vip3A, CP4-EPSPS, DMO, CspB |
| Biogenetic Services Inc., United States | Sandwich ELISA kit | Cry1Ab, Cry1F, Cry1Ac, Cry2A, Cry3A, Cry3Bb, Cry9C, CP4-EPSPS |
| | Immunostrips | Cry1Ab, Cry1Ac, Cry1F, Cry2A, Cry3Bb, Cry9C, CP4-EPSPS |
| EnviroLogix Inc., United States | Sandwich ELISA kit | Cry1A, Cry1Ab, Cry1Ac, Cry1C, Cry1F, Cry2A, Cry3A, Cry3B, Cry34, Vip3A, eCry3.1Ab, CP4-EPSPS, PAT/BAR, 2MEPSPS |
| | Dipstick (Quickstix) | Cry1A, Cry1Ab, Cry1Ac, Cry1F, Cry2A, Cry2AE, Cry34, Cry3A, Cry3B, Vip3A, eCry3.1Ab, CP4-EPSPS, PAT/BAR, 2MEPSPS, DMO, CspB |
| Romer Labs, Austria | Sandwich ELISA (AgraQuant®) | Cry1Ab, Cry1Ac, eCry3.1Ab, CP4 EPSPS, Vip3A |
| | Dipstick (AgraStrip®) | Cry1Ab, Cry1Ac, Cry1A.105, Cry1F, Cry2Ab, Cry3Bb, Cry3Bb1, Cry34Ab1, eCry3.1Ab, CspB, CP4 EPSPS, PAT, Vip3A |

*(Continued)*

TABLE 3.2 (*Continued*) Commercially Available Protein Based Kits for Testing of GM Crops

| Company | Test Format | Test Kit for Transgenic Proteins |
|---|---|---|
| Amar Immunodiagnostics, India | Sandwich ELISA kit | Cry1Ab, Cry1Ac, Cry1C, Cry1F, Cry2A, Cry1EC, Cry3A, Cry3Bb, eCry3.1Ab, Vip3A, CP4-EPSPS, PAT/BAR, HPPD |
| | Dipstick | Cry1Ab, Cry1Ac, Cry1F, Cry2A, Cry3A, Cry3Bb, Vip3A, CP4-EPSPS, PAT/BAR, HPPD |
| Abraxis, Inc., United States | Sandwich ELISA kit | Cry1Ab, Cry1Ac, Cry1F, CP4-EPSPS |
| | Dipstick | Cry1Ab, Cry1Ac, CP4-EPSPS |
| Desigen Diagnostics, India | Sandwich ELISA kit | Cry1Ac/Ab, Cry2Ab, CP4EPSPS |
| | Dipstick | Cry1Ac, Cry2Ab, CP4EPSPS |

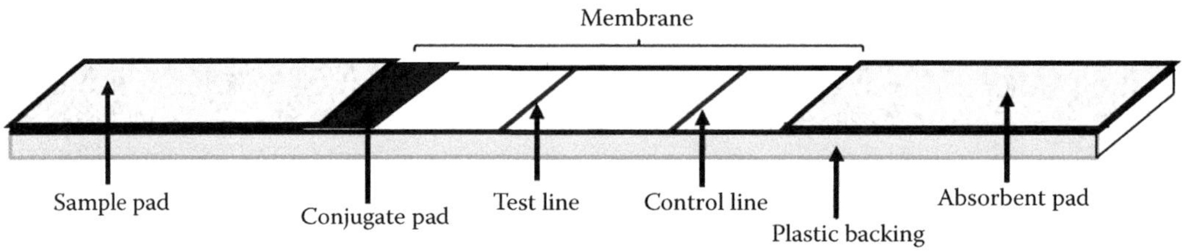


FIGURE 3.5 Schematic representation of typical dipstick strip consists of a sample pad, a conjugate pad, a NC membrane, and an absorption pad. The conjugate pad contains gold-conjugated antibody. Anti-protein IgG is immobilized at the test line (T) and anti-species IgG is immobilized at the control line (C).

## 3.4 DIPSTICK OR IMMUNOCHROMATOGRAPHIC STRIP

Another important transgenic protein-based detection method is dipstick or immunochromatographic strip or lateral flow immunoassay, which is a variant of ELISA using nitrocellulose (NC) membrane-based strips rather than microtiter wells. For the past few decades, this membrane-based technology is frequently being used for screening purpose of various analytes from the fields of food, agriculture, and health care (Ngom et al. 2010, Dzantiev et al. 2014, Sajid et al. 2014). Now, dipstick technology has become an important tool for routine, rapid, and on-site testing of GM contents. The format of the dipstick is very simple and easy to use; however, some advancement in conventional dipstick has also been reported to improve its detection limit.

### 3.4.1 Components of Dipstick

Generally, a dipstick strip consists of an NC membrane and three pads, namely, sample, absorbent, and conjugate pads, all of which are pasted onto the plastic backing. The schematic diagram of a typical dipstick strip is shown in Figure 3.5.

#### 3.4.1.1 Sample Pad

The sample pad placed at the upstream of the strip generally made up of cellulosic fiber, exhibits high absorption capacity and does not allow the protein to bind to it. The pad accepts the sample and makes it compatible with the assay format. It controls movement as well as the pH of the sample and facilitates the liquid to enter the conjugate pad uniformly. The sample pad completes the process without destabilizing the transgenic proteins and thus delivers high efficiency to the assay.

#### 3.4.1.2 Conjugate Pad (Release Pad)

The conjugate pad usually made up of glass fiber, accepts conjugated antibodies (probes). It is placed between sample pad and NC membrane overlapping toward both sides and acts as a connecting link between the two and maintains the flow toward downstream. The release pad keeps the conjugate stable and releases it efficiently with reproducibility. Sometimes, desired additives may be included in the pad based on the user's requirement.

#### 3.4.1.3 Membrane

The membrane is an important part of the dipstick strip that contains the properties such as immobilizing molecules firmly, allowing short- and long-term storage, and letting the solution phase interact with the immobilized phase without affecting the antigen–antibody chemistry. Some membranes having such important properties employed in different testing strips are NC, cellulose acetate, polyethersulfone, and nylon (Posthuma-Trumpie et al. 2009), in which NC is the most commonly used membrane. The NC membrane is cheap and easy to handle, with inherent characteristics such as good capillary flow and high protein-binding capacity, making its use more advantageous to dipstick technology over other membranes (O'Farrell and Bauer 2006). It is attached to the plastic backing card and capture zones are assigned to a separation of approximately 1 cm from each other. Then, antibodies are immobilized onto respective capture zones.

#### 3.4.1.4 Absorbent Pad (Sink Pad)

An absorbent pad is made up of cellulosic fiber with excellent absorption capacity and hydrophilic in nature, which is located downstream at end of strip. It has the ability to control sample flow through the device by pulling excess conjugates from the capture zone in the assay. Basically, it increases the volume of the liquid absorbed depending on the size and capacity of the pad.

#### 3.4.1.5 Labels (Probes)

Conjugate (probe) preparation is required for the visualization of results, which develops color over the assigned capture lines. The conjugates are prepared by combining the anti-protein antibody with optimal size and amount of labeling agent. Several choices of labeling agents have been used for the development of dipsticks such as carbon, gold, selenium, fluorescent labels, up-converting phosphor, magnetic nanoparticles, and enzymes (Song and Knotts 2008, Posthuma-Trumpie et al. 2009, Maiolini et al. 2014, Huang et al. 2016). However, colloidal gold is used as a label in most of the dipstick tests owing to its greater stability, sensitivity, and precision, which makes it suitable for use in membrane-based tests over other labeling agents (Chandler et al. 2000). The preparation of conjugates is given in the flowchart (Figure 3.6). In this chapter, the dipstick assay procedure has been described using colloidal gold as a labeling agent.

Take freshly prepared 1 ml colloidal gold solution

↓

Adjust pH 8.5 with freshly prepared 1% $K_2CO_3$ solution

↓

Add about 35 μg anti-antigen lgG

↓

Incubate mixture for 1 h at room temperature

↓

Add BSA to a final concentration of 0.1% and keep for 30 min for stabilisation

↓

Centrifuge mixture at 10,000 rpm for 30 min at 4°C.

↓

Disperse a loose pellet laden conjugated antibody in 500 μl of phosphate buffered saline (10 mM PBS, pH 7.4)

↓

Spin again to remove free unconjugated antibody and colloidal gold particles.

↓

Redissolve the resultant pellet in 100 μl conjugate storage buffer (10 mM PBS containing 0.1% BSA, pH 7.4)

↓

Store at 4°C.

FIGURE 3.6 Flow chart for conjugation of antibody to colloidal gold particles.

### 3.4.2 Principle of Dipstick Test

Sandwich type and competitive type of dipstick are being used for screening of samples, depending on the size of analytes; sandwich format is followed for larger analytes having multiple antigenic sites such as proteins and transgenic proteins, bacterial pathogens, and viruses, whereas competitive format is followed for smaller analytes with a single antigenic determinant such as pesticides (O'Farrell 2009).

In the sandwich type of assay, the procedural steps are given in the flow chart (Figure 3.7). The anti-transgenic protein antibody and the anti-species antibody are immobilized on the test line (zone 1) and control line (zone 2), respectively, as illustrated in Figure 3.8a. After drying the strip, the unoccupied site of NC membrane is blocked with a suitable blocking buffer. Concurrently, the conjugate pad is treated with colloidal gold-conjugated antibody. Then, conjugate, sample, and absorbent pads are pasted onto their respective places.

Now, take the small piece of GM leaf or seed sample and crush in the extraction buffer. Then, the strip is placed in a vial containing an extract; the sample migrates up the strip by the capillary force of the strip material. The strip can also be placed horizontally, then the extracted sample will be dropped over the sample pad, and it will migrate by capillary action toward the absorbent pad side. The absorbent pad wicks the liquid to the end of the strip, thus maintaining the flow. As the sample flows sequentially through the conjugate pad, test lines, and control line, the transgenic protein is captured/accumulated

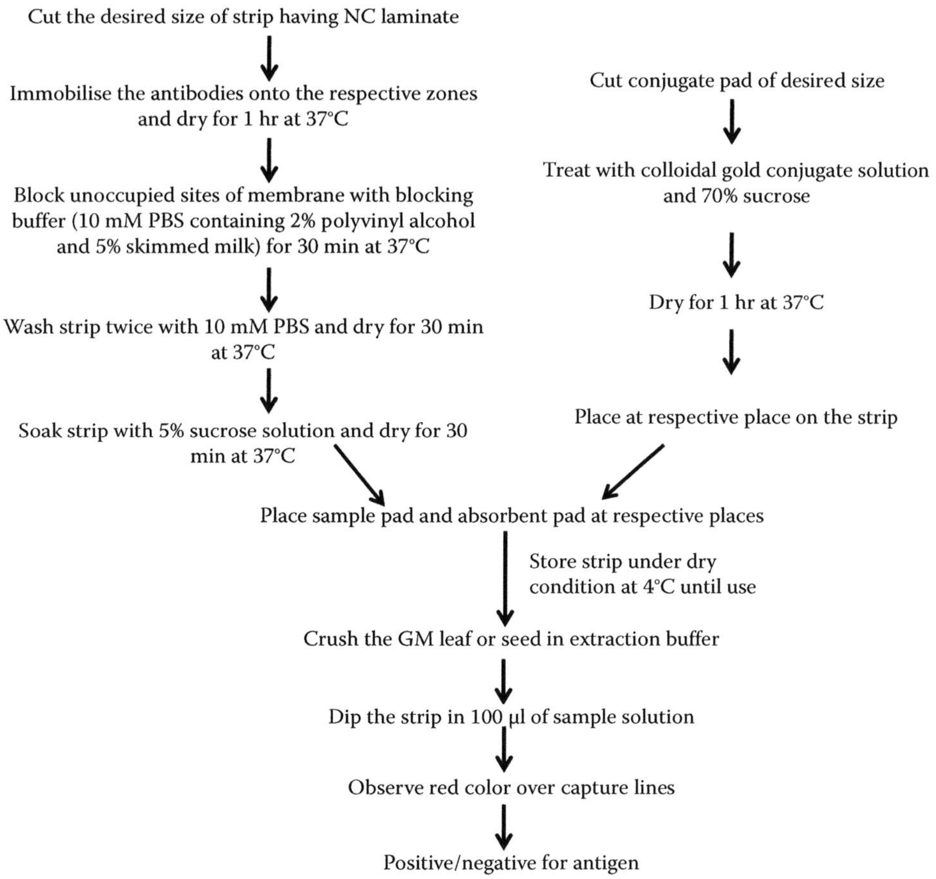


FIGURE 3.7 Flow chart for dipstick strip assay procedure.

on test lines and red-colored bands develop due to the accumulation of conjugates. The results can be visualized and interpreted within 10 min as "yes" or "no" for the presence of target protein. A red-colored line is also observed on the control line, generated by surplus gold conjugates, indicating the proper test performance. A negative test sample yields no color on the test lines, indicating the absence of target transgenic protein in the sample (Figure 3.8b). The colored band must always be visualized on the control line; the test should be considered invalid if there is no red color developed in the control region. The semiquantitative analysis can also be done by measuring the intensity of developed red band on the test line, which is directly proportional to a certain concentration range of protein present in the test sample.

### 3.4.3 Dipsticks for Detection of GM Content

The dipstick provides a qualitative test (yes or no for transgenic protein) or semiquantitative test for GMOs. This strip can suitably detect transgenic proteins in leaves, seeds, and grains of different GM crops. Such strips for detection of many transgenic proteins such as Vip, Cry toxins, CspB, CP4-EPSPS, PAT/BAR, DMO, etc., are commercially

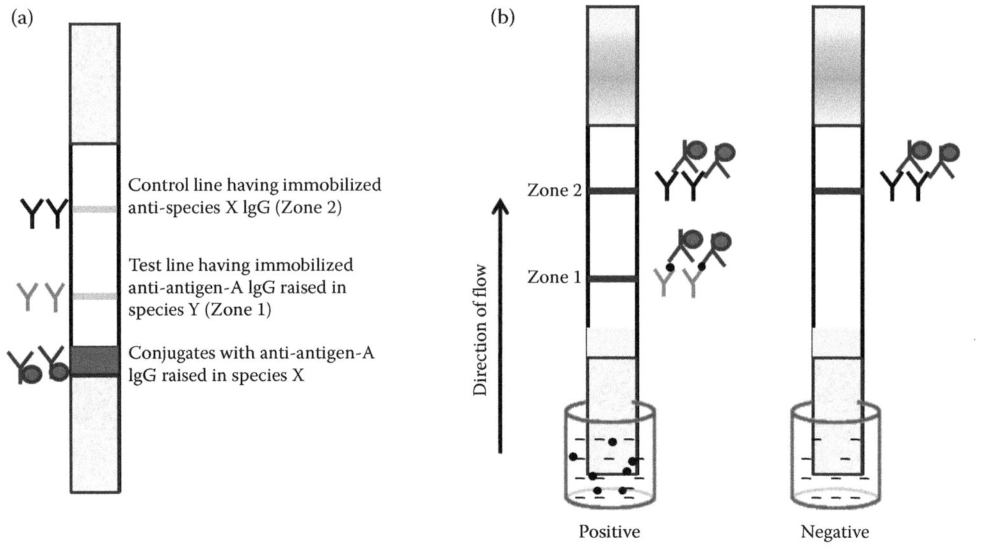


FIGURE 3.8 The illustration of dipstick assay: (a) Immobilization of antibodies on strip in sandwich format. (b) Interpretation of result: The positive result is judged by the appearance of red (assumed) line in test region (zone 1) while no red line in zone 1 in non-GM sample; red line in control region should always visible showing valid test assay.

available in the market. Currently, several manufacturers such as Agdia, (Elkhart, IN), EnviroLogix, Inc. (Portland, ME), Amar Immunodiagnostics (Hyderabad, AP, India), Romer Labs (Austria), Abraxis, Inc. (Warminster, PA), Biogenetic Services, Inc. (Aurora, SD), and DesiGen diagnostics (Maharashtra, India) are producing dipstick test kits for the screening of several transgenic proteins in GM crops (Table 3.2). Kumar et al. (2010) have developed dipstick for detection of transgenic Vip3A protein in GM crops with LOD of 100 ng/ml. Further, Kumar (2012b) developed dipstick for detection Cry1Ac/Ab with LOD of 50 ng/ml of pure protein. The purpose of these strips is to provide a rapid test for the farmer to monitor and identify GM content. The test can be performed with a kit and does not require any major equipment. Farmers can use these strips suitable for on-site testing with minimal training required. Sample can be prepared simply by crushing the leaf sample in protein extraction solutions generally provided in the kit. However, dipstick has some disadvantages such as it provides qualitative results and sometimes results in controversial readout in case of weak signal (Table 3.3).

### 3.4.4 Multiplex Dipsticks for Simultaneous Detection of Transgenic Proteins

In the multiplex analysis, specific antibodies are immobilized on test and control lines as shown in the Figure 3.9a. When this strip is placed in a vial containing a test sample, the colored bands can be visualized and results can be interpreted within 10 min as yes or no for a particular protein (Figure 3.9b).

Several commercial strips have been available for simultaneous detection of two or more transgenic proteins, such as Cry1Ac, CP4EPSPS, and Cry2A/Cry1F (Agdia; EnviroLogix; Romer Labs, Abraxis, DesiGen, Biogenetic Services). Recently, Kumar (2012b) developed

TABLE 3.3 Advantages and Disadvantages of Dipstick Assay

| | |
|---|---|
| | **Advantages** |
| 1 | The dipstick is economical, more suitable for on-site application, and can be used for initial screening method early in the food chain. |
| 2 | These test strips are fast, cheap and require minimal training and equipment. |
| 3 | The dipstick kit gives qualitative, one-step, rapid results that are interpreted by visual observation of the probe color. |
| 4 | These kits are user-friendly and available at affordable price, and do not involve complex instruments and sophisticated laboratory setup. |
| | **Disadvantages** |
| 1 | Provide qualitative or semiquantitative results. It does not give a clear picture of the exact amount of transgenic protein present in the sample. |
| 2 | Variation in results may be obtained by naked-eye interpretation, especially for colorimetric detection. This visual judgment from operators can lead to controversial readouts, especially when the detection signal is very weak or close to threshold. |
| 3 | A dipstick is sometimes criticized for its accuracy. It may cause false-negative and false-positive results, which could lead to incorrect interpretation of results, thus providing poor test performance. |
| 4 | A dipstick is preferred to take the advantage of providing cost-effective results; however, to improve sensitivity of detection, it can be linked to optical and electrochemical sensing devices, which may increase the total cost of detection. |

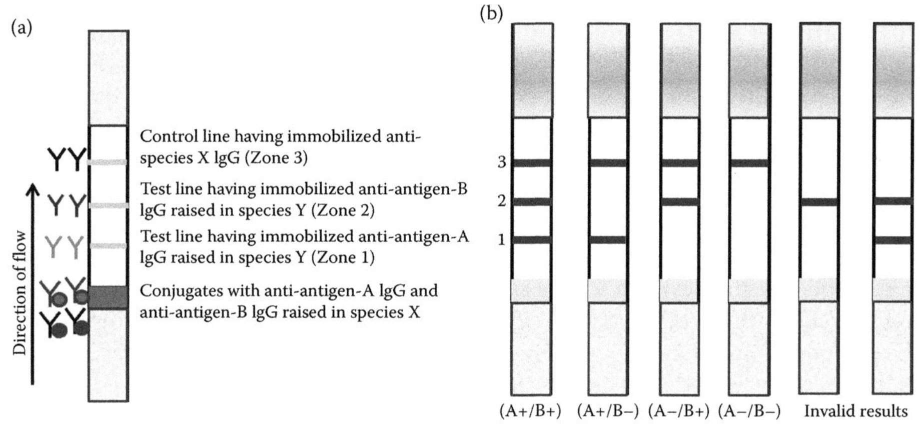


FIGURE 3.9 The illustration of multiplex dipstick assay: (a) Immobilization of antibodies on strip in sandwich format. (b) Interpretation of result: The positive result is judged by the appearance of red (assumed) line in test regions (zone 1 and/or 2) for respective protein (A or B); red line in control region should always visible showing valid test assay. + indicates protein present and – indicates protein absent.

dipsticks for simultaneous detection of Vip3A and Cry1Ab/Cry1Ac transgenic proteins suitable for on-site simultaneous screening of GM crops bearing two proteins. The multiplex dipstick has some advantages over single protein detection. First, it provides cost-effective screening results. Several target proteins can be tested simultaneously with one strip; thus, the total cost of screening of the sample costs less compared with single protein detection, making it affordable to use. Second, it reduces the consumption of assay time for the screening. Maximum results can be obtained in a short time and a speedy result is delivered. Third, the multiplex format will be valuable in increasing the flexibility of such kits and can expand measurement of a range of compounds, which provide more amounts of information per sample. The multiplex dipstick format is very useful in clinical diagnoses where multiple antigens are interdependent in deciding the stage of a disease.

### 3.4.5 Advances in Development of Dipsticks

In a conventional dipstick test, the results can be visualized by the naked eye, distinguishing color on the bands to yield a yes/no answer. However, visually distinguishing the faint-colored bands on the strip with the naked eye among end-users is prone to human error; therefore, use of strip readers helps in digitalizing the results (Glynou et al. 2003, Mao et al. 2009). The strip readers determine and analyze the results of the assays more accurately and remove subjective factors that cause human error. These strips are also able to provide semiquantitative results by the visual determination by the naked eye based on the strip cut-off value, which further can provide quantitative on-site data using a portable colorimeter. In recent, the use of biosensors is also providing more accurate result by enhancing the signal-to-noise ratio and reducing analysis time, which, in turn, is much helpful in analyzing multiple proteins simultaneously.

Recent developments in the dipstick are mainly focused on multianalyte analysis, improvement in sensitivity of detection, and quantitative output. To improve the sensitivity of detection, various strategies are generally being followed, such as enzyme (He et al. 2011, Parolo et al. 2013), gold (Kaur et al. 2007, Choi et al. 2010, Kumar et al. 2010, Rohrman et al. 2012), and silver (Shyu et al. 2002, Chiao et al. 2004, Rohrman et al. 2012). For quantitative output, visual colorimetric measurement by the naked eye is not sufficient because of the variation in visual interpretation of color. To achieve quantitative analysis in dipstick, optical strip readers are used to recording the color intensity by its relationship with the amount of protein. This is achieved by inserting the strips into a strip reader; color intensity is recorded simultaneously by imaging software (Kim and Park 2004, Zhang et al. 2009, Mudanyali et al. 2012). Optical images of the strips can also be recorded by the desktop scanner, portable scanner, and a digital camera and then processed by using suitable software. In addition, a handheld optical colorimeter has been developed for quantifying colorimetric assays in microfluidic paper-based analytical devices by the analysis of the transmission of light through the paper (Ellerbee et al. 2009). However, using this advancement makes detection by dipstick costly; therefore, employment of inexpensive readout devices can make the total cost of detection affordable.

### 3.4.6 Factors Affecting Dipstick Assay

Many factors that affect the development and performance of a dipstick assay include specificity and cross-reactivity of antibodies, blocking agents and buffers, stability of labels and probes, the pore size of the membrane, and effect of biological matrixes. Sometimes, these crucial factors cause its poor performance resulting in the generation of false-positive and false-negative signals.

Because a dipstick is an immunological assay that relies on the specific binding of protein and antibody, the specificity of such antibodies must be carefully checked to elucidate any possible cross-reaction with similar transgenic proteins that otherwise might cause false-positive results. In the multiplex analysis, cross-reactivity is an important factor, thus antibodies should be properly checked for any possible cross-reaction to the nontarget proteins; otherwise, this could provide an incorrect result. Either the combination of two types of polyclonal antibodies or polyclonal and monoclonal antibody may be used for the preparation of strips, but it should be highly specific and purified. A good-quality dipstick provides higher sensitivity results with high detection limits for the protein, which mainly depends on the quality of antibodies.

The results may sometimes be observed due to nonspecific binding in the assay that can be reduced with the use of a suitable blocking agent. A range of blocking reagents has been used in the membrane-based assay, such as polymers [PVP, polyvinyl alcohol (PVA), and polyethylene glycol], gelatin, casein, and bovine serum albumin. However, before the strip development, it should be optimized accordingly.

The shape, size, and stability of the colloidal gold label are key factors for the success of the dipstick test. The shape of colloidal gold particles should be spherical and of appropriate size. A range from 10 to 40 nm colloidal gold particles has been used in the dipstick assay to achieve sensitive results (Shyu et al. 2002, Xiulan et al. 2005, Zhao et al. 2008, Shim et al. 2009, Zhou et al. 2009). Better sensitivity is observed with larger particles, but the stability is diminished with the particle size larger than 40 nm (Laitinen and Vuento 1996). If necessary, the conjugate may be treated with sucrose solution, which provides a consistent release of the conjugate. The excess gold conjugates will also create several problems in the test, which will increase the possibility of false-positive signals.

Further, the selection of membrane and its pore size also affects the performance of the test by influencing the wicking rate, which in turn determines the reaction kinetics. Pore sizes of the NC membrane ranging from 8 to 15 μ may be used in the dipstick assay as per assay requirement. The increase in the membrane nominal pore size increases the speed of capillary flow; however, assay sensitivity suffers as a result (Henderson and Stewart 2002, Merck Millipore Corp 2016). The highest sensitivity is obtained with smaller pore size but it slows the wicking rate, which, thus, provides sufficient time for antibody and protein interaction and vice versa (Henderson and Stewart 2002, Merck Millipore Corp 2016).

Before the commercial release of the dipstick, it must be validated with the specific GM samples to minimize the matrix effect. Sometimes the red color on test lines is masked by the sample color, thereby reducing the effectiveness of the probe. The matrix sometimes also affects the specific binding of antibody and protein during the assay progress. These effects can be minimized or neutralized using the specific sample buffers according to the need of the assay condition to obtain good test results.

## 3.5 IMMUNO-PCR METHOD

The most sensitive transgenic protein-based detection is Immuno-PCR (IPCR) which is very much similar to sandwich ELISA except that the detection antibody is linked to the short reporter DNA sequences instead of a conventional enzyme which further is amplified by either conventional PCR or real-time (RT) PCR machine (Figure 3.10a). It combines the advantages of specificity of immunoassays and sensitivity of PCR. In conventional IPCR, the amplified reported DNA can be analyzed by agarose gel electrophoresis, but sometimes, the nonspecific results would also be observed. To minimize this nonspecific results, RT-IPCR is employed, which involves the RT-PCR technology. All the

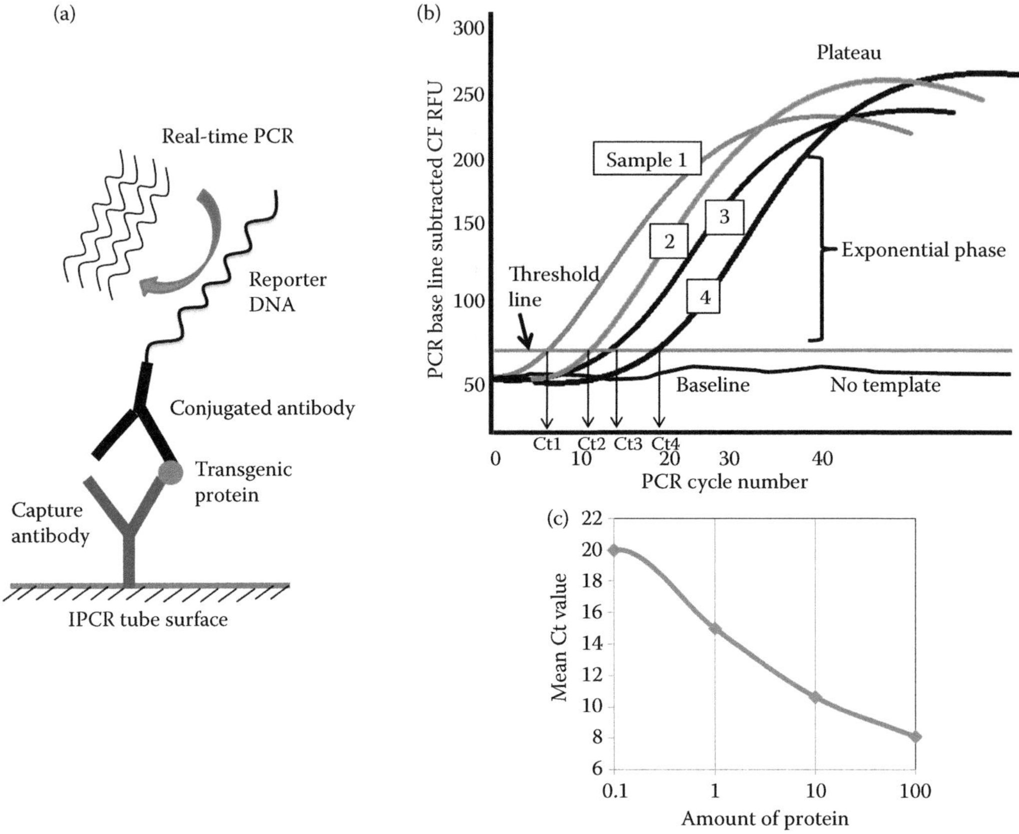


FIGURE 3.10 Illustration of sandwich type RT-IPCR assay. (a) Bound reporter DNA is amplified by RT-PCR. (b) Amplification curves for four sample of transgenic protein with negative control. (c) Representative graph plot between protein and mean Ct values.

steps can be performed in the same IPCR tube including the addition of capture antibody, transgenic protein, and conjugated antibody linked to reporter DNA. After washing with buffer, reporter DNA is amplified by RT-PCR in the same well of tube utilizing PCR reaction mixture and SYBR green dye. Then, mean threshold cycle (Ct) value is calculated for each sample from placing the threshold line at the exponential amplification curve (Figure 3.10b), and the graph is plotted against a range of transgenic protein concentration to determine the amount of transgenic protein in unknown samples (Figure 3.10c).

The RT-IPCR assay has been extensively used in the fields of immunological research and clinical diagnostics to increase the sensitivity of detection where complex biological matrices and small amounts of sample are available. Due to some limitations such as high cost, time-consuming, and requirement of expensive instruments, this technique is not routinely being utilized for transgenic detection. However, still, we find some progress in transgenic detection and quantification such as Cry1Ac protein (Allen et al. 2006), Cry1Ab protein (Kumar 2012a), and Vip3A protein (Kumar 2011) owing to the high sensitivity and the requirement of small amounts of protein over other protein-based methods. The sensitivity of detection in a RT-IPCR assay for Cry1Ab has been reported up to 0.1 ng/ml of protein (Kumar 2012a).

TABLE 3.4 Advantages and disadvantages of immunoassays

| | |
|---|---|
| | **Advantages** |
| 1 | It offers qualitative and/or quantitative results. |
| 2 | Less skill is required by personal compared to DNA based methods. |
| 3 | Equipment setup is cheaper compared to DNA based methods. |
| 4 | It is robust, specific, and has simple assay formats. |
| 5 | It is suitable and cost-effective for batch analysis of GM samples. |
| 6 | It can be used on-site for GM sample verification. |
| | **Disadvantages** |
| 1 | These methods are generally less sensitive than DNA detection methods. |
| 2 | Production of specific antibodies against transgenic proteins is a slow and difficult task that requires a great deal of skill and experience. |
| 3 | False positives may sometimes occur due to cross-reaction with other components in the sample. |
| 4 | Some GM crops do not express detectable levels of the target protein. |
| 5 | The assays are not readily conducive for quantitative analysis of multiple transgenic proteins in single reaction. |
| 6 | It is difficult to detect transgenic proteins in processed samples. |

## 3.6 ADVANTAGES AND DISADVANTAGES OF IMMUNOASSAYS

All immunoassays take advantage of an antibody's binding specificity to provide specific results. Immunoassays provide robust, specific, and cost-effective qualitative and quantitative results. However, despite the advantages immunoassay offers, many limitations/drawbacks need to be considered when it comes to their application for detection of GM crops (Table 3.4).

## 3.7 CONCLUDING REMARKS

Immunoassays are frequently being used for the detection of GM content in leaf, seed, and their food and feed produces. It is essential that such methods are demonstrated to be reliable and give consistent results. This includes the need for a proper validation of the test methods with appropriate reference GM material, which may also influence the reliability and accuracy of the analytical results. It is also important to keep in mind the possible effect of specific matrices on the methods during the assay. In addition, numerous other biological and analytical factors need to be taken into account when deciding qualitative and quantitative results. Generally, immunoassays have been proven to be fast, reliable, specific, and economic test methods.

## REFERENCES

Allen, R.C., S. Rogelj, S.E. Cordova, and T.L. Kieft. 2006. An immuno-PCR method for detecting *Bacillus thuringiensis* Cry1Ac toxin. *Journal of Immunological Methods* 308(1–2): 109–115.

Chandler, J., T. Gurmin, and N. Robinson. 2000. The place of gold in rapid tests. *In Vitro Diagnostics* 6: 37–49.

Chiao, D.J., R.H. Shyu, C.S. Hu, H.Y. Chiang, and S.S. Tang. 2004. Colloidal gold-based immunochromatographic assay for detection of botulinum neurotoxin type B. *Journal of Chromatography B* 809: 37–41.

Choi, D.H., S.K. Lee, Y.K. Oh, B.W. Bae, S.D. Lee, S. Kim, Y.B. Shin, and M.G. Kim. 2010. A dual gold nanoparticle conjugate-based lateral flow assay (LFA) method for the analysis of troponin I. *Biosensors and Bioelectronics* 25(8): 1999–2002.

Clapper, G.M., and L. Kurman. 2011. Immunoassay applications in grain products and food processing. In *Immunoassays in Agricultural Biotechnology*; Shan, G., Ed., 241–256. Hoboken, NJ: John Wiley and Sons.

Dong, S., C. Zhang, X. Zhang, Y. Liu, J. Zhong, and Y. Xie. 2016. Production and characterization of monoclonal antibody broadly recognizing Cry1 toxins using designed polypeptide as hapten. *Analytical Chemistry* 88: 7023–7032.

Dong, S., X. Zhang, Y. Liu, C. Zhang, Y. Xie, J. Zhong, C. Xu, and X. Liu. 2017a. Establishment of a sandwich enzyme-linked immunosorbent assay for specific detection of *Bacillus thuringiensis* (Bt) Cry1Ab toxin utilizing a monoclonal antibody produced with a novel hapten designed with molecular model. *Analytical and Bioanalytical Chemistry* 409: 1985.

Dong, S., C. Zhang, Y. Liu, X. Zhang, Y. Xie, J. Zhong, C. Xu, and X. Liu. 2017b. Simultaneous production of monoclonal antibodies against (Bt) Cry1 toxins using a mixture immunization, *Analytical Biochemistry* 531: 60–66.

Dzantiev, B.B., N.A. Byzova, A.E. Urusov, and A.V. Zherdev. 2014. Immunochromatographic methods in food analysis. *Trends in Analytical Chemistry* 55: 81–93.

Ellerbee, A.K., S.T. Phillips, A.C. Siegel, K.A. Mirica, A.W. Martinez, P. Striehl, N. Jain, M. Prentiss, and G.M. Whitesides. 2009. Quantifying colorimetric assays in paper-based microfluidic devices by measuring the transmission of light through paper. *Analytical Chemistry* 81: 8447–8452.

Ermolli, M., A. Prospero, B. Balla, M. Querci, A. Mazzeo, and G. Van Den Eede. 2006. Development of an innovative immunoassay for CP4EPSPS and Cry1AB genetically modified protein detection and quantification. *Food Additives and Contaminants* 23: 876–882.

Fantozzi, A., M. Ermolli, M. Marini, D. Scotti, B. Balla, M. Querci, S.R.H. Langrell, and G. Van den Eede. 2007. First application of a microsphere-based immunoassay to the detection of genetically modified organisms (GMOs): Quantification of Cry1Ab protein in genetically modified maize. *Journal of Agricultural and Food Chemistry* 550(4): 1071–1076.

Fejes, A., E. Takacs, G. Fekete, B. Darvas, B.S. Ferguson, D. Saxena, and A. Szekacs. 2012. Aquatic effect duration study of Cry4 toxin with immunoassay and *Aedes aegypti* larval biotest. *Aquatic Insects* 34: 207–222.

Garet, E., A.G. Cabado, J.M. Vieites, and A. González-Fernández. 2010. Rapid isolation of single-chain antibodies by phage display technology directed against one of the most potent marine toxins: Palytoxin. *Toxicon* 55: 1519–1526.

Gegenheimer, P. 1990. Preparation of extracts from plants. *Methods in Enzymology* 182: 174–193.

Glynou, K., P.C. Ioannou, T.K. Christopoulos, and V. Syriopoulou. 2003. Oligonucleotide-functionalized gold nanoparticles as probes in a dry-reagent strip biosensor for DNA analysis by hybridization. *Analytical Chemistry* 75: 4155–4160.

Golchin, M., and R. Aitken. 2008. Isolation by phage display of recombinant antibodies able to block adherence of Escherichia coli mediated by the K99 colonisation factor. *Veterinary Immunology and Immunopathology* 121(3–4): 321–331.

Gruber, H., V. Paul, H.H. Meyer, and M. Muller. 2012. Determination of insecticidal Cry1Ab protein in soil collected in the final growing seasons of a nine-year field trial of Bt-maize MON810. *Transgenic Research* 21: 77–88.

Guertler, P., V. Paul, C. Albrecht, and H.H. Meyer. 2009. Sensitive and highly specific quantitative real-time PCR and ELISA for recording a potential transfer of novel DNA and Cry1Ab protein from feed into bovine milk. *Analytical and Bioanalytical Chemistry* 393: 1629–1638.

Henderson, K., and J. Stewart. 2002. Factors influencing the measurement of oestrone sulphate by dipstick particle capture immunoassay. *Journal of Immunological Methods* 270: 77–84.

He, Y., S. Zhang, X. Zhang, M. Baloda, A.S. Gurung, H. Xu, and G. Liu. 2011. Ultrasensitive nucleic acid biosensor based on enzyme-gold nanoparticle dual label and lateral flow strip biosensor. *Biosensors Bioelectronics* 26: 2018–2024.

Head, G., J.B. Surber, J.A. Watson, J.W. Martin, and J.J. Duan. 2002. No detection of Cry1Ac protein in soil after multiple years of transgenic Bt cotton (Bollgard) use. *Environmental Entomology* 31: 30–36.

Helassa, N., A. M'Charek, H. Quiquampoix, S. Noinville, P. Déjardin, R. Frutos, and S. Staunton. 2011. Effects of physicochemical interactions and microbial activity on the persistence of Cry1Aa Bt (*Bacillus thuringiensis*) toxin in soil. *Soil Biology and Biochemistry* 43: 1089–1097.

Huang, X., Z.P. Aguilar, H. Xu, W. Lai, and Y. Xiong. 2016. Membrane-based lateral flow immunochromatographic strip with nanoparticles as reporters for detection: A review. *Biosensors Bioelectronics* 75: 166–180.

Jha, S., and B. Chattoo. 2009. Transgene stacking and coordinated expression of plant defensins confer fungal resistance in rice. *Rice* 2: 143–154.

Kamle, S., A. Ojha, and A. Kumar. 2011. Development of an enzyme linked immunosorbant assay for the detection of Cry2Ab Protein in transgenic plants. *GM Crops* 2(2): 118–125.

Kaur, J., K.V. Singh, R. Boro, K.R. Thampi, M. Raje, G.C. Varshney, and C.R. Suri. 2007. Immunochromatographic dipstick assay format using gold nanoparticles labeled protein-hapten conjugate for the detection of atrazine. *Environmental Science & Technology* 41: 5028–5036.

Kim, S., and J.K. Park. 2004. Development of a test strip reader for a lateral flow membrane-based immunochromatographic assay. *Biotechnology and Bioprocess Engineering* 9: 127–131.

Kumar R., C.K. Singh, S. Kamle, R.P. Sinha, R.K. Bhatnagar, and D.N. Kachru. 2010. Development of nanocolloidal gold based immunochromatographic assay for rapid detection of transgenic vegetative insecticidal protein in genetically modified crops. *Food Chemistry* 122(4): 1298–1303.

Kumar, R. 2011. A quantitative immuno-PCR method for detection of vegetative insecticidal protein in genetically modified crops. *Journal of Agricultural and Food Chemistry* 59(19): 10448–10453.

Kumar, R. 2012a. A real-time immuno-PCR assay for the detection of transgenic Cry1Ab protein. *European Food Research Technology* 234: 101–108.

Kumar R. 2012b. Development of dipsticks for simultaneous detection of Vip3A and Cry1Ab/Cry1Ac transgenic proteins. *Journal of AOAC International* 95(4): 1131–1137.

Laitinen, M.P.A., and M. Vuento. 1996. Affinity immunosensor for milk progesterone: Identification of critical parameters. *Biosensors & Bioelectronics* 11: 1207–1214.

Lipp, M., E. Anklam, and J.W. Stave. 2000. Validation of immunoassay for detection and quantification of a genetically modified soybean in food and food fractions using reference materials: Interlaboratory study. *Journal of AOAC International* 83(4): 919–927.

Loomis, W.D. 1974. Overcoming problems of phenolics and quinines in the isolation of plant enzymes and organelles. In *Methods in Enzymology*; Colowick, S.P., Kaplan, N.O., Eds., 528–545. New York: Academic Press.

Maiolini, E., E. Ferri, A.L. Pitasi, A. Montoya, M. Di Giovanni, E. Errani, and S. Girotti. 2014. Bisphenol A determination in baby bottles by chemiluminescence enzyme-linked immunosorbent assay, lateral flow immunoassay and liquid chromatography tandem mass spectrometry. *Analyst (Lond.)* 139: 318–324.

Mao, X., Y. Ma, A. Zhang, L. Zhang, L. Zeng, and G. Liu. 2009. Disposable nucleic acid biosensors based on gold nanoparticle probes and lateral flow strip. *Analytical Chemistry* 81: 1660–1668.

Merck Millipore Corp. 2016. Rapid Lateral Flow Test Strips: Considerations for Product Development, Lit. No. TB500EN00EMM. Darmstadt, Germany, www.researchgate.net/file.PostFileLoader.html.

Mire, B., H.N. Baker, T. Copa, and M.R. Hoffmeyer. 2010. Multiplexed sandwich assay for quantitation of transgenic proteins in genetically modified plants using the luminex® FLEXMAP 3D® system. BioTechniques Poster Hall 2010 (p.3). www.BioTechniques.com/posters/113596.

Mudanyali, O., S. Dimitrov, U. Sikora, S. Padmanabhan, I. Navruz, and A. Ozcan. 2012. Integrated rapid-diagnostic-test reader platform on a cellphone. *Lab Chip* 12: 2678–2686.

Ngom, B., Y. Guo, X. Wang, and D. Bi. 2010. Development and application of lateral flow test strip technology for detection of infectious agents and chemical contaminants: A review. *Analytical and Bioanalytical Chemistry* 397: 1113–1135.

O'Farrell, B., and J. Bauer. 2006. Developing highly sensitive, more-reproducible lateral-flow assays. *In Vitro Diagnostics* 7: 41–49.

O'Farrell, B. 2009. In *Lateral Flow Immunoassay*, Wong, R.C., Tse, H.Y. Eds., Chapter 1: Evolution in Lateral Flow–Based Immunoassay Systems–33. New York: Humana Press.

Parolo, C., M. Medina-Sánchez, A. dela Escosura-Muniz, and A. Merkoçi. 2013. Simple paper architecture modifications lead to enhanced sensitivity in nanoparticle based lateral flow immunoassays *Lab Chip* 13: 386–390.

Paul, V., K. Steinke, and H.H. Meyer. 2008. Development and validation of a sensitive enzyme immunoassay for surveillance of Cry1Ab toxin in bovine blood plasma of cows fed Bt-maize (MON810). *Analytica Chimica Acta* 607: 106–113.

Posthuma-Trumpie, G.A., J. Korf, and A. van Amerongen. 2009. Lateral flow (immuno) assay: Its strengths, weaknesses, opportunities and threats. A literature survey. *Analytical and Bioanalytical Chemistry* 393: 569–582.

Roda, A., M. Mirasoli, M. Guardigli, E. Michelini, P. Simoni, and M. Magliulo. 2006. Development and validation of a sensitive and fast chemiluminescent enzyme immunoassay for the detection of genetically modified maize. *Analytical and Bioanalytical Chemistry* 384(6): 1269–1275.

Rogan, G.J., Y.A. Dudin, T.C. Lee, K.M. Magin, J.D. Astwood, N.S. Bhatka, J.N. Leach, P.R. Sanders, and R.L. Fuchs. 1999. Immunodiagnostic methods for detection of 5 enolpyruvylshikimate-3-phosphate synthase in Roundup Ready soybeans. *Food Control* 10: 407–414.

Rohrman, B.A., V. Leautaud, E. Molyneux, and R.R. Richards-Kortum. 2012. A lateral flow assay for quantitative detection of amplified HIV-1 RNA. *PLoS One* 7: e45611.

Sajid, M., A.N. Kawde, and M. Daud. 2014. Designs, formats and applications of lateral flow assay: A literature review. *Journal of Saudi Chemical Society* 19: 689–705.

Shan, G., S.K. Embrey, and B.W. Schaffer. 2007. A highly specific enzyme-linked immunosorbent assay for the detection of Cry1Ac insecticidal crystal protein in transgenic Wide Strike cotton. *Journal of Agricultural and Food Chemistry* 55: 5974–5979.

Shim, Y.Y., W.S. Shin, G.S. Moon, and K.H. Kim. 2007. Quantitative analysis of phosphinothricin-N-acetyltransferase in genetically modified herbicide tolerant pepper by an enzyme-linked immunosorbent assay. *Journal of Microbiology and Biotechnology* 17(4): 681–684.

Shim, W.B., K.Y. Kim, and D.H. Chung. 2009. Development and validation of a gold nanoparticle immunochromatographic assay (ICG) for the detection of zearalenone. *Journal of Agricultural and Food Chemistry* 57: 4035–4041.

Shyu, R.H., H.F. Shyu, H.W. Liu, and S.S. Tang. 2002. Colloidal gold-based immunochromatographic assay for detection of ricin. *Toxicon* 40: 255–258.

Song, X., and M. Knotts. 2008. Time-resolved luminescent lateral flow assay technology. *Analytica Chimica Acta* 626: 186–192.

Strain, K.E., S.A. Whiting, and M.J. Lydy. 2014. Laboratory and field validation of a Cry1Ab protein quantitation method for water. *Talanta* 128: 109–116.

Walschus, U., S. Witt, and C. Wittman. 2002. Development of monoclonal antibodies against Cry1Ab protein from *Bacillus thuringiensis* and their application in an ELISA for detection of transgenic BT-maize. *Food and Agricultural Immunology* 14: 231–240.

Wang, Y., X. Zhang, C. Zhang, Y. Liu, and X. Liu. 2012. Isolation of single chain variable fragment (scFv) specific for Cry1C toxin from human single fold scFv libraries. *Toxicon* 60(7): 1290–1297.

Wang, S., Y.A. Guo, W.Z. Zheng, Y. Zhang, H. Qiao, and I.R. Kennedy. 2007. Development of ELISA for the determination of transgenic Bt-cottons using antibodies against cry1Ac protein from bacillus Thruingiensis HD-73. *Journal of Engineering in Life Sciences* 7(2): 1–7.

Wright, T.R., G. Shan, T.A. Walsh, J.M. Lira, C. Cui, and P. Song. 2010. Robust crop resistance to broadleaf and grass herbicides provided by aryloxyalkanoate dioxygenase transgenes. *Proceedings of the National Academy of Sciences USA* 107: 20240–20245.

Xiulan, S., Z. Xiaolian, T. Jian, J. Zhou, and F.S. Chu. 2005. Preparation of gold-labeled antibody probe and its use in immunochromatography assay for detection of aflatoxin B1. *International Journal of Food Microbiology* 99: 185–194.

Xu, C., X. Zhang, X. Liu, Y. Liu, X. Hu, J. Zhong, C. Zhang, and X. Liu. 2016. Selection and application of broad-specificity human domain antibody for simultaneous detection of Bt Cry toxins. *Analytical Biochemistry* 512: 70–77.

Xu, C., C. Zhang, J. Zhong, H. Hu, S. Luo, X. Liu, X. Zhang, Y. Liu, and X. Liu. 2017. Construction of an Immunized Rabbit Phage Display Library for Selecting High Activity against *Bacillus thuringiensis* Cry1F Toxin Single-Chain Antibodies. *Journal of Agricultural and Food Chemistry* 65(29): 6016–6022.

Zhang, M.Z., M.Z. Wang, Z.L. Chen, J.H. Fang, M.M. Fang, J. Liu, and X.P. Yu. 2009. Development of a colloidal gold-based lateral-flow immunoassay for the rapid simultaneous detection of clenbuterol and ractopamine in swine urine. *Analytical and Bioanalytical Chemistry* 395: 2591–2599.

Zhang, X., Y. Liu, C. Zhang, Y. Wang, C. Xu, and X. Liu. 2012. Rapid isolation of single-chain antibodies from a human synthetic phage display library for detection of *Bacillus thuringiensis* (Bt) Cry1B toxin. *Ecotoxicology and Environmental Safety* 81: 84–90.

Zhang, X., C. Xu, C. Zhang, Y. Liu, Y. Xie, and X. Liu. 2014. Established a new double antibodies sandwich enzyme linked immunosorbent assay for detecting *Bacillus thuringiensis* (Bt) Cry1Ab toxin based single-chain variable fragments from a naïve mouse phage displayed library. *Toxicon* 81: 13–22.

Zhang, Y., W. Zhang, Y. Liu, J. Wang, G. Wang, and Y. Liu. 2016. Development of monoclonal antibody-based sensitive ELISA for the determination of Cry1Ie protein in transgenic plant. *Analytical and Bioanalytical Chemistry* 408(28): 8231–8239.

Zhao, Y., G. Zhang, Q. Liu, M. Teng, J. Yang, and J. Wang. 2008. Development of a lateral flow colloidal gold immunoassay strip for the rapid detection of enrofloxacin residues. *Journal of Agricultural and Food Chemistry* 56: 12138–12142.

Zhou, Y., F.G. Pan, Y.S. Li, Y.Y. Zhang, J.H. Zhang, S.Y. Lu, H.L. Ren, and Z.S. Liu. 2009. Colloidal gold probe-based immunochromatographic assay for the rapid detection of brevetoxins in fishery product samples. *Biosenors and Bioelectronics* 24: 2744–2747.

CHAPTER 4

# PCR Techniques for Detection and Quantification of GMOs

*Frédéric Debode and Gilbert Berben*
Walloon Agricultural Research Center (CRA-W)

CONTENTS

## 4.1 INTRODUCTION

Different DNA-based detection techniques can be used in the framework of genetically modified organism (GMO) detection (Kok et al., 2002; Holst-Jensen et al., 2003; Morisset et al., 2008; Marmiroli et al., 2008). For good sensitivity, these techniques first involve the extraction of DNA still contained in the food or feed products (even if direct amplification is feasible, Kermekchiev et al., 2009; Kitpipit et al., 2014), followed by the detection of a well-defined DNA target within a fraction of the DNA extract. Currently, this requires amplifying the target. There is a large variety of genetic amplification techniques (e.g., loop-mediated isothermal amplification, nucleic acid sequence-based amplification, etc.); some of which were used in GMO detection (e.g., Morisset et al., 2008; Zhang et al., 2010) but the most commonly utilized one is the polymerase chain reaction (PCR). This chapter is specifically devoted to PCR and will consider its different formats aimed at the detection of GMOs or genetically modified (GM)-derived products.

### 4.1.1 Classical PCR

PCR entails the enzymatic multiplication of a precise DNA fragment (Mullis et al., 1987). Detection is possible, thanks to the exponential effect of the reaction, which permits the synthesis of several billion copies from a single copy of the segment and allows highlighting the searched DNA even if the number of copies present in the DNA extract is very low.

In the context of GMO detection, the targeted DNA can be a promoter, a terminator, or a gene in case of a screening, or even a specific junction between elements. Many classical PCR methods are available for GMO detection. Available methods are listed (Database, Dong et al., 2008; GMOMETHODS, Bonfini et al., 2012; EUginius, www.euginius.eu) and regularly updated. To set up an amplification, at least some knowledge of the sequence of the fragment of interest is mandatory to enable the design of a pair of complementary oligonucleotides (primers) located at the extremities of the fragment to be amplified. The primers have two functions: identify (by hybridization) the region of DNA to be amplified and serve as a starting point for DNA synthesis given that the DNA polymerase can only add new nucleotides to an already existing strand of DNA.

PCR capitalizes on the ability of a double-stranded DNA fragment to denature and rehybridize as a function of temperature, the hybridization properties between complementary DNA sequences, and the ability of DNA polymerase to synthesize a new strand from a primer hybridized to a DNA template. The DNA extract to be analyzed is added to the reaction mixture containing a buffer (placing the products under optimum pH conditions for amplification), $MgCl_2$ (co-factor necessary for the enzyme), nucleotides (dATP, dGTP, dCTP and dTTP, or optionally dUTP), primers, and *Taq* DNA polymerase. The amplification effect is the result of a chain reaction fed by various thermal cycles, including the denaturation of the DNA strands, the hybridization of the primers, and the elongation (synthesis) of new strands from the primers. The use of *Taq* polymerase as DNA polymerase makes it unnecessary to add enzyme to the reaction mixture after each denaturation step. *Taq* polymerase indeed has a built-in tolerance to high temperatures required for denaturation. At each amplification cycle, the number of newly synthesized copies (amplicons) will theoretically be doubled. At least during the first cycles of the run, this will lead to an exponential amplification rate. Once enough cycles have been completed, consumption of the reagents in the mixture will progressively slow down the reaction rate until a plateau is reached. The result of the whole process is that, starting from only one copy of the target, the amplification can give rise to several billion copies of that target. In classical PCR, only the end products of the reaction are analyzed. This is known as the "end-point" PCR.

The products of amplification can be visualized after migration on agarose gel in the presence of an intercalating agent such as ethidium bromide. This reagent has a high affinity for DNA. When intercalated between the nucleic acid bases, an orange fluorescence is visible under ultraviolet light. The presence of a band of the expected size indicates that the target has been amplified. Capillary electrophoresis (García-Cañas et al., 2004; Heide et al., 2008) is a faster and more precise alternative to agarose gels.

Conventional PCR tends to be less effective than real-time PCR; the latter is faster because it does not require migration on agarose gel. Real-time PCR is more specific due to the use of a hybridization probe and gives access to quantitative data.

### 4.1.2 Nested PCR

Nested PCR is a variant of classical PCR where the product of a first PCR is amplified again through a second pair of primers hybridizing to an inner part (nested) of the amplified sequence. The sensitivity is considerably increased as two successive PCRs are performed. This technique was already successfully used for GMO detection (Zimmermann et al., 1998; Brod et al., 2007a; Brod and Arisi 2007b; Jinxia et al., 2011). The specificity of the reaction is also increased given that two pairs of primers are used. However, the risk of contamination has to be taken into account. Indeed, to proceed with the second PCR, the tubes must be opened, and a fraction of the PCR product must be removed to use as substrate for the amplification with the second couple of primers (Picó, 2007).

### 4.1.3 Real-Time PCR

Real-time PCR, also called quantitative PCR (qPCR), consists of following the progress of amplification reaction from start to finish. This can be measured through the emission of fluorescence which is proportional to the quantity of amplicon produced (Higuchi et al., 1993).

This fluorescence can be provided by using an intercalating reagent, the most commonly used being SYBR® Green. SYBR Green shows a high affinity for double-stranded DNA; its fluorescence is largely enhanced once it is bound to the major groove of a DNA molecule (Higuchi et al., 1993, Figure 4.1). During the denaturation step, all SYBR Green

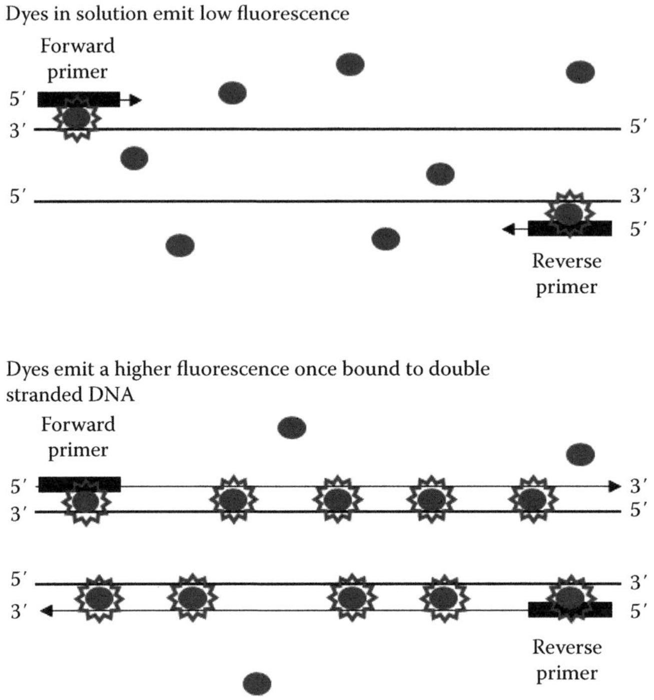


FIGURE 4.1 Real-time PCR using SYBR Green molecules. The number of integrated SYBR Green molecules will depend on the length of the amplicon. The fluorescent signal is reconstituted at each cycle.

molecules intercalated between the two strands are released and used again at the next amplification cycle. SYBR Green permits to rapidly transform an end-point PCR test into a real-time PCR test. However, because the molecules are intercalating between all double-stranded DNA, a non specific amplifications or primer-dimers will also generate a fluorescent signal. This can result in a lack of specificity, which is why in such a format checking, the melting temperature (Tm) of amplicons (Figures 4.2 and 4.3) is mandatory at the end of the amplification run. Tm is defined as the temperature at which half of the DNA strands (oligonucleotides acting as primers and probes or products of amplification) are hybridized or in a single-stranded state. Therefore, the thermocyclers for real-time PCR are able to perform a dissociation protocol at the end of the thermal profile used for the amplification of the target. The melting temperature is a parameter influenced by the GC per cent, length, and sequence of the amplicon.

A better specificity is generally obtained by real-time PCR using hybridization probes (Figure 4.4). The two most widely used hybridization probes for GMO detection are hydrolysis probes: the TaqMan® probe (Holland et al., 1991) and the MGB probe (Tyagi and Kramer, 1996; Afonina et al., 1997). TaqMan probes are oligonucleotides of about 25–35 bases, single-stranded, linear, and labeled with two fluorophores: one at the 5'end of the probe (reporter dye) and the other at the 3'end of the probe (quencher dye). As long as the probe remains intact and the reporter is close to the quencher, the fluorescence signal emitted by the reporter will be captured by the quencher and the device will not be able to detect a signal of that wavelength. The probe will hybridize to its complementary sequence between the primers after the denaturation phase. It cannot be elongated, as the

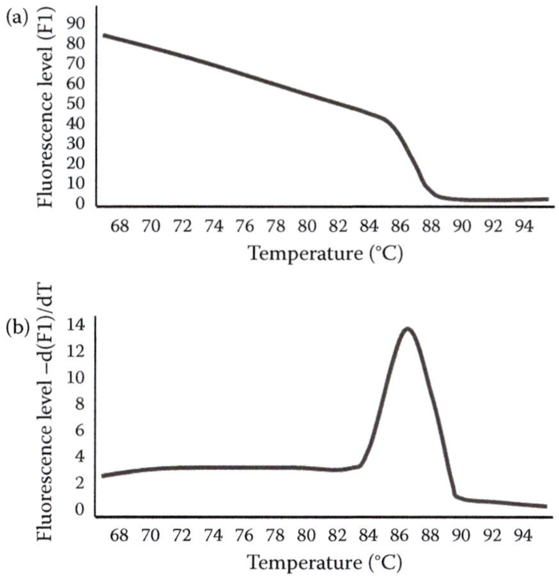


FIGURE 4.2 Example of dissociation curves observed in SYBR Green. (a) Dissociation curve for an amplicon. (b) First derivative of the dissociation curve.

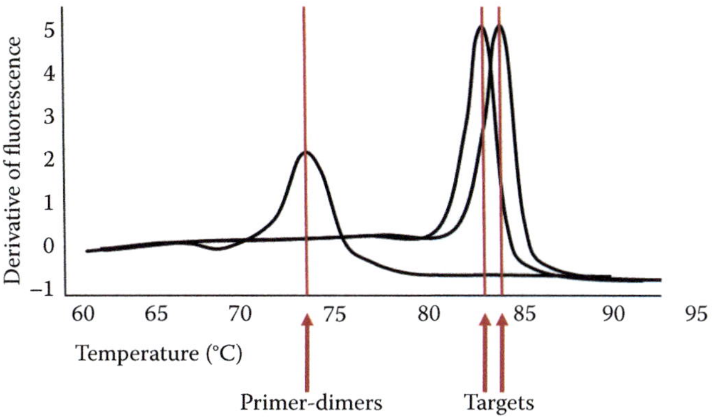


FIGURE 4.3 The first derivative of the dissociation curves allows to calculate the melting temperature (Tm) of the amplicon and to identify primer-dimers. Slight differences between Tm could indicate some variations in the sequence of the amplicons.

hydroxyl at its 3'end has been suppressed. During the elongation phase of the primer on the same strand, the *Taq* polymerase will reach the hybridized probe and through its exonuclease activity cleave the probe. The reporter fluorophore dissociates and moves away from the quencher, thus allowing the emitted fluorescence to be measured by the instrument. Double-dye probes cannot be reused once they are degraded by the exonuclease activity of the *Taq* polymerase. The fluorescence produced by the cleavage of new probes is added to the fluorescence acquired during previous cycles. Fluorescence is therefore an indirect measurement of the number of amplicons of the last cycle, but cumulatively it reflects the number of amplicons generated by all the previous cycles.

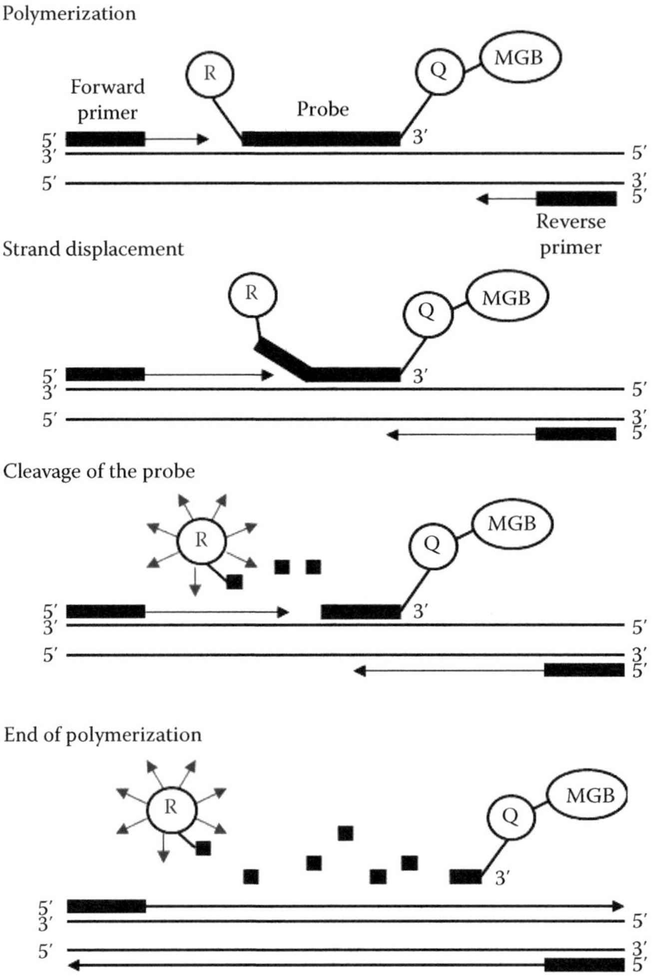


FIGURE 4.4 Real-time PCR using double dye probes. Dyes will be released at the end of each amplification cycle. The signal is cumulative. R: reporter dye, Q: quencher dye, MGB: Minor Groove binder used in MGB probes to reduce the length of the double dye probe.

MGB probes have a shorter length than the TaqMan probes but a similar melting temperature. This is possible because of the addition of a "minor groove binder" (MGB) linked to the oligonucleotide, which will permit a stronger hybridization and compensate for the decrease in length. MGB probes are particularly appreciated when the sequence between the two primers is short-sized or offers a reduced possibility of designing a probe with a sufficiently high melting temperature. The price of MGB probes is however higher than the price of TaqMan probes.

The advantages of hydrolysis probes compared with intercalating reagents are an increased specificity thanks to the presence of a third oligonucleotide complementary to the sequence used in the system, the absence of interfering fluorescence linked to primer-dimers, and the possibility of multiplexing by using reporter dyes emitting at distinguishable wavelengths.

#### *4.1.3.1 The Cq concept*

The Cq term (*quantitation Cycle*) corresponds to the number of amplification cycles necessary to reach a given level of fluorescence (Figure 4.5). Once this level is reached, the signal can be considered positive (provided there is an actual amplification). The Cq is inversely proportional to the quantity of fluorescence emitted and, therefore, to the initial number of copies. The lower the number of cycles required to produce a detectable fluorescence, the higher the initial copy number of the target into the reaction vial.

At the beginning of the PCR, given the small number of fragments present, the emitted fluorescence will not exceed the background noise. As the cycles progress, the number of fragments synthesized increases exponentially and the fluorescence becomes measurable.

The fluorescence threshold corresponds to a level of fluorescence located above the background noise but always remains in the exponential phase of the curve. Depending on the equipment used, the Cq may also be called Ct (Cycle threshold) or Cp (Crossing point-PCR-cycle).

By comparing the amplification curves reflecting the quantity of amplicons (through the emitted fluorescence) as a function of the number of cycles with those obtained from reference materials with certified GM levels or standards containing a known copy number of the target, it is possible to assign a quantitative value to the signals of samples. That is why real-time PCR is generally abbreviated as qPCR for quantitative PCR, but this is only valid if an appropriate calibration is included in the run of reactions.

Currently, qPCR is the reference technique for the detection and quantification of GMOs. Numerous methods validated by the European Reference Laboratory for GMO detection (JRC-IHCP, Ispra, Italy) are available in an online database (Bonfini et al., 2012). How to use PCR in the quantification of a GM content is detailed in a separate section of this chapter.

### 4.1.4 Multiplex PCR

Multiplex PCR is used to amplify several targets together in a same reaction. For instance, it can amplify simultaneously a target focused on the plant species and a

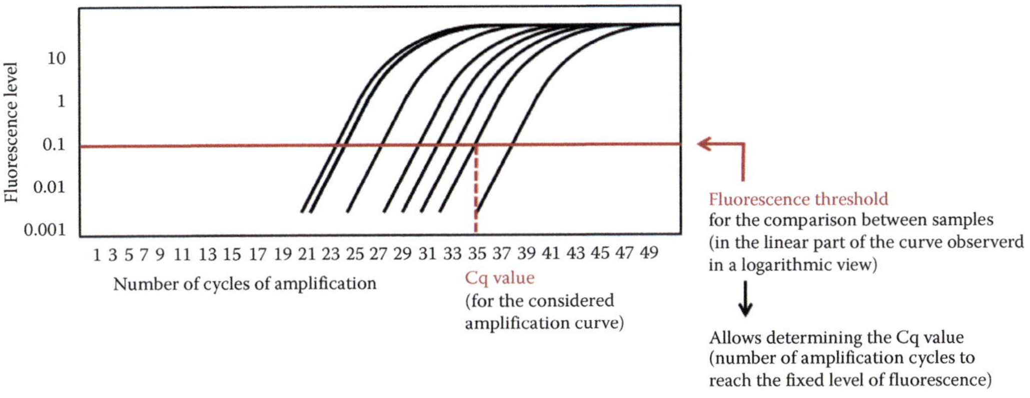


FIGURE 4.5 Real-time PCR: "Fluorescence threshold" (set at a given level) and "Cycle threshold" (Cq).

second one on the transgenic constructs. Another possibility is to amplify several screening targets or different identification targets in the same reaction. It is important to be aware of the competition between targets, which may decrease the sensitivity of the detection. That is why in the validation of such assays, the asymmetric limit of detection (Broeders et al., 2014) is a crucial concept. It examines the lower levels where a target is still detectable even if the other targets of the multiplex are present at higher levels. The multiplex PCR requires a more complex optimization in the concentrations of primers and probes introduced into the reaction mixture and the use of suitable buffers and polymerases (Pansiot et al., 2011). Targets amplified together in a multiplex assay can be differentiated on the basis of their respective amplicon sizes in the case of conventional PCR (James et al., 2003; García-Cañas, 2004; Hernández et al., 2005a; Cheah et al.,2011; Fidan and Arican, 2014) or by the use of probes labeled with dyes having different emission spectra in real-time PCR (Höhne et al., 2002; Huang et al., 2004; Waiblinger et al., 2008; Pansiot et al., 2011) or on the basis of the Tm of each signal (Van den Bulcke et al., 2010).

Multiplex PCR gained renewed interest due to the increasing number of transgenic constructs that require testing. By amplifying several targets within the same tube and the same reaction mixture, multiplex PCR should save considerable time. The trend is to amplify an increasing number of targets within the same reaction mixture (Heide et al., 2008; Shrestha et al., 2008; Bahrdt et al., 2010; Cottenet et al., 2013; Kim et al., 2014). However, the analysis of the results may be more complex in terms of attributing the positive result to the corresponding target as fluorescence emission peaks may overlap. Generally, no more than five targets can be amplified together due to the number of channels on the qPCR devices, although this number can be increased by using alternative approaches (Bahrdt et al., 2010; Spilsberg et al., 2015).

### 4.1.5 Digital PCR

In digital PCR, one assay involves a huge number of PCR because the reaction mix of the sample is divided into a high number of small volumes, called partitions (Table 4.1). This procedure can be carried out by distributing the reaction mixture in hundreds or thousands of chambers of a nanofluidic plate (digital chamber PCR or dcPCR) or via an emulsion leading to a very high number of droplets (digital droplet PCR or ddPCR). All the partitions are submitted to thermal cycling which will lead to an amplification reaction in the chambers or droplets where the targeted DNA is present. It is again an end-point approach because what is important is to determine the number of partitions wherein the PCR took place. It is this presence/absence of a reaction that is reflected in the name "digital."

A sample is usually tested at several levels of dilutions so that each partition contains, if possible, close to one copy of the target (some partitions could however contain several copies). By counting the partitions giving positive and negative results, the number of copies present in the used DNA extract may be accurately quantified. Since the distribution of DNA templates over the several partitions is assumed to follow a Poisson process, the analysis of results includes Poisson statistics.

Currently, this technique has elicited great interest because it allows the detection and quantification of low numbers of copies and appears less susceptible to the presence of inhibitors (Rački et al., 2014; Nixon et al., 2014; Iwobi et al. 2016). Many see it as a technique that will replace real-time PCR for the quantification of GMOs (Corbisier et al., 2010;

TABLE 4.1 Comparison of the Capacities of the Digital PCR Devices on the Market (January 2018)

| dPCR platform | BioMark HD | | QX100 QX200 | Quant Studio 12kflex | Quant Studio 3D dPCR | Constellation | | RainDrop | Naica |
|---|---|---|---|---|---|---|---|---|---|
| Company | Fluidigm | | BioRad | Life Technologies | | Formulatrix | | RainDance | Stilla |
| Mode of partition | chamber | | droplet | Chamber | | chamber | | droplet | droplet |
| Number of partitions per sample | 765 (Array 12) | 770 (Array 48) | 20000 | 64 (48 subarrays) | 20000 | 8000 | 36 000 | 10 000 000 | 30 000 |
| Number of partitions per array | 9180 | 36960 | / | 3072 | 20000 | 768 000 | 864 000 | / | / |
| Visualization of the amplification curve | Yes | | No | Yes | | No | | No | No |
| Volume per partition | 6.075nl | 0.85nl | 1 nl | 33 nl | 755 pl | 4.4 nl | 0.22 nl | 5 pl | 0.44 nl |
| Reaction volume ($\mu$l) | 8 | 4 | 20 | 5 | 14.5 | 2.2 | 1.8 | 50 | 25 |
| Number of fluorescent channels that can be analyzed | 4 | | 2 | 2 | | 5 | | 5 | 3 |

Sanders et al., 2011; Urquiza et al., 2014; Demeke et al., 2014; Köppel et al., 2015; Dobnik et al., 2015), but issues involving the possible number of partitions and the range of copy numbers that can be encountered in the DNA extracts still need to be addressed (Pecoraro et al., 2018). One of the difficulties associated with digital PCR is that it is not always straightforward to determine if a partition gives a positive or negative response. For instance, samples A01 and B01 in Figure 4.6 provide clear results while sample C01 is not as clear. It results in what is known as "rain" and the problem becomes defining what is positive and what is negative within the rain's partitions. In Figure 4.6, the vertical line for a defined fluorescence level separates positive from negative partitions.

The design of primers and probes follow the same rules governing real-time PCR (Degen et al., 2006; Pecoraro et al., 2018). However, primers and probe concentrations for digital PCR are usually higher than for real-time PCR and an optimization is necessary even if a transposition of the conditions for real-time PCR is feasible. Higher primer and probe concentrations increase the intensity of the end-point fluorescence signal and permit a better separation of the background noise from specific signals (Pecoraro et al., 2018). This observation is more visible with digital PCR devices that allow visualizing the amplification curves. Digital PCR is useful for the detection of GMOs at low levels (Fu et al., 2015; Iwobi et al., 2016), GMO quantification (Köppel et al., 2015; Dalmira et al., 2015; Dobnik et al., 2016; Gerdes et al., 2016) and the determination of copy numbers for sensitivity studies (Burns et al., 2010; Yu et al., 2014; Urquiza et al., 2014; Xu et al., 2016).

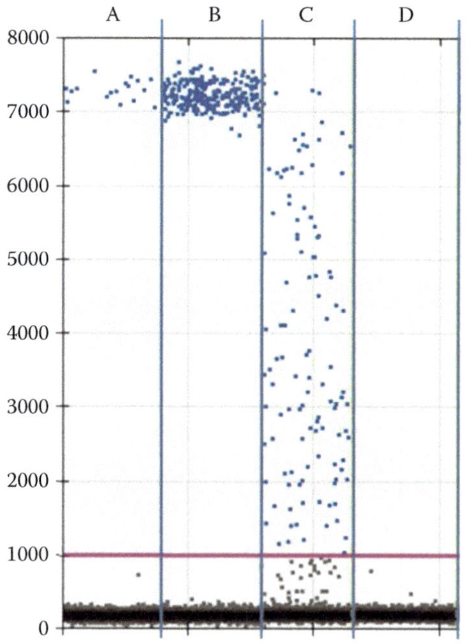


FIGURE 4.6 Example of digital PCR result. Abscissa: samples, Ordinate: fluorescence level. Droplets below the fixed decision level (in pink) are considered negative. Sample A contains less positive droplets than sample B. Sample C illustrates the rain effect linked to a nonoptimal amplification (poor efficiency of the amplification or inhibitory effect linked to the sample). Sample D is negative.

Currently, six different companies are proposing digital PCR devices and numerous publications are providing evidence of the growing interest in this technology for GMO detection and quantification (Morisset et al., 2013; Köppel et al., 2017; Dobnik et al., 2018). Even though the number of fluorescent markers that can be used together is sometimes more limited than in real-time PCR, multiplexing is nevertheless possible (Spilsberg et al., 2015; Dalmira et al., 2015).

The price of the instrument and of consumables can vary significantly from one company to another. Most digital PCR machines can use the same reagents (primers and probes) as qPCR, but specific consumables (chips, cartridges, gaskets, holders) are required for each instrument. Note that high quality tips for micropipettes are needed as plastic particles in suspension can obstruct nanofluidic capillaries.

## 4.2 GMO ANALYSIS AND TYPES OF TARGETS AMPLIFIED

Within the framework of GMO detection, different categories of targets can be highlighted: universal plant targets to check whether it is possible to amplify the extracted DNA; plant-specific targets used to identify the plant species involved; screening targets to detect the presence of GMOs; donor organism targets designed to ensure that the signal with the screening target is not due to the natural presence of the donor organism; and event-specific targets to identify the GMOs or for quantitation purposes (in combination with the plant-specific targets). These different targets are presented in more detail in the following sections.

### 4.2.1 Universal Plant Targets

The goal of universal plant primers is to highlight the DNA of any plant species. Their main use is to check if plant DNA is still amplifiable in a DNA extract. In the presence of a large quantity of inhibitors, no signal will be generated by PCR and no additional analyses can be performed without an additional purification or a dilution of the DNA extract to remove this inhibition. Highly processed products containing very few DNA or degraded DNA must also be tested with universal plant primers to avoid carrying out unnecessary PCR tests targeting specific plants or transgenic constructs. On the other hand, plant DNA can be highlighted with a multicopy plant target.

The search for DNA sequences that may be used for the development of universal plant primers must meet several criteria. The targeted segments must have conserved regions to allow the hybridization of consensus primers that will permit amplifying a maximum number of plant species. If the tests are developed for an application in real-time PCR with hybridization probes, a part of the internal region between the primers must also be conserved in order to allow the positioning of a hybridization probe. Ideally, the produced amplicons must not exceed a certain size (≤120 bp), so the methods are applicable to processed products (Debode et al., 2007).

Targets can have a high copy number (mitochondrial or chloroplast DNA, repeated sequences) or a low number of copies per cell. Having a larger number of copies per cell increases the possibilities of detection even in processed products. Conserved areas could, however, present some variability in different species. In this case, primers with degenerate bases or inosine bases, which can match indifferently with A, C, G, or T, should be used. Table 4.2 shows an overview of several universal plant primers given in the literature.

TABLE 4.2 Universal Targets for Plant DNA Detection

| Target | Target Origin | Method | Amplicon size (bp) | Reference |
|---|---|---|---|---|
| 18S | rDNA (high copy number) | real-time PCR | 137 | Chinese standard (SNT 1199-2010) |
| 5.8S | rDNA (high copy number) | real-time PCR | 77 | Debode et al., 2012 |
| 5.8S–18S | rDNA (high copy number) | PCR | +/–350 (according to plant species) | |
| rbcL | chloroplast DNA (high copy number) | real-time PCR | 106 | |

### 4.2.2 Targets Specific to Plant Species

The determination of plant species in agri-food products is an essential information for the detection, identification, and quantification of GMOs. The plant-specific PCR tests aim to detect the presence of genomic material of specific plant species (maize, soybean, rapeseed, etc.) by means of endogenous plant targets. What is interesting about these targets is that they also permit checking if the DNA of the searched plant species is still detectable. If it is no longer possible to detect the presence of the soybean *lectin* gene (endogenous target for soybean), searching for the presence of transgenic equivalents of this plant by screening or event-specific tests, would be fruitless. These endogenous targets should ideally be specific to the plant species (interaction with closely related species certainly at least those with commercial value has to be considered) without significant sequence differences between the different cultivars of the species. Moreover, if the target is to be used for quantification purposes it must also have a low copy number target of nuclear origin (Taverniers et al., 2013).

In a time-saving strategy, PCR tests for plant species may be directly associated with screening targets. Whatever the strategy adopted, the combination of results yielded by the plant species and the screening tests will allow a reduction and a more rigorous selection of the identification tests.

Many endogenous targets have been published to meet the needs of GMO analysis. Articles comparing different endogenous targets have also been published for a certain number of plant species. Indeed, when many detection methods are available, it is sometimes difficult to know which target to use. Two important criteria can however be considered: the fact that the target has been validated through an international study or via the JRC-IHCP (which in this case permits to qualify the method as reference method, at least in the EU) or the fact that it was included in a comparative study. A brief presentation of the existing systems for rice, sugar beet, bean, wheat, rapeseed, maize, potatoes, soybean, flax, cotton, chicory, tomato, sunflower, papaya, and pea is discussed below. Information from comparative studies was added when available.

#### *4.2.2.1 Sugar Beet* (***Beta vulgaris***)

Two methods for the detection of sugar beet are currently available. The first one is based on the *GS* (glutamine synthetase) gene and was validated by the EURL-GMFF in 2006 (Mazzara et al., 2006). While this target presents some specificities with *Brassica rapa*, the signals obtained differ significantly from those yielded by the sugar beet on the same amount of analyzed DNA. The second method (Chaouachi et al., 2013) is focused on the *ant* (adenylate transporter) gene and appears to have good specificity. The primers are associated to an MGB probe, which increases the analytical cost.

#### 4.2.2.2 Wheat (Triticum aestivum)

The endogenous targets *PKABA*1, *ALMT*1, *Acc*1, and *waxy*-D1 for wheat detection and quantification of transgenic wheat were compared by Huang et al. (2013). The authors' preference leaned toward the *waxy*-D1 gene in view of its specificity and the coherence of signals on the different varieties tested. The *ALMT*1 and *PKABA*1 genes show some single-nucleotide polymorphisms (SNPs) depending on the selected varieties that induce a decrease in the efficiency of amplification. Recent studies carried out by Ugo Marchesi compare *SS*II (Matsuoka et al., 2011; Kitta et al., 2014) and *waxy* (from Iida et al., 2005) targets. At this stage, both targets seem to have similar performance (Ugo Marchesi, 24th plenary session, Ispra, Italy, 22–23 September 2015). However, according to Jaroslava Ovesna (Crop Research Institute, Prague, Czech Republic), the *waxy* target would not be suitable for all wheat varieties (personal communication, ENGL meeting, 23 September 2015).

#### 4.2.2.3 Chicory (Cichorium intybus)

A target based on the fructan gene was developed by Debode et al. (2017a) for the detection of chicory and quantification of transgenic chicory.

#### 4.2.2.4 Rapeseed (Brassica napus)

Five endogenous targets for the detection of rapeseed and the quantification of transgenic rapeseed were compared by Wu et al. in 2010. These targets are *BnACCg*8 (acetyl-CoA carboxylase gene), *PEP* (phosphoenolpyruvate carboxylase), *Fat*A (oleoyl hydrolase gene), *HMG-I/Y* (high mobility-group protein I/Y gene), and *Cru*A (Cruciferin A). None was found to be completely specific to all rapeseed (*Brassica napus*) but the *BnACCg*8 target had the highest specificity (Hernández et al., 2001; Weng et al., 2005). However, this target appears to have a greater variability of sequence among the different cultivars (Wu et al., 2010). This specificity problem was also encountered with targets proposed in other publications as *PEP*, Zeitler et al., 2002; *Sgt* (*S*-glucose transferase), Block and Schwartz, 2003; *PhyA* (Phytochrome A), Beilstein et al., 2008 and Allnutt et al., 2013; and *ACoAC** (acetyl-CoA carboxylase) target, Debode et al., 2017a).

Rapeseed, the result of a cross between rape and cabbage, includes both genomes (Chalhoub et al., 2014). This can explain the difficulty of developing a specific target for rapeseed. It is also important to remember that the position of the primers and probes on the genes can have an important influence on the specificity and efficiency of the PCR test. This explains why methods designed for the same gene may have different performances (Wu et al., 2010).

Other targets for the detection of rapeseed have been validated at European level as the *hmg*A (Pan et al., 2007) or *cru*A (Mazzara et al., 2007a) targets. A new *fat*A target was proposed by Henderson et al. (2016). According to the authors, this target ensures a better specificity compared to the other existing systems, and is focused on Brassica *napus*, *juncea*, and *rapa*.

---

* *ACoAC* was used for *acetyl-CoA carboxylase but other abbreviations are found in the literature such* as *ACC*, *ACAC*, or *ACACA*.

#### 4.2.2.5 Cotton (*Gossypium hirsutum*)

Three targets have been validated by the EURL-GMFF for the detection of cotton and the quantification of transgenic cottons. Methods focused on the *adh*C, *acp*1, and *SAH7* genes have been validated in combination with methods for the quantification of transgenic events in cotton (Compendium of Reference Methods, 2010). A fourth method for the *SAD*1 gene was proposed by Yang et al. (2005a). There is currently no comparative study on the performance of these different targets.

#### 4.2.2.6 Bean (*Phaseolus vulgaris*)

An endogenous target for bean was developed by Dinon et al. (2012). The method is based on the *Pvsrp* (*Phaseolus vulgaris* stress related protein) gene and generates an amplicon of 183 bp. This size seems relatively high for real-time PCR. The test uses an MGB probe. The specificity was also tested on a limited number of species. A second target was proposed by Venturelli et al., 2014 and is focused on the *lectin* gene of bean.

#### 4.2.2.7 Flax (*Linum usitatissimum*)

A method developed by Genetic Id and spread by the EURL-GMFF (Charles-Delobel et al., 2009) during the FP967 flax crisis is based on the *SAD* gene as endogenous target. A second method developed by Debode et al. (2012) focuses on the *conlinin* gene. No comparison was made between the two targets.

#### 4.2.2.8 Maize (*Zea mays*)

Four targets (*Adh*1, *hmga*, *invertase*, and *zein*) were compared by Hernández et al., 2004. Five targets corresponding to two genes (three targets for *adh* and two targets for *hmg*) were compared by Paterno et al., 2009, and six targets corresponding to five genes (*SSII*B, *adh*, *hmg*, *zein*, and *invertase*) were identified by Scholdberg et al., 2009. These targets appear to have similar performances in terms of quantifying GM maize. The most widely used targets for the validation of quantitative methods for GM maize are the *SSII*b, *adh*1, and *hmga* genes. However, according to Broothaerts et al. (2008), the target *adh*1 is not recommended because, depending on the maize varieties, the targeted region can present a polymorphism at the level of the reverse primer that can result in a loss of efficiency.

#### 4.2.2.9 Papaya (*Carica papaya*)

Two genes are used to detect papaya, *papain* (Goda et al., 2001; Xu et al., 2008) and *chymopapain* (Guo et al., 2009). Only the target for *chymopapain* (Wei et al., 2013) was the subject of an interlaboratory study (conducted in various Chinese laboratories).

#### 4.2.2.10 Pea (*Pisum sativum*)

A pea target, based on the *lectin* gene, was developed by Debode et al. (2017b) and validated through an interlaboratory study at the European level. There are currently no genetically modified peas commercially available, but transgenic lines are under study (herbicide tolerance, protein content change). The interest behind such a target lies more in the fact that some structural elements used in transgenic constructs originate from the pea. Such a method is then necessary to avoid false positives and verify if the detection of a structural element used in transgenic constructs (e.g., terminator E9) is not linked to the presence of pea in food or feed products.

#### *4.2.2.11 Potato **(Solanum tuberosum)***

There is currently no comparative study for the different endogenous targets for potato detection. The method referenced by the JRC-IHCP (EURL, Savini et al., 2006) is focused on the UGPase gene but this target is present in high copy numbers (more than a thousand copies per haploid genome) that can vary largely from one variety to another one (Isabel Taverniers, ILVO, personal communication). This is a disadvantage for quantitation purposes.

A target was developed by Chaouachi et al. (2008a) and uses the differences within the *β-fructosidase* gene to propose PCR tests for the detection and differentiation between potato, tomato, and eggplant (all three are Solanaceae and amplified with the same primers). To maximize the differences, Chaouachi uses MGB probes. The gene for *patatin* is sometimes cited as a gene of interest for the selection of primers and probes; however, its multicopy character and the presence of pseudogenes (Stupar et al., 2006) make it an unsuitable candidate.

An alternative, the *StSL* (Light-inducible leaf-stem specific protein of *Solanum tuberosum*) gene has been proposed (Debode et al., 2018). The target was considered as single copy number per haploid genome (Eckes et al., 1986; Stockhaus et al., 1987) and no specificities with other plant species were observed. It should be noted that the primers alone give a positive signal with tomato and eggplant and that the probe is necessary to eliminate these specificities.

#### *4.2.2.12 Rice **(Oryza sativa)***

The genes *gos9*, *ppi-PPF* (ppi phosphofructokinase), *PLD* (phospholipase D), *RBE4* (starch branching enzyme), and *SPS* (sucrose phosphate synthase) were compared (Wang et al., 2011; Zhang et al., 2012) for detection and quantification of GM rice. The study conducted by Zhang et al. (2012) shows that both are equivalent for quantitative analyses. Nevertheless, the *PLD* and *ppi-PPF* targets present some specificity problems in the presence of sugar cane or sorghum DNA. The target focused on the *RBE4* gene is considered the most suitable target because it is specific to the plant species tested and no SNP were observed among the cultivars tested.

#### *4.2.2.13 Soybean **(Glycine max)***

Soybean can be detected through a large number of targets based on the *lectin* gene sequence (Kuribara et al., 2002; Moens et al., 2005; Mazzara et al., 2007b; Wang et al., 2011). These targets are specific to soybean and are adapted for GMO quantitation.

Surprisingly, few alternative genes are used. Three alternative targets were developed (glycinin, conglycinin, and hmg soya) in order to provide alternatives to the *lectin* gene (Debode et al., 2008).

#### *4.2.2.14 Tomato **(Solanum lycopersicum)***

The most referenced gene for the detection of tomato is *LAT52*. To this end, a target was developed (Yang et al., 2005b) and validated in an interlaboratory study (Yang et al., 2008). Two other methods are referenced: a method based on the *β-fructosidase* gene (Chaouachi et al., 2008a) and a method based on the *apx* gene (Mason et al., 2002). The LAT52 target is currently recommended by the EURL-GMFF.

#### *4.2.2.15 Sunflower **(Helianthus annuus)***

To our knowledge, the only existing target for the detection of the sunflower was developed by Hernández et al. (2005b), who amplified a 60 bp amplicon of the *helianthin* gene.

Endogenous targets are proposed for the 15-plant species listed above as they can be genetically modified and the probability of finding them in food and feed products is large. These plants were therefore considered a priority. Currently, (January 2018), test fields exist for 71 other plant species (www.GMO-Compass.org) having different traits such as herbicide tolerance; protection against insect; resistance to bacterial, viral, or fungal diseases; compositional modification; or production of molecules for pharmaceutical purposes. Depending on the plant considered, the arrival of these plants on the market can be planned in the short, medium, or long term. The identification of endogenous targets specific to all plant species is therefore still far from being fully realized.

### 4.2.3 Screening Targets

The screening targets are focused on elements commonly observed in transgenic constructs such as promoters, terminators, or gene coding sequences (Figure 4.7). These elements are not specific to a defined transgenic line; in fact, what we intend to exploit is their common characteristics.

Construct-specific targets are focused on junctions between elements (Figure 4.7) and can also be considered as screening targets if the association between elements is frequently met. The system can be considered safer to detect an artificial construct as the detection of a junction between two elements of distinct origins has less chance of occurring naturally. Now, this kind of association could be present in different GM constructs or the same construct could be introduced in different plants, and so even if this system permits orientating the identification of GM lines, it is insufficient for the identification of a transgenic event. Different construct-specific targets have already been developed for screening purposes, namely: p35S-pat (real-time PCR, Anonymous, 2006); p35S-bar (real-time PCR, Bayer CropScience, 2006); LY-SAMS (real-time PCR, Bahrdt et al., 2010); p35S-nptII (real-time PCR, Reiting et al., 2010); pNOS-nptII (real-time PCR, Reiting et al., 2010); gat-tpinII (SYBRGreen, Broeders et al., 2015; and real-time

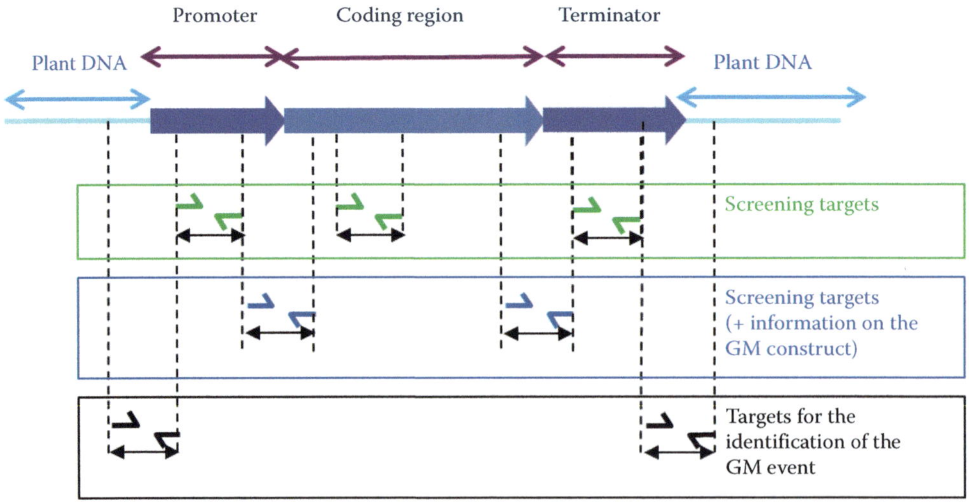


FIGURE 4.7 Schematic illustration of the different types of targets used for GMO detection.

PCR with double dye probes, Prins et al., 2017). However, these are generally less used than screening targets based on promoters, terminators, and gene coding sequences.

Screening is the first step in determining the presence or absence of GMOs. If the result is positive, additional analyses must be performed to check for the potential presence of GM material. The screening should be as broad as possible to cover the different GMOs encountered on the market.

#### *4.2.3.1 Screening Focused on Promoters and Terminators*

Toward the end of 2004, it was possible to detect most of the transgenic constructs with the p35S promoter and the tNOS terminator targets. The sequence of the p35S originates from the cauliflower mosaic virus (CaMV) and the sequence of the tNOS from *Agrobacterium tumefaciens*. Since then, the number and diversity of transgenic constructs has increased and the coverage rate of these two targets in combination is no longer sufficient. If we look at the GMO listed in the GMOseek Matrix (Block et al., 2013), a screening with both the p35S and tNOS targets can detect 53 per cent of the GM events (the stacked events are not considered in this evaluation).

Numerous PCR tests for p35S and tNOS were developed successfully both for classical PCR (Vollenhofer et al., 1999; Wolf et al., 2000; Matsuoka et al., 2002; Mattarucchi et al., 2005) and real-time PCR (Mattarucchi et al., 2005; Höhne et al., 2002; Zeitler et al., 2002; Alary et al., 2002; Kuribara et al., 2002; Kimio et al., 2005; Fernandez et al., 2005; Reiting et al., 2007).

The fact that an increasing number of new constructions are completely free of these elements has made it necessary to implement new screening methods.

Checked on the GMOseek database, the promoters and terminators having an occurrence ≥2 per cent were highlighted (Figure 4.8).

The most widely used promoters after p35S are the Rice Actin promoter from rice, the Ubiquitin promoter from maize, the promoter of the Figwort Mosaic Virus (pFMV), the promoter of Nopaline synthase from *Agrobacterium tumefaciens*, the SSuAra promoter from Arabidopsis thaliana, the TA29 promoter from tobacco, and the manopine synthase

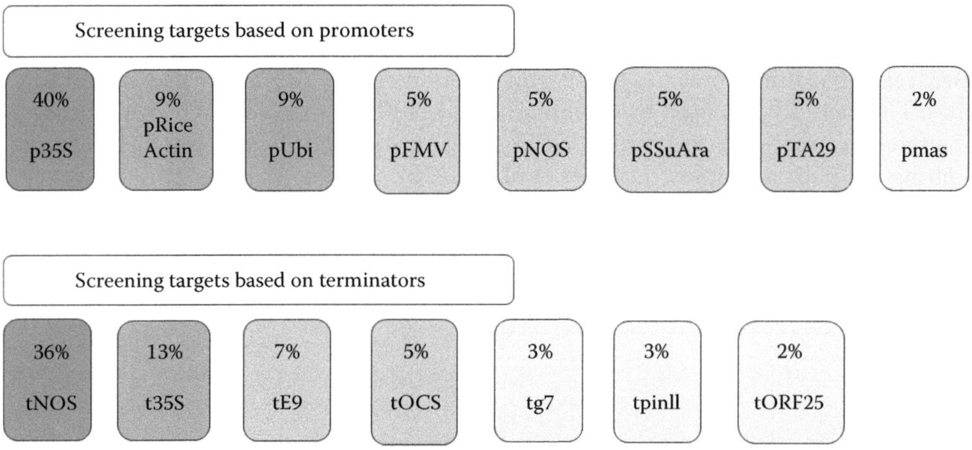


FIGURE 4.8 Most used promoters and terminators in GM constructs (stacked events excluded) as calculated from the GM events listed in the GMOseek database (Block et al., 2013).

promoter from *Agrobacterium tumefaciens*. The literature reports real-time PCR tests for pRice actin (Debode et al., 2013), pUbi (Babekova et al., 2008; Debode et al., 2013), pFMV (Dörries et al., 2010; Debode et al., 2013), pNOS (Pansiot et al., 2011; Debode et al., 2013), pSSuAra (Debode et al., 2013), and pTA29 (Debode et al., 2013).

Concerning the terminators, the ones most used in GM constructs after the tNOS are the terminator 35S of the CaMV, the E9 terminator from pea, the octopine synthase terminator, and g7 terminator from *Agrobacterium tumefaciens*, the protease inhibitor II terminator from potato, and the ORF25 terminator from *Agrobacterium tumefaciens*. Real-time PCR tests were already proposed for the t35S (Pansiot et al., 2011; Debode et al., 2013), tE9 (Debode et al., 2017b), tOCS (Debode et al., 2013), tg7 (Debode et al., 2013), and tpinII (Debode et al., 2018).

#### *4.2.3.2 Screening Focused on Gene Coding Sequences*

New gene coding sequences were introduced in GM constructs to develop a new trait. The most used genes in GM constructs are those enabling transformant selection, tolerance to herbicides or protection against insects. Considering their coverage rate (Figure 4.9), they also are excellent screening elements and complete the panel of screening elements based on promoters and terminators.

Marker genes like neomycin phosphotransferase II (*npt*II), betalactamase (*bla*), or beta-D-glucuronidase gene (also called *gus*, *gus*A, or *uid*A) are unfit for detection because the *Taq* polymerase used in PCR is itself a recombinant structure, and therefore, traces of DNA of these genes can be present in the master mix. Some methods were, however, developed in classical PCR for *npt*II (Lipp et al., 1999; ISO 21569, 2005) and *bla* (Holst-Jensen et al., 2003), and in classical and real-time PCR for *gus* (Randhawa et al., 2010; Debode et al., 2017a).

The most widely used methods for GMO screening based on gene coding sequences are focused on *pat*, *bar*, and *cp4-EPSPS*.

The *bar* gene of *Streptomyces hygroscopicus* codes for the phosphinothricin acetyltransferase and confers tolerance to glufosinate, an organophosphorus compound present in many nonselective systemic herbicides. Many primers were proposed for the detection of the *bar* gene by classical PCR (Ehlers et al., 1997; Matsuoka et al., 2002; James et al., 2003, Demeke et al., 2008; Guo et al. 2011; Kim et al., 2013). Few methods are available for real-time PCR (Barbau-Piednoir et al., 2014) for monitoring amplification with SYBRGreen, (Grohmann et al., 2009 and Debode et al., 2017a), to use with TaqMan probes. The method proposed by Grohmann et al. 2009 is an excellent method being part of the reference methods recommended by the JRC-IHCP. It is also the method used in validating the pat/bar duplex (Debode et al., 2017b).

The *pat* gene has a similar function to the *bar* gene. It allows tolerance to herbicides containing glufosinate as an active ingredient. However, it originates from *Streptomyces*

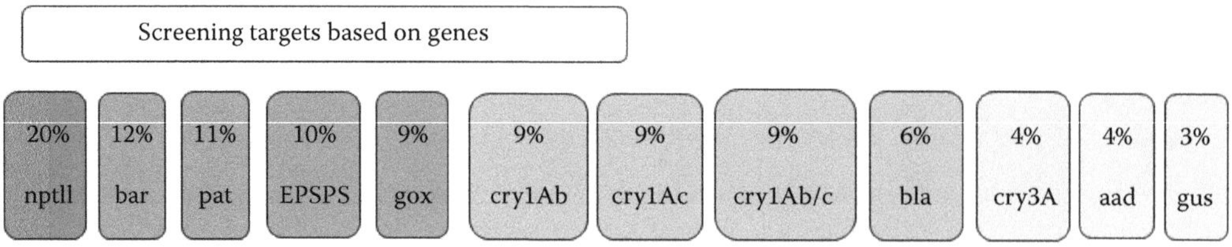


FIGURE 4.9 Most used genes in GM constructs (stacked events excluded) as calculated from the GM events listed in the GMOseek database (Block et al., 2013).

*viridochromogenes*, a different organism. Primers were already proposed for classical PCR by Matsuoka et al. (2002), Permingeat et al. (2002), and Lu et al. (2010). Due to variations in the sequence of the *pat* gene in the different GM plants, the primers so far developed are not always able to detect different variants of the *pat* gene (Lu et al., 2010). Ideally, the specificity should be verified experimentally. A target for the detection of the *pat* by real-time PCR was proposed by Weighardt et al. (2004) but is specific to the T25 maize. A target allowing a better coverage was developed by Zeitler et al. (2002) and validated in a pat/bar duplex (Debode et al., 2013).

The *EPSPS* gene introduced in GM plants confers tolerance to glyphosate through a better distinction between its natural substrate (phosphoenolpyruvate or PEP) and glyphosate. This naturally modified *EPSPS* gene comes from a defined strain of *Agrobacterium tumefaciens*. Its sequence was adapted in terms of codon use before introduction into plants, but homologies remain with the natural sequence. There is variability in the *EPSPS* sequence of genes introduced into GM plants. This causes difficulties for the development of primers and probes. In some genetically modified plants, the integration of a truncated version of the gene is clearly announced (e.g., GA21 maize with the introduction of the *mEPSPS* gene with "m" for "modified"), whereas for other GM plants, a little information is known.

Many targets relative to the *EPSPS* already exist. However, existing primers seem all focused on the junction between CTP2-*EPSPS* and *CTP4-EPSPS*. When the CTP2-*EPSPS* region is targeted, GM plants having the CTP4-*EPSPS* sequence, such as Roundup Ready soybean (GTS 40-3-2), will not be detected. Indeed, the sequences of the "chloroplast transit peptide" of *Petunia* (CTP4) and *Arabidopsis* (CTP2) present some differences. Among the existing PCR tests, some were proposed for a use in classical PCR (Vaïtilingom et al., 1999; Demeke et al., 2002; Matsuoka et al., 2002; Wang et al., 2011; Kim et al., 2013) or in real-time PCR (Zhang et al., 2003; Kuribara et al., 2002; Corbisier et al., 2005, Wang et al., 2011; Köppel et al., 2014). Most of these targets are specific to some particular GM events. The published primers that currently offer the best coverage are those of Grohmann et al., 2009 (88 bp). They are able to detect the GT73 rapeseed; the MON1445 cotton; the MON809, NK603, and MON88017; MON89788 soybean; and the GTSB77 and H7-1 sugar beet (data experimentally checked). However, the real-time PCR test of Grohmann et al. is based on the CTP2-*EPSPS* junction and is thus not able to detect the Roundup Ready soya (CTP4-*EPSPS*). Real-time PCR tests focusing exclusively on the *EPSPS* gene as target were proposed by Debode et al. (2017a).

The *gox* gene is less interesting for screening purposes as it is mainly integrated in the same constructions than the *EPSPS* gene. The *gox* gene codes for a modified version of the glyphosate oxidase, a bacterial enzyme derived from *Ochrobactrum anthropi* that inactivates the herbicidal effect of glyphosate through oxidation. Tests were developed in classical PCR (Matsuoka et al., 2002) and real-time PCR (Weng et al., 2005; Debode et al. 2017a).

The *cry* genes are part of a widely used gene family in transgenic constructs developed to provide protection against insects. More than 200 *cry* toxins are referenced (Crickmore et al., 1998) as insecticidal proteins produced by *Bacillus thuringiensis* (Bt), a soil bacterium. The crystals synthesized by the bacteria are made up of protoxins, which, when ingested by the insect, are transformed into active toxic polypeptides. Poisoning occurs very quickly in the form of extensive damage to the intestine and paralysis of the digestive tract, causing feeding to stop immediately. In the case of genetically modified plants, the gene sequence has been truncated to produce toxins readily available in their active form.

Depending on the type of *cry* proteins, their actions may be more oriented toward lepidopterans, dipterans, or coleopterans (Tohidfar and Khosravi, 2015). Therefore, it is not unusual to find transgenic constructs that include several *cry* genes that provide wider spectrum of action against insects.

The genes introduced in the transgenic constructs are generally modified versions of the original sequences, the so-called "truncated" versions showing the greatest level of change. To increase the spectrum of action against insects, some genes assemble parts originating from various genes (e.g., the fusion gene *cry*1Ab/Ac, where a first part of its sequence is derived from the *cry*1Ab gene and the second part from a portion of the *cry*1Ac gene). The homologies between the different *cry* genes are highly variable (Maciel et al., 2014), ranging from 19 to 90 per cent (Höfte et al., 1989). For this reason, a single target cannot be used to detect all the cry genes introduced in GM constructs.

The most common *cry* genes are *cry*1Ab and *cry*1Ac. Initially, the PCR assays proposed for the detection of *cry*1Ab focused were only able to detect the *cry*1Ab of the Bt176 maize (Ehlers et al., 1997; Vollenhofer et al., 1999; Vaïtilingom et al., 1999; Germini et al., 2004). Their detection potential was later expanded to Bt11 and MON810 maize (Matsuoka et al., 2002; Permingeat et al., 2002). Proposals for PCR assays were also formulated for *cry*1Ac and *cry*1F (Choi et al., 2011, run tests on cotton 281 x 3006 exclusively), *Cry*9C (Windels et al., 2003, run tests on just corn CBH-351), and *cry*2Ab (Kamle et al., 2011, on MON15985 cotton, Bt rice, Bt okra—*Hibiscus esculentus*, Bt maize, Bt eggplant, Bt potato, and Bt tomato).

Methods for real-time PCR detection were developed for *cry*1A105 (Dinon et al., 2011), *cry*2Ab2 (Dinon et al., 2011), the fusion gene *cry*1Ab/Ac (Guan et al., 2011) for the detection of Bt cotton (although the target was only tested on plasmid DNA, which indicates a rather theoretical potential of use) and *cry*3A (Rho et al., 2004) able to detect SEMT15-15, SPBT02-5, and RBMT21-350 potato. However, most of the available targets are based on classical PCR.

Despite the urgent need to perform effective monitoring of Asian imported rice (Reiting et al., 2013), targets for the simultaneous detection by real-time PCR of the most frequent *cry* genes, *cry*1Ab and *cry*1Ac, have not been identified for years. A method was developed using SYBRGreen (Barbau-Piednoir et al., 2012), a second method using TaqMan probes was validated in 2015 (Grohmann et al., 2015), and a third method was proposed by Debode et al. (2017c).

Most of the tests proposed share similar amplification conditions (or eventually would require some adaptations) and could be used on a same PCR plate. This methodology is also relevant because, after proposing ready-to-use plates containing identification tests for all the GMOs authorized in Europe (pre-spotted plates, Querci et al., 2008), the EURL -GMFF aims to develop a similar approach focused on screening tests (Rosa et al., 2016) capable of dealing with the arrival of new GMOs into the market.

#### *4.2.3.3 Screening and Donor Organisms*

Signals obtained with a screening target used for GMO detection may originate from the donor organism of the targeted element if the organism, or the biological entity, is present in the product to be analyzed. The aim of targets highlighting the presence of donor organisms is to confirm or invalidate the hypothesis of the presence of GMOs after a positive screening.

If we look at the origin of promoters used in transgenic constructs, 61 per cent come from plants, 22 per cent from bacteria (or hybrids assimilated to bacteria), and 17 per cent from viruses. For their part, 50 per cent of terminators have a vegetable origin, 43 per cent a bacterial origin, and 7 per cent a viral origin. These values are based on the 55 promoters and 31 terminators listed in the GMOseek database (Block et al., 2013).

*Agrobacterium tumefaciens* is the donor organism of the pNOS and pmas promoters, and of the tNOS, tOCS, tg7 and tORF25 terminators. The natural presence of *Agrobacterium tumefaciens* had already been observed in rapeseed (Spiridonova et al., 2009; Weller et al., 2002). Qualitative detection tests had been proposed by Sachadyn and Kur (1997) and Kuznetsov (Spiridonova et al., 2009). The *Agrobacterium* group is polyphyletic, which implies that the similarities within this taxon are not necessarily inherited from a common ancestor. Based on biochemical, phenotypic, and more recently on sequence comparisons, the taxonomic classification between *Agrobacterium* and *Rhizobium* is confusing. Therefore, several targets could be needed to detect the presence of *Agrobacterium tumefaciens* (Debode et al., 2017a).

The CaMV is the most widely used viral donor organism as it has contributed to two major structural elements: p35S and t35S. CaMV may contaminate several plant species, especially Brassicaceae. A number of tests were developed in an attempt to perform a more specific detection of this virus (Wolf et al., 2000; Cankar et al., 2008; Chaouachi et al., 2008b; Debode et al., 2017a).

In terms of donor organisms from vegetal origin, we can cite rice for pRice Actin, maize for pUbi, *Arabidopsis thaliana* for pSSuAra, tobacco for pTA29, pea for tE9, potato for tpinII, and soybean for t7S. In this case, the detection methods are identical to the endogenous targets used for the detection of plant species.

#### *4.2.3.4 Event-Specific Targets*

When the primers used to amplify a DNA segment are located on either side of the junction between the DNA of the plant and the GM construct, we talk about event-specific methods (Figure 4.7). Only this type of target will allow a univocal identification of the transgenic lines.

When a GMO is developed, many transformants are produced. They contain the same construct but integrated at different locations in the plant genome. Each of these transformants are called "events." Only one will be chosen for approval and commercialization. The junctions between the plant genome and the GM construct will be quite characteristic of the GM event.

The GMOMETHODS database (http://gmo-crl.jrc.ec.europa.eu/gmomethods) provides 79 (January 2018) recommended event-specific methods for the identification of GMOs. Additionally, the GMDD (http://gmdd.shgmo.org/index/search) lists existing event-specific methods.

## 4.3 GMO QUANTIFICATION

For the quantification of GMOs, event-specific targets and endogenous targets are needed. Quantification is done by relating the content of an event-specific target to an endogenous target. Several approaches can be used to determine the GMO content, depending not only on how the GMO percentage was calculated but also on the type of calibrators used.

### 4.3.1 Quantification by qPCR

Quantification by real-time PCR is possible by comparing values obtained in the respective standard curves for transgenic and specific targets. Several strategies are available for this procedure.

#### *4.3.1.1 Delta Cq Method*

The amplification curves obtained from a transgenic and an endogenous target are used to determine a Cycle threshold (Ct) or a Quantitative cycle (Cq) value for each target. The Cq is the cycle number required to reach a defined amount of fluorescence within the range of the exponential amplification phase. The difference between both Cqs, i.e., the ones yielded by the transgenic and specific targets, respectively, gives a parameter called ΔCq (Figure 4.10), which can be linearly correlated to the logarithm of the GMO content (Vaïtilingom et al., 1999). Quantification is possible once a calibration curve is made with DNA extracts obtained out of the reference material with certified GMO amounts expressed in mass fractions (Figure 4.10).

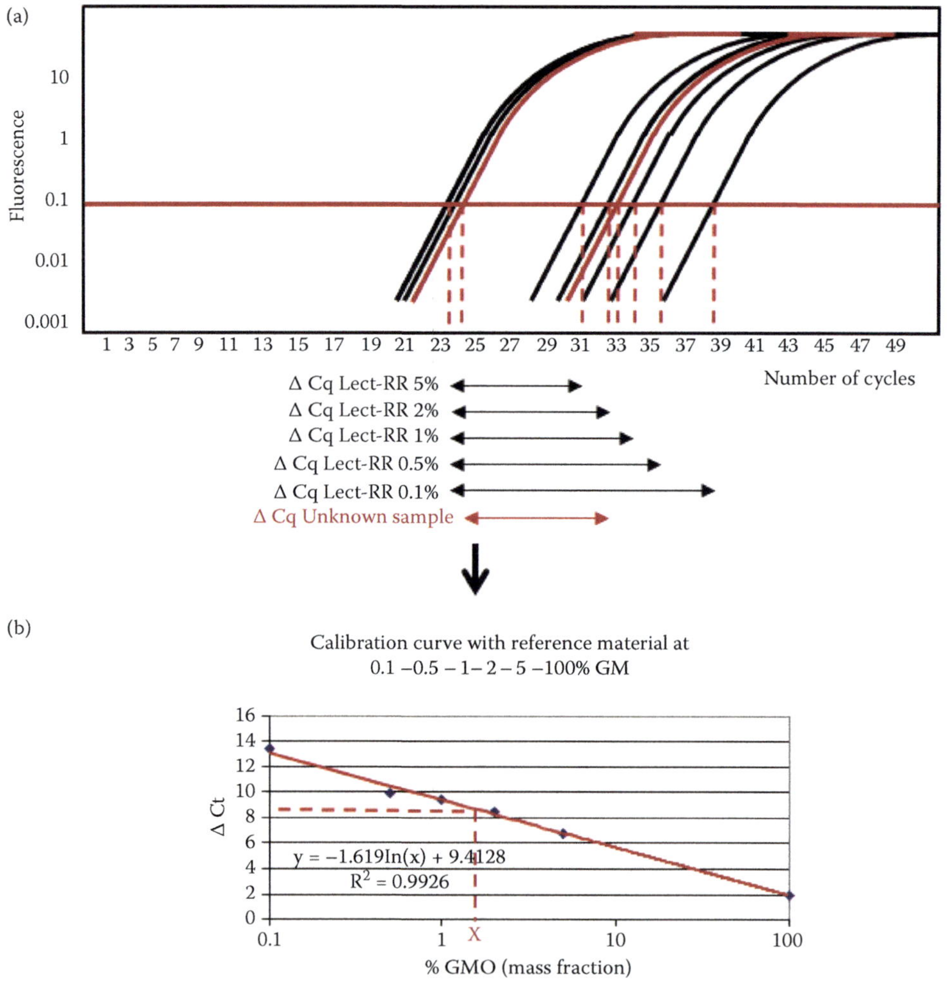


FIGURE 4.10 (a) Visualization of the ΔCq values between the Cq values for the lectin target (endogenous target for soybean detection) and the transgenic target on reference flours of Roundup Ready soybean at 5, 2, 1, 0.5, and 0.1 per cent. (b) Example of calibration curve for GM quantification base on the ΔCq method. The ΔCq value obtained for a sample will give the GM per cent once introduced in the calibration curve. Amplification curves represented in red originate from the sample to be quantified.

The establishment of such a calibration curve requires the ability to obtain reference material at different mass fractions. In this method, only one calibration curve is needed. An advantage of this method is being able to automatically proceed to a correction if one of the targets used is present more than once per haploid genome. This method can provide a quantification in mass fraction directly which, however, could involve some bias depending on the suitability of the reference material used for the sample to be analyzed (see Section 4.3.4)

### 4.3.1.2 Dilutions of Calibrants

In this second method, calibration curves are established for each target: one for the endogenous target and one for the transgenic target. In each case, this is done by relating the logarithm of the copy number of the target to the Cq value (Figure 4.11). The Cq values obtained for both targets of the unknown samples are introduced in the respective calibration curves. By dividing, the copy number of the event-specific target thus obtained by that of the endogenous target, and multiplying this number by 100, we can define the GM percentage which is expressed as a percentage of the event-specific target per haploid genome equivalent. The calibration curves can be obtained from the dilution of a DNA extracted from a certified reference material or from plasmid DNA (Burns et al., 2006; Taverniers et al., 2004), but in most cases, what is considered is the copy number of the target.

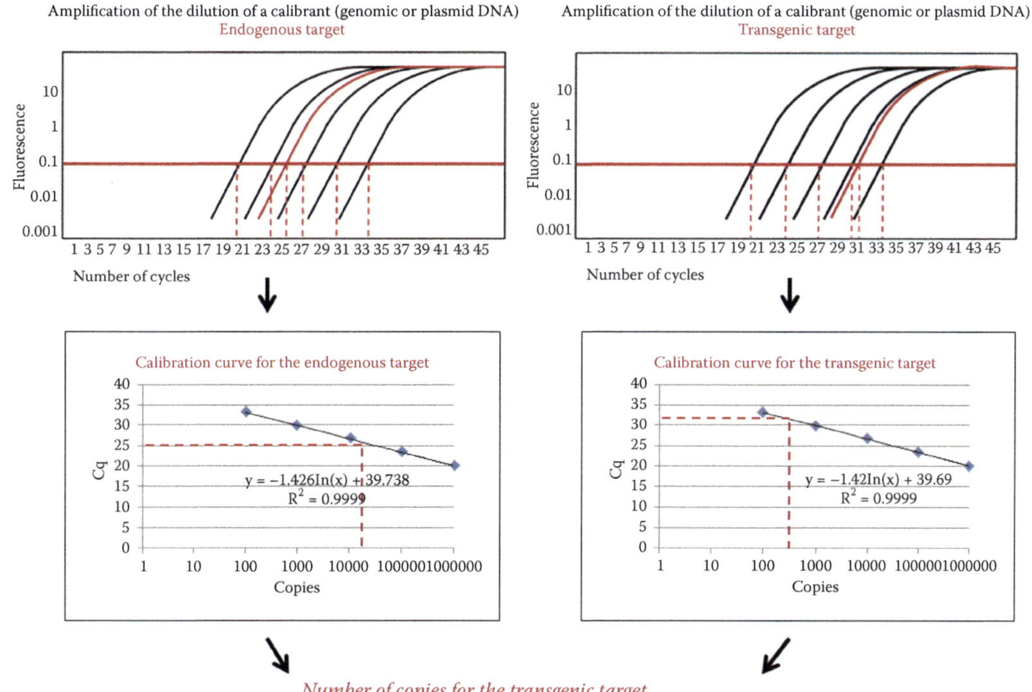


$$\left(\frac{\textit{Number of copies for the transgenic target}}{\textit{Number of copies for the endogenous target}}\right) \times 100 = \text{GM \%}$$

FIGURE 4.11 GMO quantification with calibrations curves obtained from the dilutions of two standards: one for the endogenous target and one for the transgenic target. Amplification curves in red correspond to the sample being quantified.

The precise determination of the copy number of the DNA that needs to be diluted for building the calibration curves is not always necessary as we proceed to a relative quantification. If care is taken to set up both calibration curves in such a way that the ratio of targets is consistent with the mass fraction of the certified reference material, then one can safely ignore the number of copies per haploid genome of the endogenous target. When plasmid DNA is used as calibrator, the recommendation is that the plasmid contains both the transgenic and the endogenous targets as this will reduce the risk of errors since the estimation of the plasmid copy number will be identical for both the targets and subsequent dilutions (Kuribara et al., 2002; Mattarucchi et al., 2005; Burns et al., 2006; Debode et al., 2010). A condition for this approach is that the endogenous and transgenic targets must have similar efficiencies both in the reference material and in the samples under investigation (Cankar et al., 2005; Demeke and Jenkins, 2010; Caprioara-Buda et al., 2012). This being the case, the use of linearized plasmids is also important (Mattarucchi et al., 2005).

If care is taken to set up the calibration curves of the two targets in a way such that the ratio between figures is consistent with the mass fraction of the certified reference material from which the genomic DNA is obtained, then the fact that one of the targets may be present more than once per haploid genome would not pose a potential problem. On the other hand, if one of the targets is present more than once per haploid genome equivalent and the calibration curves are set up in copy numbers, for instance, with plasmids, then a simple ratio of the targets might not reflect the actual quantity. Other parameters linked to the zygosity and the ploidy should also be considered. A more in-depth discussion about this is provided in a separate section of this chapter. The advantage of the calibration curves obtained from genomic DNA is that they directly integrate an eventual correction factor if one of the targets is present several times per haploid genome (if expressed in mass fraction and estimated with a reference material comparable to the sample being analyzed). This is not the case for plasmid DNA where an eventual correction factor must be defined and applied if necessary (Zhang et al., 2014; Corbisier et al., 2017). However, genomic DNA is not available for all the GM events. The expression "unit" will depend on the way it is used for relative quantification and on the calibrators selected. With the ΔCq method, using several independent calibrators, the results of analysis will directly give the GM percentage expressed in mass fraction. When a diluted calibrator is used, results will be expressed in mass fraction if a genomic DNA is used (as the reference material is expressed in mass percentage) and in copy number when a diluted plasmid is used. The characteristics of the reference material used for quantification must also be indicated next to the evaluated GM percentage.

### 4.3.2 Quantification by Digital PCR

Nowadays, digital PCR is increasingly being used for GMO quantification. Much like real-time PCR, the copy number of a transgenic target is compared to the copy number of an endogenous target. The positive and negative signals for each partition are counted by fluorescence measurement. Considering that the rationale for counting is linked to an endpoint detection (results are considered either positive or negative), a decrease of efficiency or the presence of PCR inhibitors will have less of an impact on the results, leading to a higher precision and trueness. In contrast to quantification by real-time PCR, the DNA can be quantified without resorting to standard curves at every run. This is a great advantage if we take into account the increasing number of authorized and un-authorized

GM events on the market and the limited number of reference materials needed for quantification purposes. However, this does not exclude checking the equipment with reference material to prevent important biases. Direct quantification procedures will also allow minimizing the differences in PCR efficiencies that could be linked to the difference of matrix effect between calibrants and samples.

The main problem of quantification by digital PCR is still the range that can be covered with the number of partitions generated by most state-of-the-art digital PCR devices. So, for a sample at 0.1 per cent GM, we have 1000 times less transgenic than endogenous targets. This implies that the quantification of low copy numbers can be affected and that not all the digital PCR devices are appropriate for GMO quantification. The procedure devised to test several dilutions must guarantee that all targets will be tested in an acceptable range of copy number. Ideally, to obtain the greatest achievable precision and optimize quantification, the mean amount of target per partition should approach 1.6 (Majumdar et al., 2015). This is achievable for the endogenous target but maybe more tricky for the transgenic one in case of a low GMO presence. Several laboratories have successfully tested the potential of cdPCR (Corbisier et al., 2010; Urquiza et al., 2014) and ddPCR (Dobnik et al., 2016; Gerdes et al., 2016; Iwobi et al., 2016; Košir et al., 2017; Köppel et al., 2017) for GMO quantification. As for real-time PCR, multiplexing in digital PCR is possible but more complex (Gerdes et al., 2016), and at low GM content, the precision and trueness are affected if the endogenous and transgenic targets are tested in the same partition.

The Unit of measurement by digital PCR is necessarily expressed in copy number and does not provide an estimate of the amount of GM in mass fraction. The conversion of copy number ratio into mass fraction can be done via one single conversion factor (CF) per event. A recent guideline explains how to report traceable and comparable results expressing GM content in accordance with EU legislation (Corbisier et al., 2017).

### 4.3.3 Considerations on the Targets Used for Quantification

To carry out quantification by PCR reliably, it is advised to follow the MIQE (Bustin et al., 2009) or digital MIQE (Huggett et al., 2013) guidelines. Next to this, we would like to insist on two other important aspects. When the matrix on which the quantification has to be done contains highly degraded DNA, it is important that the transgenic target and the endogenous one have similar sizes in order to avoid a bias in the calculated ratio (Debode et al., 2007). As a rule of thumb try always to get rather short targets as in real-time PCR their efficiency is better (Debode et al., 2017d).

### 4.3.4 Considerations on the Unit of Measurement

When quantifying a GMO content in a matrix this one may either be expressed in terms of copy number of the transgenic target expressed in percentage of a haploid genome equivalent or in percentage of mass fraction. A third possibility exists for seeds by expressing the results in percentage of seeds. The most natural unit for PCR is in copy number as this is basically the parameter that is measured in real-time PCR or in digital PCR. Therefore, to obtain other units, a conversion maybe required. Generally, the GMO content for soybean kernels will be identical if expressed in mass fraction or in copy number. In corn, transgenic plants are most generally heterozygote for the transgenic trait. This means that if leaf material of such transgenic plants is collected and measured for its GMO content by PCR it would reach a result in copy number of 50 per cent. Such a result arises from the zygosity of the material. In some instances, next to the zygosity, the ploïdy of the material will also affect the result. For instance in maize kernels, the endosperm is triploid with one paternal haploid genome and two maternal ones. This has consequences on the result expressed in copy number because according to the variety and the paternal or maternal origin of the transgenic trait in the heterozygote, the mean content will respectively be close to 40 per cent or 60 per cent (Trifa and Zhang, 2004). For enforcement purposes, the mass fraction unit is the one to be considered. It is advised to apply the CF that one will derive from the use of a well-defined certified reference material for which the mass fraction is known (Corbisier et al., 2017) and measuring what it provides in copy number. This approach has the advantage that whatever the technique of quantification is used, several labs should arrive to similar results on a given matrix when using the same reference material even though the so obtained content of the sample may in fact be a biased figure with respect to its real content.

## 4.4 CONCLUSION

PCR in several formats is presently the best technique for screening and detection of GMO's or GM derived products. Moreover, with real-time PCR or digital PCR, it allows the quantification of the content in genetically modified material. However, the approach is dependent on what one is looking for. New techniques linked to next generation sequencing are now in development to enable detection without any preliminary knowledge of what should be searched.

## REFERENCES

Afonina, I., Zivarts, M., Kutyavin, I., Lukhtanov, E., Gamper, H., Meyer, R.B. (1997). Efficient priming of PCR with short oligonucleotides conjugated to a minor groove binder. *Nucleic Acids Research*, *25*(13), 2657–2660.

Alary, R., Serin, A., Maury, D., Jouira, H.B., Sirven, J.P., Gautier, M.F., Joudira, P. (2002) Comparison of simplex and duplex real-time PCR for quantification of GMO in maize and soybean. *Food Control*, *13*, 235–244.

Allnutt, T., Blackburn, J., Copeland, J., Dennis, C., Dixon, J., Laybourn, R., Wontner-Smith, T., Hugo, S., Henry, C. (2013). Estimates of genetically modified oilseed in shared farming machinery. *Annals of Applied Biology*, *162*(1), 119–130.

Anonymous. (2006). Real-time PCR for the quantification of genetically modified rapeseed lines using the 35S/pat-construct. *Journal fur Verbraucherschutz und Lebensmittelsicherheit*, *3*, 111–114.

Babekova, R., Funk, T., Pecoraro, S., Engel, K.H., Baikova, D., Busch, U. (2008). Duplex polymerase chain reaction (PCR) for the simultaneous detection of cryIA (b) and the maize ubiquitin promoter in the transgenic rice line KMD1. *Biotechnology and Biotechnological Equipment*, *22*(2), 705–708.

Bahrdt, C., Krech, A. B., Wurz, A., Wulff, D. (2010). Validation of a newly developed hexaplex real-time PCR assay for screening for presence of GMOs in food, feed and seed. *Analytical and Bioanalytical Chemistry*, *396*(6), 2103–2112.

Barbau-Piednoir, E., Lievens, A., Vandermassen, E., Mbongolo-Mbella, E.G., Leunda-Casi, A., Roosens, N., Sneyers, M., Van den Bulcke, M. (2012). Four new SYBR Green qPCR screening methods for the detection of Roundup Ready®, LibertyLink®, and CryIAb traits in genetically modified products. *European Food Research and Technology*, *234*(1), 13–23.

Barbau-Piednoir, E., Stragier, P., Roosens, N., Mazzara, M., Savini, C., Van den Eede, G., Van den Bulcke, M. (2014). Inter-laboratory testing of GMO detection by combinatory SYBR Green PCR screening (CoSYPS). *Food Analytical Methods*, 7(8), 1719–1728.

Bayer CropScience-BioScience (2006). Grain testing method for detection of rice GM events containing P35S:bar sequences using RT-PCR protocols PGS0494 and PGS0476. Protocol. Bayer CropScience, Gent, Belgium.

Beilstein, M.A., Al-Shehbaz, I.A., Mathews, S., Kellogg, E.A. (2008). Brassicaceae phylogeny inferred from phytochrome A and ndhF sequence data: Tribes and trichomes revisited. *American Journal of Botany*, *95*(10), 1307–1327.

Block, A., Schwarz, G. (2003). Validation of different genomic and cloned DNA calibration standards for construct-specific quantification of LibertyLink in rapeseed by real-time PCR. *European Food Research and Technology*, *216*(5), 421–427.

Block, A., Debode, F., Grohmann, L., Hulin, J., Taverniers, I., Kluga, L., Barbau-Piednoir, E., Broeders, S., Huber, I., Van den Bulcke, M., Heinze, P., Berben, G., Busch, U., Roosens, N., Janssen, E., Žel, J., Gruden, K., Morisset, D. (2013). The GMOseek matrix: a decision support tool for optimizing the detection of genetically modified plants. *BMC Bioinformatics*, *14*(1), 256.

Bonfini, L., Van den Bulcke, M.H., Mazzara, M., Ben, E., Patak, A. (2012). GMOMETHODS: The European union database of reference methods for GMO analysis. *Journal of AOAC International*, *95*(6), 1713–1719.

Brod, F.C.A., dos Santos Ferrari, C., Valente, L.L., Arisi, A.C.M. (2007a). Nested PCR detection of genetically modified soybean in soybean flour, infant formula and soymilk. *LWT-Food Science and Technology*, *40*(4), 748–751.

Brod, F. C., Arisi, A. (2007b). Recombinant DNA in meat additives: Specific detection of Roundup Ready™ soybean by nested PCR. *Journal of the Science of Food and Agriculture*, *87*(10), 1980–1984.

Broeders, S., Fraiture, M.A., Vandermassen, E., Delvoye, M., Barbau-Piednoir, E., Lievens, A., Roosens, N. (2015). New qualitative trait-specific SYBR Green qPCR methods to expand the panel of GMO screening methods used in the CoSYPS. *European Food Research and Technology*, *241*(2), 275–287.

Broeders, S., Huber, I., Grohmann, L., Berben, G., Taverniers, I., Mazzara, M., Roosens, N., Morisset, D. (2014). Guidelines for validation of qualitative real-time PCR methods. *Trends in Food Science and Technology*, *37*(2), 115–126.

Broothaerts, W., Corbisier, P., Schimmel, H., Trapmann, S., Vincent, S., Emons, H. (2008). A single nucleotide polymorphism (SNP839) in the adh1 reference gene affects the quantitation of genetically modified maize (Zea mays L.). *Journal of Agricultural and Food Chemistry*, *56*(19), 8825–8831.

Burns, M., Corbisier, P., Wiseman, G., Valdivia, H., McDonald, P., Bowler, P., Ohara, K., Schimmel, H., Charels, D., Damant, A., Harris, N. (2006). Comparison of plasmid and genomic DNA calibrants for the quantification of genetically modified ingredients. *European Food Research and Technology*, *224*(2), 249–258.

Burns, M.J., Burrell, A.M., Foy, C.A. (2010). The applicability of digital PCR for the assessment of detection limits in GMO analysis. *European Food Research and Technology*, *231*(3), 353–362.

Bustin, S.A., Benes, V., Garson, J.A., Hellemans, J., Huggett, J., Kubista, M., Mueller, R., Nolan, T., Pfaffl, M.W., Shipley, G.L., Vandesompele, J., Wittwer, C.T. (2009). The MIQE guidelines: Minimum information for publication of quantitative real-time PCR experiments. *Clinical Chemistry*, 55(4), 611–22.

Cankar, K., Ravnikar, M., Žel, J., Gruden, K., Toplak, N. (2005). Real-time polymerase chain reaction detection of cauliflower mosaic virus to complement the 35S screening assay for genetically modified organisms. *Journal of AOAC International*, *88*(3), 814–822.

Cankar, K., Chauvensy-Ancel, V., Fortabat, M.N., Gruden, K., Kobilinsky, A., Zel, J., Bertheau, Y. (2008). Detection of nonauthorized genetically modified organisms using differential quantitative polymerase chain reaction: Application to 35S in maize. *Analytical Biochemistry, 376*, 189–199.

Caprioara-Buda, M., Meyer, W., Jeynov, B., Corbisier, P., Trapmann, S., Emons, H. (2012). Evaluation of plasmid and genomic DNA calibrants used for the quantification of genetically modified organisms. *Analytical and Bioanalytical Chemistry*, *404*(1), 29–42.

Chalhoub, B., Denoeud, F., Liu, S., Parkin, I.A., Tang, H., Wang, X., Chiquet, J., Belcram, H., Tong, C., Samans, B., Sidebottom, C.H. (2014). Early allopolyploid evolution in the post-Neolithic Brassica napus oilseed genome. *Science*, *345*(6199), 950–953.

Chaouachi, M., El Malki, R., Berard, A., Romaniuk, M., Laval, V., Brunel, D., Bertheau, Y. (2008a). Development of a real-time PCR method for the differential detection and quantification of four solanaceae in GMO analysis: Potato (*Solanum Tuberosum*), tomato (*Solanum Lycopersicum*), eggplant (*Solanum Melongena*), and pepper (*Capsicum Annuum*). *Journal of Agricultural and Food Chemistry, 56*(6), 1818–1828.

Chaouachi, M., Fortabat, M.-N., Geldreich, A., Yot, P., Kerlan, C., Kebdani, N., Audeon, C., Romaniuk, M., Bertheau, Y. (2008b). An accurate real-time PCR test for the detection and quantification of cauliflower mosaic virus (CaMV) applicable in GMO screening. *European Food Research and Technology*, *227*, 789–798.

Chaouachi, M., Alaya, A., Ali, I.B.H., Hafsa, A.B., Nabi, N., Bérard, A., Romaniuk, M., Skhiri, F., Saïd, K. (2013). Development of real-time PCR method for the detection and the quantification of a new endogenous reference gene in sugar beet "Beta vulgaris L.": GMO application. *Plant Cell Reports*, *32*(1), 117–128.

Charles-Delobel, C., Foti, N., Savini, C, Patak, A., Van den Bulcke, M., Ermolli, M., Folloni, S., Pinski, G., Mazzara, M., Van den Eede, G. (2009). Report on the verification of the performance of a construct-specific assay for the detection of flax CDC triffid event FP967 using real-time PCR. *EUR* 24154

Cheah, Y.K., Chong, Y.T., Khoo, S.P., Radu, S. (2011). Development of multiplex-PCR for genetically modified organism (GMO) detection targeting EPSPS and Cry1Ab genes in soy and maize samples. *International Food Research Journal*, *18*(2), 515–522.

Choi, S.H. (2011). Hexaplex PCR assay and liquid bead array for detection of stacked genetically modified cotton event 281-24-236×3006-210-23. *Analytical and Bioanalytical Chemistry*, *401*(2), 647–655.

Compendium of reference methods for GMO analysis. (2010). JRC reference reports. European union reference laboratory for GM food and feed (EURL-GMFF) European network of GMO laboratories (ENGL). *EUR* 24526 *EN*.

Corbisier, P., Trapmann, S., Gancberg, D., Hannes, L., Van Iwaarden, P., Berben, G., Schimmel, H., Emons, H. (2005). Quantitative determination of Roundup Ready soybean (Glycine max) extracted from highly processed flour. *Analytical and Bioanalytical Chemistry*, *383*(2), 282–290.

Corbisier, P., Bhat, S., Partis, L., Xie, V.R.D., Emslie, K.R. (2010). Absolute quantification of genetically modified MON810 maize (Zea mays L.) by digital polymerase chain reaction. *Analytical and Bioanalytical Chemistry, 396*(6), 2143–2150.
Corbisier, P., Barbante, A., Berben, G., Broothaerts, W., De Loose, M., Emons, H., Georgieva, Tz., Lievens, A., Mazzara, M., Papazova, N., Perri, E., Sowa, S., Stebih, D., Terzi, V., Trapmann, S. (2017). Recommendation for the unit of measurement and the measuring system to report traceable and comparable results expressing GM content in accordance with EU legislation. EUR28536 EN, doi:10.2760/177516.
Cottenet, G., Blancpain, C., Sonnard, V., Chuah, P.F. (2013). Development and validation of a multiplex real-time PCR method to simultaneously detect 47 targets for the identification of genetically modified organisms. *Analytical and Bioanalytical Chemistry, 405*(21), 6831–6844.
Crickmore, N., Zeigler, D.R., Feitelson, J., Schnepf, E., Van Rie, J., Lereclus, D., Baum, J., Dean, D.H. (1998). Revision of the nomenclature for the Bacillus thuringiensis pesticidal crystal proteins. *Microbiology and Molecular Biology Reviews, 62*(3), 807–813.
Dalmira, F.U., Melina, P.U., José-Benigno, V.T., Josefina, L.F., Raymundo, G.E., Abraham, A.S. (2015). Development, optimization, and evaluation of a duplex droplet digital PCR assay to quantify the T-nos/hmg copy number ratio in genetically modified maize. *Analytical Chemistry, 88*(1), 812–819.
Debode, F., Janssen, E., Berben, G. (2007). Physical degradation of genomic DNA of soybean flours does not impair relative quantification of its transgenic content. *European Food Research and Technology, 226*, 273–280.
Debode, F., Marien, A., Janssen, E., Taverniers, I., De Loose, M., Berben, G. (2008). Spiking products with a cloned endogenous target can significantly influence the GM content determined by PCR. Proceedings in 1st Global conference on GMO analysis, Villa Erba - Como (Italy), 24–27 June, p 65.
Debode, F., Marien, A., Janssen, E., Berben, G. (2010). Design of multiplex calibrant plasmids, their use in GMO detection and the limit of their applicability for quantitative purposes owing to competition effects. *Analytical and Bioanalytical Chemistry, 396*(6), 2151–2164.
Debode, F., Janssen, E., Marien, A., Berben, G. (2012). DNA detection by conventional and real-time PCR after extraction from vegetable oils. *Journal of the American Oil Chemists' Society, 89*(7), 1249–1257.
Debode, F., Janssen, E., Berben, G. (2013). Development of 10 new screening PCR assays for GMO detection targeting promoters (pFMV, pNOS, pSSuAra, pTA29, pUbi, pRice actin) and terminators (t35S, tE9, tOCS, tg7). *European Food Research and Technology, 236*(4), 659–669.
Debode F. (2017a). Développement de méthodologies pour la détection des plantes génétiquement modifiées. Thèse de doctorat, AGRO, UCL, 367/2017, 391 p. http://hdl.handle.net/2078.1/186329
Debode, F., Huber, I., Macarthur, R., Rischitor, P.E., Mazzara, M., Herau, V., Sebah, D., Dobnik, D., Broeders, S., Roosens, N.H., Busch, U., Berben, G., Morisset, D., Zel, J. (2017b). Inter-laboratory studies for the validation of two singleplex (tE9 and pea lectin) and one duplex (pat/bar) real-time PCR methods for GMO detection. *Food Control, 73*, 452–461.
Debode, F., Janssen, E., Bragard, C., Berben, G. (2017c). Detection by real-time PCR and pyrosequencing of the *cry*1Ab and *cry*1Ac genes introduced in GM constructions. *Food Additives and Contaminants: Part A, 34*(8), 1398–1409.

Debode F., Marien A., Janssen E., Bragard C., Berben G. (2017d). Influence of the amplicon length on real-time PCR results. *Biotechnologie, Agronomie, Société et Environnement, 21*, 3–11.

Debode, F., Zdeňková, K., Janssen, E., Tizolova, A., du Jardin, P., Berben, G., Demnerova, K. (2018). Development of real-time PCR assays for the detection of the *pin* II terminator (*tpin*II) used in GM constructs and its donor organism, potato (*solanum tuberosum*). *Food Analytical methods, 11*(8), 2172 -2180.

Degen, H.J., Deufel, A., Eisel, D., Grunewald-Janho, S., Keesey, J., editors. (2006). PCR applications manual. 3rd edition. Roche, Mannheim, Germany. www.gene-quantification.com/ras-pcr-application-manual-3rd-ed.pdf (last consultation 10 October 2017).

Demeke, T., Giroux, R.W., Reitmeier, S., Simon, S.L. (2002). Development of a polymerase chain reaction assay for detection of three canola transgenes. *Journal of the American Oil Chemists' Society, 79*(10), 1015–1019.

Demeke, T., Ratnayaka, I. (2008). Multiplex qualitative PCR assay for identification of genetically modified canola events and real-time event-specific PCR assay for quantification of the GT73 canola event. *Food Control, 19*(9), 893–897.

Demeke, T., Jenkins, G.R. (2010). Influence of DNA extraction methods, PCR inhibitors and quantification methods on real-time PCR assay of biotechnology-derived traits. *Analytical and Bioanalytical Chemistry, 396*(6), 1977–1990.

Demeke, T., Gräfenhan, T., Holigroski, M., Fernando, U., Bamforth, J., Lee, S.J. (2014). Assessment of droplet digital PCR for absolute quantification of genetically engineered OXY235 canola and DP305423 soybean samples. *Food Control, 46*, 470–474.

Dinon, A.Z., Prins, T.W., van Dijk, J.P., Arisi, A.C.M., Scholtens, I.M., Kok, E.J. (2011). Development and validation of real-time PCR screening methods for detection of cry1A.105 and cry2Ab2 genes in genetically modified organisms. *Analytical and Bioanalytical Chemistry, 400*(5), 1433–1442.

Dinon, A., Brod, F., Mello, C., Oliveira, E., Faria, J., Arisi, A. (2012). Primers and probes development for specific PCR detection of genetically modified common bean (*Phaseolus vulgaris*) Embrapa 5.1. *Journal of Agricultural and Food Chemistry, 60*, 4672–4677.

Dobnik, D., Spilsberg, B., Bogožalec Košir, A., Holst-Jensen, A., Žel, J. (2015). Multiplex quantification of 12 European union authorized genetically modified Maize lines with Droplet Digital Polymerase Chain reaction. *Analytical Chemistry, 87*(16), 8218–8226.

Dobnik, D., Štebih, D., Blejec, A., Morisset, D., Žel, J. (2016). Multiplex quantification of four DNA targets in one reaction with Bio-Rad droplet digital PCR system for GMO detection. *Scientific Reports, 6*, 35451.

Dobnik, D., Demšar, T., Huber, I., Gerdes, L., Broeders, S., Roosens, N., Debode, F., Berben, G., Žel, J. (2018). Inter-laboratory analysis of selected genetically modified plant reference materials with digital PCR. *Analytical and Bioanalytical Chemistry, 410*(1), 211–221.

Dong, W., Yang, L., Shen, K., Kim, B., Kleter, G.A., Marvin, H.J., Guo, R., Liang, W., Zhang, D. (2008). GMDD: A database of GMO detection methods. *BMC Bioinformatics, 9*(1), 260.

Dörries, H.H., Remus, I., Grönewald, A., Grönewald, C., Berghof-Jäger, K. (2010). Development of a qualitative, multiplex real-time PCR kit for screening of genetically modified organisms (GMOs). *Analytical and Bioanalytical Chemistry, 396*(6), 2043–2054.

Eckes, P., Rosahl, S., Schell, J., Willmitzer, L. (1986). Isolation and characterization of a light-inducible, organ-specific gene from potato and analysis of its expression after tagging and transfer into tobacco and potato shoots. *Molecular and General Genetics*, *205*(1), 14–22.

Ehlers, B., Strauch, E., Goltz, M., Kubsch, D., Wagner, H., Maidhof, H., Bendiek, J., Appe, L. B., Buhk, H.J. (1997). Nachweis gentechnischer veränderungen in Mais mittels PCR. *Bundesgesundheitsblatt*, *40*(4), 118–121.

Fernandez, S., Charles-Delobel, C., Geldreich, A., Berthier, G., Boyer, F., Collonnier, C., Coué-Philippe, G., Diolez, A., Duplan, M.-N., Kebdani, N., Romaniuk, M., Feinberg, M., Bertheau, Y. (2005). Quantification of the 35S promoter in DNA extracts from genetically modified organisms using real-time polymerase chain reaction and specificity assessment on various genetically modified organisms, Part I: Operating procedure. *Journal of AOAC International*, *88*, 547–573.

Fidan, S., Arican, E. (2014). Transgenic investigation of Canola (*Brassica napus* L.). *Annual Research & Review in Biology*, *4*(24), 4293.

Fu, W., Zhu, P., Wang, C., Huang, K., Du, Z., Tian, W., Wang, Q., Wang, H., Xu, W., Zhu, S. (2015). A highly sensitive and specific method for the screening detection of genetically modified organisms based on digital PCR without pretreatment. *Scientific reports*, *5*, 12715.

García-Cañas, V., González, R., Cifuentes, A. (2004). Sensitive and simultaneous analysis of five transgenic maizes using multiplex polymerase chain reaction, capillary gel electrophoresis, and laser-induced fluorescence. *Electrophoresis*, *25*(14), 2219–2226.

Gerdes, L., Iwobi, A., Busch, U., Pecoraro, S. (2016). Optimization of digital droplet polymerase chain reaction for quantification of genetically modified organisms. *Biomolecular Detection and Quantification*, *7*, 9–20.

Germini, A., Zanetti, A., Salati, C., Rossi, S., Forré, C., Schmid, S., Marchelli, R. (2004). Development of a seven-target multiplex PCR for the simultaneous detection of transgenic soybean and maize in feeds and foods. *Journal of Agricultural and Food Chemistry*, *52*(11), 3275–3280.

Goda, Y., Asano, T., Shibuya, M., Hino, A., Toyoda, M. (2001). Detection of recombinant DNA from genetically modified papaya. *Shokuhin eiseigaku zassh. Journal of the Food Hygienic Society of Japan*, *42*(4), 231–236.

Grohmann, L., Brünen-Nieweler, C., Nemeth, A., Waiblinger, H.U. (2009). Collaborative trial validation studies of real-time PCR-based GMO screening methods for detection of the bar gene and the ctp2-cp4epsps construct. *Journal of Agricultural and Food Chemistry*, *57*(19), 8913–8920.

Grohmann, L., Reiting, R., Mäde, D., Uhlig, S., Simon, K., Frost, K., Randhawa G.J., Zur, K. (2015). Collaborative trial validation of cry1Ab/Ac and Pubi-cry TaqMan-based real-time PCR assays for detection of DNA derived from genetically modified Bt plant products. *Accreditation and Quality Assurance*, *20*(2), 85–96.

Guan, Q., Wang, X., Teng, D., Yang, Y., Tian, F., Yin, Q., Wang, J. (2011). Construction of a standard reference plasmid for detecting GM cottonseed meal. *Applied Biochemistry and Biotechnology*, *165*(1), 24–34.

Guo, J., Yang, L., Liu, X., Zhang, H., Qian, B., Zhang, D. (2009). Applicability of the chymopapain gene used as endogenous reference gene for transgenic Huanong No. 1 papaya detection. *Journal of Agricultural and Food Chemistry*, *57*, 6502–6509.

Guo, J., Yang, L., Chen, L., Morisset, D., Li, X., Pan, L., Zhang, D. (2011). MPIC: A high-throughput analytical method for multiple DNA targets. *Analytical Chemistry*, *83*(5), 1579–1586.

Heide, B.R., Heir, E., Holck, A. (2008). Detection of eight GMO maize events by qualitative, multiplex PCR and fluorescence capillary gel electrophoresis. *European Food Research and Technology, 227*(2), 527–535.

Henderson, N., Harmon, M., Zhong, C.X. (2016). PCR-based detection and quantification of a transgenic glyphosate-tolerant canola using a novel reference gene system. *Food Analytical Methods, 9*(2), 353–361.

Hernández, M., Río, A., Esteve, T., Prat, S., Pla, M. (2001). A rapeseed-specific gene, acetyl-CoA carboxylase, can be used as a reference for qualitative and real-time quantitative PCR detection of transgenes from mixed food samples. *Journal of Agricultural and Food Chemistry, 49*(8), 3622–3627.

Hernández, M., Duplan, M.N., Berthier, G., Vaïtilingom, M., Hauser, W., Freyer, R., Pla, M., Bertheau, Y. (2004). Development and comparison of four real-time polymerase chain reaction systems for specific detection and quantification of Zea mays L. *Journal of Agricultural and Food Chemistry, 52*(15), 4632–4637.

Hernández, M., Rodríguez-Lázaro, D., Zhang, D., Esteve, T., Pla, M., Prat, S. (2005a). Interlaboratory transfer of a PCR multiplex method for simultaneous detection of four genetically modified maize lines: *Bt*11, MON810, T25, and GA21. *Journal of Agricultural and Food Chemistry, 53*(9), 3333–3337.

Hernández, M., Esteve, T., Pla, M. (2005b). Real-time polymerase chain reaction based assays for quantitative detection of barley, rice, sunflower, and wheat. *Journal of Agricultural and Food Chemistry*, 53(18), 7003–7009.

Higuchi, R., Fockler, C., Dollinger, G., Watson, R. (1993). Kinetic PCR analysis: Real-time monitoring of DNA amplification reactions. *Biotechnology, 11*, 1026–1030.

Höfte, H., Whiteley, H. R. (1989). Insecticidal crystal proteins of Bacillus thuringiensis. *Microbiological Reviews, 53*(2), 242–255.

Höhne, M., Santisi, C., Meyer, R. (2002). Real-time multiplex PCR: An accurate method for the detection and quantification of 35S-CaMV promoter in genetically modified maize-containing food. *European Food Research and Technology, 215*(1), 59–64.

Holst-Jensen, A., Rønning, S.B., Løvseth, A., Berdal, K.G. (2003). PCR technology for screening and quantification of genetically modified organisms (GMOs). *Analytical and Bioanalytical Chemistry, 375*(8), 985–993.

Holland, P.M., Abramson, R.D., Watson, R., Gelfand, D.H. (1991). Detection of specific polymerase chain reaction product by utilizing the 5'----3'exonuclease activity of Thermus aquaticus DNA polymerase. *Proceedings of the National Academy of Sciences, 88*(16), 7276–7280.

Huang, H.Y., Pan, T.M. (2004). Detection of genetically modified maize MON810 and NK603 by multiplex and real-time polymerase chain reaction methods. *Journal of Agricultural and Food Chemistry, 52*(11), 3264–3268.

Huang, H., Cheng, F., Wang, R., Zhang, D., Yang, L. (2013). Evaluation of four endogenous reference genes and their real-time PCR assays for common wheat quantification in GMOs detection. *Plos One, 8*, e75850.

Huggett, J.F., Foy, C.A., Benes, V., Emslie, K., Garson, J.A., Haynes, R., Hellemans, J., Kubista, M., Mueller R.D., Nolan, T., Pfaffl, M.W., Shipley, G.L., Vandesompele, J., Wittwer, C.T., Bustin, S.A. (2013). The digital MIQE guidelines: Minimum information for publication of quantitative digital PCR experiments. *Clinical Chemistry, 59*, 892–902.

Iida, M., Yamashiro, S., Yamakawa, H., Hayakawa, K., Kuribara, H., Kodama, T., Furui, S., Akiyama, H., Maitani, T., Hino, A. (2005). Development of taxon-specific

sequences of common wheat for the detection of genetically modified wheat. *Journal of Agricultural and Food Chemistry*, *53*(16), 6294.
ISO 21569. (2005). *Foodstuffs—Methods of Analysis for the Detection of Genetically Modified Organisms and Derived Products—Qualitative Nucleic Acid Based Methods*. International Organization for Standardization, Geneva, Switzerland.
Iwobi, A., Gerdes, L., Busch, U., Pecoraro, S. (2016). Droplet digital PCR for routine analysis of genetically modified foods (GMO)–A comparison with real-time quantitative PCR. *Food Control*, *69*, 205–213.
James, D., Schmidt, A.M., Wall, E., Green, M., Masri, S. (2003). Reliable detection and identification of genetically modified maize, soybean, and canola by multiplex PCR analysis. *Journal of Agricultural and Food Chemistry*, *51*(20), 5829–5834.
Jinxia, A., Qingzhang, L., Xuejun, G., Yanbo, Y., Lu, L., Minghui, Z. (2011). A multiplex nested PCR assay for the simultaneous detection of genetically modified soybean, maize and rice in highly processed products. *Food Control*, *22*(10), 1617–1623.
Kamle, S., Kumar, A., Bhatnagar, R.K. (2011). Development of multiplex and construct specific PCR assay for detection of cry2Ab transgene in genetically modified crops and product. *GM Crops*, *2*(1), 74–81.
Kermekchiev, M.B., Kirilova, L.I., Vail, E.E., Barnes, W.M. (2009). Mutants of Taq DNA polymerase resistant to PCR inhibitors allow DNA amplification from whole blood and crude soil samples. *Nucleic Acids Research*, *37*(5), e40–e40.
Kim, J.H., Kim, E.H., Yea, M.C., Kim, H.Y. (2013). Validation of A multiplex PCR detection kit for screening of herbicide-tolerant genes in genetically modified crops. *Journal of the Korean Society for Applied Biological Chemistry*, *56*(2), 251–254.
Kim, J. H., Zhang, D., Kim, H. Y. (2014). Detection of sixteen genetically modified maize events in processed foods using four event-specific pentaplex PCR systems. *Food Control*, *35*(1), 345–353.
Kimio, M., Rie, A., Naoki, S., Masaki, S., Hisatsugu, I., Kazue, S., Takashi, T., Kunihiro, K., Akihiro, H., Kazuo, S. (2005) Detection of genetically modified organisms in foreign-made processed foods containing corn and potato. *Journal of Food Hygiene Society of Japan, 46*, 79–85.
Kitpipit, T., Sittichan, K., Thanakiatkrai, P. (2014). Direct-multiplex PCR assay for meat species identification in food products. *Food Chemistry*, *163*, 77–82.
Kitta, K., Furui, S., Mano, J., Matsuoka, Y., Arami, S., Sato, M., Haragushi, H., Kurimoto, Y., Imai, S., Tanaka, K. (2014). *U.S. Patent No. 8,865,433*. Washington, DC: U.S. Patent and Trademark Office.
Kok, E.J., Aarts, H.J., Hoef, A.M., Kuiper, H.A. (2002). DNA methods: Critical review of innovative approaches. *Journal of AOAC International*, *85*(3), 797–800.
Köppel, R., Sendic, A., Waiblinger, H.U. (2014). Two quantitative multiplex real-time PCR systems for the efficient GMO screening of food products. *European Food Research and Technology*, *239*(4), 653–659.
Köppel, R., Bucher, T., Frei, A., Waiblinger, H.U. (2015). Droplet digital PCR versus multiplex real-time PCR method for the detection and quantification of DNA from the four transgenic soy traits MON87769, MON87708, MON87705 and FG72, and lectin. *European Food Research and Technology*, *241*(4), 521–527.
Köppel, R., Bucher, T., Bär, D., van Velsen, F., Ganeshan, A. (2017). Validation of 13 duplex droplet digital PCR systems for quantitative GMO analysis of most prevalent GMO traits. *European Food Research and Technology*, *244*(2), 313-321.

Košir, A. B., Spilsberg, B., Holst-Jensen, A., Žel, J., Dobnik, D. (2017). Development and inter-laboratory assessment of droplet digital PCR assays for multiplex quantification of 15 genetically modified soybean lines. *Scientific Reports*, 7(1), 8601.

Kuribara, H., Shindo, Y., Matsuoka, T., Takubo, K., Futo, S., Aoki, N., Hirao, T., Akiyama, H., Goda, Y., Toyada, M., Hino, A. (2002). Novel reference molecules for quantitation of genetically modified maize and soybean. *Journal of AOAC International*, *85*(5), 1077–1089.

Lipp, M., Brodmann, P., Pietsch, K., Pauwels, J., Anklam, E. (1999). IUPAC collaborative trial study of a method to detect genetically modified soy beans and maize in dried powder. *Journal-AOAC International*, *82*, 923–928.

Lu, I.J., Lin, C.H., Pan, T.M. (2010). Establishment of a system based on universal multiplex-PCR for screening genetically modified crops. *Analytical and Bioanalytical Chemistry*, *396*(6), 2055–2064.

Maciel, H., Zingaretti, S., Maciel, G. (2014). Comparative analysis of the amino acid sequence of the Cry protein of Bacillus thuringiensis codify the toxic protein to insects of the orders Lepidoptera, Diptera and Lepidoptera/Diptera. *BMC Proceedings*, *8*(4), P120.

Majumdar, N., Wessel, T., Marks, J. (2015). Digital PCR modeling for maximal sensitivity, dynamic range and measurement precision. *PLoS One*, *10*(3), e0118833.

Marmiroli, N., Maestri, E., Gullì, M., Malcevschi, A., Peano, C., Bordoni, R., De Bellis, G. (2008). Methods for detection of GMOs in food and feed. *Analytical and Bioanalytical Chemistry*, *392*(3), 369–384.

Mason, G., Provero, P., Vaira, A.-M., Accotto, G.P. (2002). Estimating the number of integrations in transformed plants by quantitative real-time PCR. *BMC Biotechnology*, *2*, 20.

Matsuoka, T., Kuribara, H., Takubo, K., Akiyama, H., Miura, H., Goda, Y., Kusakabe, Y., Isshiki, K., Toyoda, M., Hino, A. (2002). Detection of recombinant DNA segments introduced to genetically modified maize (Zea mays). *Journal of Agricultural and Food Chemistry*, *50*(7), 2100–2109.

Matsuoka, Y., Arami, S.I., Sato, M., Haraguchi, H., Kurimoto, Y., Imai, S., Tanaka, K., Mano, J., Furui, S., Kitta, K. (2011). Development of methods to distinguish between durum/common wheat and common wheat in blended flour using PCR. *Shokuhin eiseigaku zassh.. Journal of the Food Hygienic Society of Japan*, *53*(5), 195–202.

Mattarucchi, E., Weighardt, F., Barbati, C., Querci, M., Van den Eede, G. (2005). Development and applications of real-time PCR standards for GMO quantification based on tandem-marker plasmids. *European Food Research and Technology*, *221*, 511–519.

Mazzara, M., Foti, N., Savini, C., Van den Eede, G. (2006). Event-specific method for the quantitation of sugarbeet Line H7-1 using real-time PCR -validation report and protocol. EUR 22134 EN. 2006. JRC32190 (ISBN 92-79-01536-2).

Mazzara, M., Bogni, A., Savini, C., Van Den Eede, G. (2007a). Event-specific method for the quantification of oilseed rape line Ms8 using real-time PCR—validation report and protocol- seeds sampling and DNA extraction of oilseed rape. EUR 22917 EN. Luxembourg (Luxembourg): OPOCE 2007. JRC37545 (ISBN 978-92-79-06934-5).

Mazzara, M., Charles-Delobel, C., Grazioli, E., Larcher, S., Savini, C., Van Den Eede, G. (2007bc). Event-specific method for the quantification of soybean line A2704–12 using real-time PCR- validation report and protocol—soybean seeds sampling and DNA extraction. EUR 22910. JRC37483 (ISBN 978-92-79-06928-4).

Moens, W., Deloose, M., Remacle, J., Callebaut, A., Berben, G. (2005). Tracing and authentication of GMOs and derived products in the food-processing area, www.belspo.be/belspo/organisation/publ/pub_ostc/CPagr/rappCP32_en.pdf (last consultation 14 March2014).

Morisset, D., Stebih, D., Cankar, K., Zel, J., Gruden, K. (2008). Alternative DNA amplification methods to PCR and their application in GMO detection: a review. *European Food Research and Technology, 227*(5), 1287–1297.

Morisset, D., Štebih, D., Milavec, M., Gruden, K., Žel, J. (2013). Quantitative analysis of food and feed samples with droplet digital PCR. *PloS one, 8*(5), e62583.

Mullis, K.B., Faloona, F.A. (1987). Specific synthesis of DNA in vitro via a polymerase-catalyzed chain reaction. *Methods in Enzymology, 155*, 335.

Nixon, G., Garson, J.A., Grant, P., Nastouli, E., Foy, C.A., Huggett, J.F. (2014). Comparative study of sensitivity, linearity, and resistance to inhibition of digital and nondigital polymerase chain reaction and loop mediated isothermal amplification assays for quantification of human cytomegalovirus. *Analytical Chemistry, 86*(9), 4387–4394.

Pan, L., Zhang, S., Yang, L., Broll, H., Tian, F., Zhang, D. (2007). Interlaboratory trial validation of an event-specific qualitative polymerase chain reaction-based detection method for genetically modified RT73 rapeseed. *Journal of AOAC International, 90*(6), 1639–1646.

Pansiot, J., Chaouachi, M., Cavellini, L., Romaniuk, M., Ayadi, M., Bertheau, Y., Laval, V. (2011). Development of two screening duplex PCR assays for genetically modified organism quantification using multiplex real-time PCR master mixes. *European Food Research and Technology, 232*(2), 327–334.

Paterno, A., Marchesi, U., Gatto, F., Verginelli, D., Quarchioni, C., Fusco, C., Zepparoni, A., Amaddeo, D., Ciabatti, I. (2009). Finding the joker among the maize endogenous reference genes for genetically modified organism (GMO) detection. *Journal of Agricultural and Food Chemistry, 57*, 11086–11091.

Pecoraro, S., Berben, G., Burns, M., Corbisier, P., De Giacomo, M., De Loose, M., Dagand, E., Dobnik, D., Eriksson, R., Herau, V., Holst-Jensen, A., Kagkli, D.-M., Kreysa, J., Lievens, M., Mäde, D., Mazzara, M., Paternò, A., Peterseil, V., Savini, C., Sovová, T., Sowa, S., Spilsberg, B. (2018). Overview and recommendations for the application of digital PCR. ENGL WG on digital PCR. JRC Technical Report (in press).

Permingeat, H.R., Reggiardo, M.I., Vallejos, R.H. (2002). Detection and quantification of transgenes in grains by multiplex and real-time PCR. *Journal of agricultural and food chemistry, 50*(16), 4431–4436.

Picó, Y. (2007). *Food Toxicants Analysis: Techniques, Strategies and Developments*. Elsevier, Amsterdam. 786 p. ISBN-13: 978-0-444-52843-8.

Prins, T.W., van Hoof, R.A., Scholtens, I.M., Kok, E.J. (2017). Novel TaqMan PCR screening methods for element cry3A and construct gat/T-pinII to support detection of both known and unknown GMOs. *European Food Research and Technology, 243*(3), 481–488.

Querci, M., Van den Bulcke, M., Žel, J., Van den Eede, G., Broll, H. (2008). New approaches in GMO detection. *Analytical and Bioanalytical Chemistry, 396*, 1991–2002.

Rački, N., Dreo, T., Gutierrez-Aguirre, I., Blejec, A., Ravnikar, M. (2014). Reverse transcriptase droplet digital PCR shows high resilience to PCR inhibitors from plant, soil and water samples. *Plant Methods, 10*(1), 42.

Randhawa, G.J., Chhabra, R., Singh, M. (2010). Decaplex and real-time PCR based detection of MON531 and MON15985 Bt cotton events. *Journal of Agricultural and Food Chemistry, 58*(18), 9875–9881.

Reiting, R., Broll, H., Waiblinger, H.U., Grohmann, L. (2007). Collaborative study of a T-nos real-time PCR method for screening of genetically modified organisms in food products. *Journal für Verbraucherschutz und Lebensmittelsicherheit, 2*(2), 116–121.

Reiting, R. (2010). Real-time PCR methods for the detection of DNA constructs with the nptII gene for the detection of genetically modified plants in food, feed and seed. *Journal für Verbraucherschutz und Lebensmittelsicherheit*, 5(3–4), 377–390.

Reiting, R., Grohmann, L., Moris, G., Mäde, D. (2013). Detection and characterization of an unknown rice event in Basmati rice products. *European Food Research and Technology, 236*(4), 715–723.

Rho, J.K., Lee, T., Jung, S.I., Kim, T.S., Park, Y.H., Kim, Y.M. (2004). Qualitative and quantitative PCR methods for detection of three lines of genetically modified potatoes. *Journal of Agricultural and Food Chemistry, 52*(11), 3269–3274.

Rosa, S. F., Gatto, F., Angers-Loustau, A., Petrillo, M., Kreysa, J., Querci, M. (2016). Development and applicability of a ready-to-use PCR system for GMO screening. *Food Chemistry, 201*, 110–119.

Sachadyn, P., Kur, J. (1997). A new PCR system for Agrobacterium tumefaciens detection based on amplification of T-DNA fragment. *Acta Microbiologica Polonica, 46*, 145–156.

Sanders, R., Huggett, J.F., Bushell, C.A., Cowen, S., Scott, D.J., Foy, C.A. (2011). Evaluation of digital PCR for absolute DNA quantification. *Analytical Chemistry, 83*(17), 6474–6484.

Savini, C., Foti, N., Mazzara, M., Charles-Delobel, C., Van Den Eede, G. (2006). Event-specific method for the quantification of event EH92–527-1 potato using real-time PCR- validation report and protocol—sampling and DNA extraction of potato. *EUR 22358 EN. 2006. JRC34758.*

Scholdberg, T.A., Norden, T.D., Nelson, D.D., Jenkins, G.R. (2009). Evaluating precision and accuracy when quantifying different endogenous control reference genes in maize using real-time PCR. *Journal of Agricultural and Food Chemistry, 57*(7), 2903–2911.

Shrestha, H.K., Hwu, K.K., Wang, S.J., Liu, L.F., Chang, M.C. (2008). Simultaneous detection of eight genetically modified maize lines using a combination of event- and construct-specific multiplex-PCR technique. *Journal of Agricultural and Food Chemistry, 56*(19), 8962–8968.

SNT 1199–2010. Protocol of the polymerase chain reaction for detecting genetically modified components in cotton. www.chinesestandard.net (last consultation 26 February 2018).

Spilsberg, B., Košir, A.B., Holst-Jensen, A., Zel, J. (2015). Multiplex quantification of twelve EU authorized GM maize lines with droplet digital PCR. *Analytical Chemistry, 87*, 8218–8226.

Spiridonova, E., Bertheau, Y., Kuznetsov, B. (2009). Designing the PCR markers Agrobacterium tumefaciens gall forming strains. *Co-Extra International conference*, Paris. Book of abstracts, abstract P6: 110–111.

Stockhaus, J., Eckes, P., Blau, A., Schell, J., Willmitzer, L. (1987) Organ-specific and dosage-dependent expression of the leaf/stem specific gene from potato after tagging and transfer into potato and tobacco plants. *Nucleic Acids Research, 15*, 3479–3491.

Stupar, R.M., Beaubien, K.A., Jin, W., Song, J., Lee, M.K., Wu, C., Zhang, H.B., Han, B., Jiang, J. (2006). Structural diversity and differential transcription of the patatin multicopy gene family during potato tuber development. *Genetics*, *172*(2), 1263–1275.

Taverniers, I., Van Bockstaele, E., De Loose, M. (2004). Cloned plasmid DNA fragments as calibrators for controlling GMOs: Different real-time duplex quantitative PCR methods. *Analytical and Bioanalytical*, *378*, 1198–1207.

Taverniers, I., Papazova, N., Allnutt, T., Baumler, S., Bertheau, Y., Esteve, T., Freyer, R., Gruden, K., Kuznetzov, B., Luis La Paz, J., Nadal, A., Pla, M., Vojvoda, D., Wulff, D., Zhang, D. (2013). Harmonised reference genes and PCR assays for GMO quantification. In: *Genetically Modified and Non-Genetically Modified Food Supply Chains: Co-Existence and Traceability*, (Ed. Bertheau Y.), Wiley-Blackwell, 273–292.

Tohidfar, M., Khosravi, S. (2015). Transgenic crops with an improved resistance to biotic stresses. A review. *Biotechnologie, Agronomie, Société et Environnement*, *19*(1), 62.

Trifa, Y., Zhang, D. (2004). DNA content in embryo and endosperm of maize kernel (*Zea mays* L.): Impact on GMO quantification. *Journal of Agricultural and Food Chemistry, 52*(5), 1044–1048.

Tyagi, S., Kramer, F.R. (1996). Molecular beacons: probes that fluoresce upon hybridization. *Nature Biotechnology*, *14*(3), 303–308.

Urquiza, M.P., Silva, A.A. (2014). Copy number ratios determined by two digital polymerase chain reaction systems in genetically modified grains. *Metrologia*, *51*(1), 61.

Van den Bulcke, M., Lievens, A., Barbau-Piednoir, E., MbongoloMbella, G., Roosens, N., Sneyers, M., Casi, A.L. (2010). A theoretical introduction to "Combinatory SYBR Green qPCR Screening," a matrix-based approach for the detection of materials derived from genetically modified plants. *Analytical and Bioanalytical Chemistry*, *396*(6), 2113–2123.

Vaïtilingom, M., Pijnenburg, H., Gendre, F., Brignon, P. (1999). Real-time quantitative PCR detection of genetically modified maximizer maize and roundup ready soybean in some representative foods. *Journal of Agricultural and Food Chemistry*, *47*(12), 5261–5266.

Venturelli, G.L., Brod, F.C., Rossi, G.B., Zimmermann, N.F., Oliveira, J.P., Faria, J.C., Arisi, A.C. (2014). A specific endogenous reference for genetically modified common bean (Phaseolus vulgaris L.) DNA quantification by real-time PCR targeting lectin gene. *Molecular Biotechnology*, *56*(11), 1060–1068.

Vollenhofer, S., Burg, K., Schmidt, J., Kroath, H. (1999). Genetically modified organisms in food screening and specific detection by polymerase chain reaction. *Journal of Agricultural and Food Chemistry, 47*(12), 5038–5043.

Waiblinger, H. U., Ernst, B., Anderson, A., Pietsch, K. (2008). Validation and collaborative study of a P35S and T-nos duplex real-time PCR screening method to detect genetically modified organisms in food products. *European Food Research and Technology*, *226*(5), 1221–1228.

Wang, X., Teng, D., Yang, Y., Tian, F., Guan, Q., Wang, J. (2011). Construction of a reference plasmid molecule containing eight targets for the detection of genetically modified crops. *Applied Microbiology and Biotechnology*, *90*(2), 721–731.

Weller, S.A., Simpkins, S.A., Stead, D.E., Kurdziel, A., Hird, H., Weekes, R.J. (2002). Identification of *Agrobacterium* spp. present within *Brassica napus* seed by TaqMan PCR—implications for GM screening procedures. *Archives of Microbiology, 178*, 338–343.

Wei, J., Li, F., Guo, J., Li, X., Xu, J., Wu, G., Zhang, D., Yang, L. (2013). Collaborative ring trial of the papaya endogenous reference gene and its polymerase chain reaction assays for genetically modified organism analysis. *Journal of Agricultural and Food Chemistry, 61*(47), 11363–11370.

Weighardt, F., Barbati, C., Paoletti, C., Querci, M., Kay, S., De Beuckeleer, M., Van den Eede, G. (2004). Real-time polymerase chain reaction-based approach for quantification of the pat gene in the T25 Zea mays event. *Journal of AOAC International, 87*(6), 1342–1355.

Weng, H., Yang, L., Liu, Z., Ding, J., Pan, A., Zhang, D. (2005). Novel reference gene, high-mobility-group protein I/Y, used in qualitative and real-time quantitative polymerase chain reaction detection of transgenic rapeseed cultivars. *Journal of AOAC International, 88*(2), 577–584.

Windels, P., Bertrand, S., Depicker, A., Moens, W., Van Bockstaele, E., De Loose, M. (2003). Qualitative and event-specific PCR real-time detection methods for StarLink maize. *European Food Research and Technology, 216*(3), 259–263.

Wolf, C., Scherzinger, M., Wurz, A., Pauli, U., Hubner, P., Luthy, J. (2000). Detection of cauliflower mosaic virus by the polymerase chain reaction: testing of food components for false-positive 35S-promoter screening results. *European Food Research and Technology, 210*, 367–372.

Wu, G., Zhang, L., Wu, Y., Cao, Y., Lu, C. (2010) Comparison of five endogenous reference genes for specific PCR detection and quantification of *Brassica napus*. *Journal of Agricultural and Food Chemistry, 58*, 2812–2817.

Xu, W., Bai, W., Guo, F., Luo, Y., Yuan, Y., Huang, K. (2008) A papaya-specific gene, papain, used as an endogenous reference gene in qualitative and real-time quantitative PCR detection of transgenic papayas. *European Food Research and Technology, 228*, 301–309.

Xu, X., Peng, C., Wang, X., Chen, X., Wang, Q., Xu, J. (2016). Comparison of droplet digital PCR with quantitative real-time PCR for determination of zygosity in transgenic maize. *Transgenic Research, 25*(6), 855–864.

Yang, L., Chen, J., Huang, C., Liu, Y., Jia, S., Pan, L., Zhang, D. (2005a). Validation of a cotton-specific gene, Sad1, used as an endogenous reference gene in qualitative and real-time quantitative PCR detection of transgenic cottons. *Plant Cell Reports, 24*(4), 237–245.

Yang, L., Pan, A., Jia, J., Ding, J., Chen, J., Cheng, H., Zhang, C., Zhang, D. (2005b). Validation of a tomato-specific gene, *LAT52*, used as an Endogenous reference gene in qualitative and real-time quantitative PCR detection of transgenic tomatoes. *Journal of Agriculture and Food Chemistry, 53*, 183–190.

Yang, L., Zhang, H., Guo, J., Pan, L., Zhang, D. (2008). International collaborative study of the endogenous reference gene LAT 52 used for qualitative and quantitative analyses of genetically modified tomato. *Journal of Agricultural and Food Chemistry, 56*(10), 3438–3443.

Yu, J., JiaYing, H., LiTao, Y. (2014). Estimating the exogenous genes copy number of genetically modified organisms by droplet digital PCR. *Journal of Agricultural Biotechnology, 22*(10), 1298–1305.

Zeitler, R., Pietsch, K., Waiblinger, H.U. (2002). Validation of real-time PCR methods for the quantification of transgenic contaminations in rape seed. *European Food Research and Technology, 214*(4), 346–351.

Zhang, Y., Zhang, D., Li, W., Chen, J., Peng, Y., Cao, W. (2003). A novel real-time quantitative PCR method using attached universal template probe. *Nucleic Acids Research*, *31*(20), e123–e123.

Zhang, J.Z., Guan, X.Y., Zhang, H.B., Yang, L.T. (2010). Nucleic Acid Isothermal Amplification Technique for Genetically Modified Food Analysis. *Journal of Agricultural Science and Technology*, *4*, 007.

Zhang, L., Cao, Y., Liu, X., Wu, G., Wu, Y., Lu, C. (2012). In-depth analysis of the endogenous reference genes used in the quantitative PCR detection systems for rice. *European Food Research and Technology*, *234*(6), 981–993.

Zhang, L., Wu, Y., Wu, G., Cao, Y., Lu, C. (2014). Correction of the lack of commutability between plasmid DNA and genomic DNA for quantification of genetically modified organisms using pBSTopas as a model. *Analytical and Bioanalytical Chemistry*, *406*(25), 6385–6397.

Zimmermann, A., Hemmer, W., Liniger, M., Lüthy, J., Pauli, U. (1998). A sensitive detection method for genetically modified Maisgard™ corn using a nested PCR-system. *LWT-Food Science and Technology*, *31*(7–8), 664–667.

CHAPTER 5

# Sensors

*Beatriz López-Ruiz and Marta Sánchez-Paniagua López*
Complutense University of Madrid

*Carmen Lorena Manzanares-Palenzuela*
University of Chemistry and Technology Prague

CONTENTS

## 5.1 BIOSENSORS

According to Jarata, "chemical sensing is part of an information-acquisition process in which an insight is obtained about the chemical composition of the system in real time. In this process, an amplified electrical signal results from the interaction between some chemical species and the sensor" (Jarata, 1989). Generally, it consists of two distinct steps: "recognition" and "amplification."

Hence, a biosensor can be defined as a chemical sensor in which a biological sensing element is connected to a transducer (Figure 5.1). The biorecognition elements can be enzymes, antibodies, nucleic acids, aptamers, etc. The recognition system comprises a biochemical mechanism, such as an enzymatic reaction, antigen–antibody interaction, nucleic acid hybridization, etc. The transducer converts the magnitude of the biological reaction in a measurable signal that keeps a mathematical relationship with the analyte concentration. The signal measured by the transducer can be electrochemical, optical, or gravimetric.

Biosensors are considered as a cutting-edge technology, as they allow the development of fast and inexpensive analytical methods with desirable properties, such as specificity, sensitivity, reliability, portability, real-time analysis, ease of automation, and simplicity of operation.

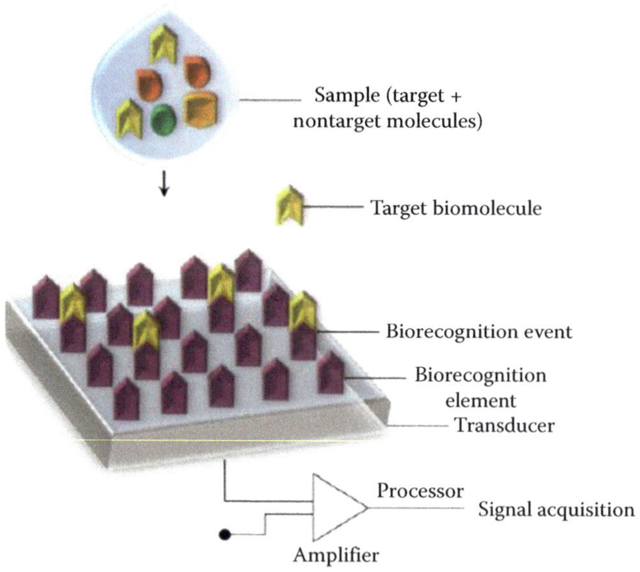


FIGURE 5.1 Classical representation of a general biosensor.

## 5.2 CLASSIFICATION OF BIOSENSORS

Biosensors can be classified according to different criteria, although the most widely used are the nature of the recognition event (scheme 1) and the physical principle of the transducer (scheme 2).

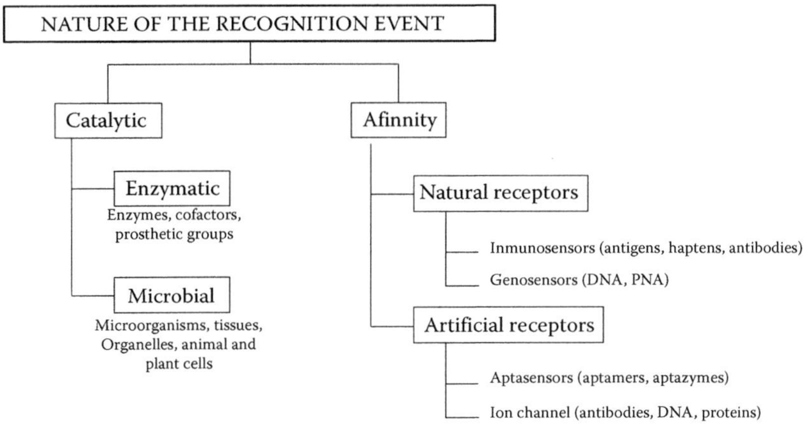


SCHEME 5.1 Classification of biosensors based on the nature of the recognition event.

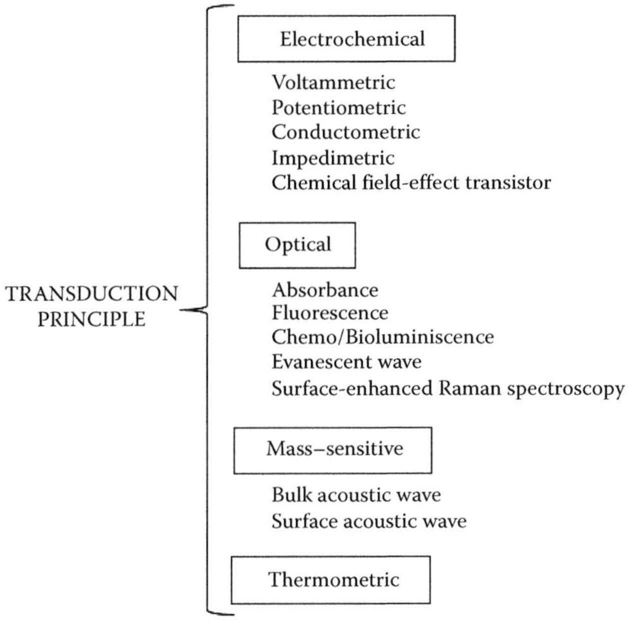


SCHEME 5.2 Classification of biosensors based on the transduction principle.

## 5.3 RECOGNITION EVENT

The biomolecules used for these purposes must comply with certain requirements to be used as sensor units; they must have affinity for the element being recognized, must be sufficiently selective to recognize this element in the presence of other compounds, and also must remain stable over time. Molecular recognition may involve the molecular bond between the receptor element and the recognized molecule (antigen-antibody) or a catalytic reaction (enzyme-substrate-product).

### 5.3.1 Catalytic Biosensors

They are based on biological catalysts, in which one or more substrates are involved, to generate one or several products. Once the process is completed, the biocatalyst is regenerated and it can be reused. These catalysts can be used to detect some of the components of the reaction, or indirectly to detect compounds that interfere in the reaction, by inhibiting the capabilities of the biocatalyst (Sánchez-Paniagua and Lopez-Ruiz, 2011; Sánchez-Paniagua et al., 2017).

### 5.3.2 Affinity Biosensors

In this case, the "analyte–recognition element" interaction involves the modification of an equilibrium in which an analyte-receptor complex is formed. In the absence of transformation of substrates into products, the monitoring of these interactions requires, in some cases, the use of markers. However, the inclusion of markers entails some drawbacks, which is why transduction systems sensitive to mass changes are increasing. Different types of bioaffinity reagents are currently used, such as antibodies, nucleic acids, aptamers, peptide nucleic acids (PNAs) receptors and ion channels, molecular imprinting polymers, etc. (Smuc et al., 2013; Patris et al., 2016).

#### *5.3.2.1 Immunosensors*

The fundamental basis of all immunosensors is the specific molecular recognition of immunogenic compounds by antibodies. Direct (non-labeled) and indirect (labeled) techniques can be employed to transduce the binding event. Potentiometry, ion-sensitive field-effect transitor (ISFET), impedance/conductance, surface plasmon resonance (SPR), and mass-sensitive techniques have been used for direct transduction. Indirect immunosensors are usually more sensitive, which involve the use of markers covalently attached to the antigen or to the antibody depending on the assay format. Competitive and noncompetitive assays can be designed. Among the latter, the most popular is the sandwich enzyme-linked immunoassay, which involves the use of two antibodies, one of them is enzyme-labeled. Competitive assays rely on the competition between ligands for a limited amount of antibody. These assays can be subdivided into homogeneous and heterogeneous depending on the need for phase separation to distinguish between labeled-reagent in excess and labeled-reagent forming the immunological complex. Homogeneous competitive assays involve a change in enzyme activity or fluorescent emission upon the binding event. Enzyme multiplied immunotechniques, fluorescent polarization immunoassay, or fluorescent energy transfer immunoassay are only a few examples of homogeneous competitive assays applicable to biosensors. In spite of the high affinity and selectivity of antibodies, their use presents several difficulties. They have to be produced in vivo by immunization of host animals, which takes time, and they can only be used under physiological or near physiological conditions due to denaturalization. The regeneration of the antibody is still a challenge because the binding is so strong that sometimes it becomes irreversible and can be reverted only at extreme (denaturating) conditions. The production of monoclonal antibodies was a breakthrough in this field due to their enhanced purity and lower cross-reactivity.

#### *5.3.2.2 Nucleic Acid-Sensors*

The advent of low-cost synthetic oligonucleotides opened the door to the use of nucleic acids as recognition elements for affinity biosensors. The recognition of a specific DNA sequence relies on the detection of the hybridization event. Ideally, these biosensors have to be able to distinguish a single mutation (a single mismatch) and be sensitive enough to detect very small amount of copies to avoid the use of amplification techniques such as polymerase chain reaction (PCR). These biosensors, also called genosensors, rely on the attachment of a single-stranded DNA (ssDNA), known as probe, onto the transducer surface to recognize its complementary sequence (target) through hybridization. The direct transduction of this event can be done by SPR, quartz crystal microbalance, (QCM), surface impedance measurements, and electrochemical oxidation of the nucleobases, which is a destructive method. Indirect transduction can be performed using the catalytic activity of nucleobases toward metal complexes, intercalation of fluorescent, or electroactive molecules into the double helix and through labeling of the target or the probe with an electroactive species, a fluorophore, or enzymes. It is also possible to carry out sandwich-type assays, which involve the use of a second, labeled probe that is complementary to part of the target. An attractive approach is the use of structured DNA such as molecular beacons. They are ssDNA molecules with hairpin secondary structure. The loop contains a sequence complementary to the target and the stem is a double-stranded sequence located at both sides of the probe sequence. The hairpin is immobilized onto the transducer by one arm and, in the opposite extreme or arm, there is usually a fluorophore, an electroactive compound or an enzyme covalently attached. In the absence of the complementary target, the hairpin remains closed and the electrochemical or optical signal is hindered. In the presence of the complementary target, the thermodynamic force leading to the formation of the double helix forces the hairpin to open and the analytical signal changes.

The hybridization event can also occur with an analog of ssDNA, the so-called peptide nucleic acid (PNA), first described in 1991. PNAs are composed of repeated peptide units linked by amido bonds that replace the sugar-phosphate backbone of nucleic acids. The nucleobases are covalently attached to the peptide skeleton at equal spacing to those in DNA. The lack of ribose makes them endonuclease-resistant and the neutral backbone stabilizes the double helix PNA-DNA because it avoids electrostatic repulsion occurring between natural single strands. Therefore, they exhibit enhanced stability at high temperatures (higher melting temperatures) and low ionic strengths and offer greater mismatch discrimination (Wang., 1998).

#### *5.3.2.3 Aptasensors*

Aptamers are a special type of ssDNA or RNA oligonucleotide sequences that recognize a specific target by adopting a different three-dimensional structure in the presence of that molecule. In that sense, they mimic the behavior of antibodies with several advantages over them, which suggests that aptasensors can rival or even replace immunosensors in the near future. These artificial nucleic acid sequences were identified in the beginning of the 90s by using a selection process called systhematic evolution of ligand by exponential enrichment (SELEX) (Ellington and Szostak., 1990). They are chemically synthesized, which ensures high purity. They can be selected to work in stringent conditions and with affinity binding constants similar to antibodies, although the most promising feature is their reversible denaturation, which permits easy regeneration. Detection strategies using aptasensors are analogous to immunosensors (Navani and Li., 2006). The detection of high molecular weight molecules is easier because the binding affinity is usually higher and causes larger conformational changes that can be exploited for transduction.

## 5.4 METHODS OF IMMOBILIZATION

The biological component has to be intimately connected to the transducer without detriment in the access of the analyte and the catalytic activity of enzymes or binding sites in the affinity sensors. It is a complex and decisive step in the development of the biosensor. Among the wide variety of immobilization methods that exist in the literature, the most common are physical adsorption, covalent attachment, entrapment inside of polymer matrices or indirect coupling by self-assembled monolayers and intermediate biomolecular species (Sassolas et al., 2012). Adsorption is undoubtedly the simplest strategy, widely used for being fast and inexpensive. Other strategies seek to increase the amount of biomolecules near the surface or have them in a more organized, stable manner. Microencapsulation, for example, involves the use of membranes to keep the receptor in close proximity to the transducer. Entrapment in polymeric matrices, gels, or pastes is a very simple and efficient method of immobilization that is also aimed at bettering receptor-to-transducer contact. Covalent attachment, on the other hand, is a common approach because the strong nature of the chemical bonds formed between the biological component and the transducer usually results in highly organized and stable layers of the biological material. Another frequently used method is the cross-linking method, in which a bifunctional reagent is used to anchor the biological component to the transducer. These methods and more specific ones will be explained in detail in the following sections.

## 5.5 TRANSDUCTION PRINCIPLE

Transducers are able to measure changes induced by the biochemical reaction in the physicochemical properties of the system. There are several types of transducers depending on the nature of these changes, which can be electrochemical, optical, piezoelectric, or thermometric. The primary signal is transduced in a secondary one that can be amplified, filtered, displayed, etc.

### 5.5.1 Electrochemical Biosensors

The transducer is an electrode in contact with the biorecognition element. There is a wide variety of electrode subtracts suitable for the development of biosensors, such as platinum, gold, carbon-based materials (pyrolytic graphite, glassy carbon, carbon paste, boron-doped diamond, and recently, carbon nanotubes and graphene), indium-tin oxide (ITO), and fluoride-doped tin oxide (FTO), among others. Other mixed materials called composites are also common. Electrodes can present any configuration, from bulk to screen-printed electrodes.

Depending on the measured electrical magnitude, electrochemical biosensors can be divided into the following subgroups (Grieshaber et al., 2008).

#### *5.5.1.1 Voltammetric*

Voltammetric techniques involve the application of a potential (E) to an electrode and the measurement of the resulting current (i) flowing through the electrochemical cell. The applied potential forces changes in the concentration of an electroactive species at the electrode surface by electrochemically reducing or oxidizing it. In some cases, a specific potential is applied and the current is monitored over a period of time (amperometric biosensors), or the potential can be varied according to some predefined waveform that is electronically modulated (voltammetric biosensors). The latter has the possibility of improving greatly the sensitivity by introducing a preconcentration step, as it is the case of voltammetric redisolution methods.

#### *5.5.1.2 Potentiometric*

These techniques are based on the monitoring of the interfacial potential difference between a reference and an indicator electrode when no significant current passes through them. Ion-selective and gas-selective electrodes are the most common examples.

#### *5.5.1.3 Conductimetric/Impedimetric*

In this type of transduction, an alternating voltage is applied across two electrodes and the alternating current response is measured. Conductance or impedance is currently calculated using a frequency response analyzer. This transduction is used when changes in ionic strength are produced as consequence of the biological reaction.

Electrochemical impedance spectroscopy (EIS) is a powerful tool for monitoring changes in interfacial properties of the electrode surface upon a biorecognition event. This technique requires the presence of a redox probe in the electrolyte solution. The working electrode is biased at the formal potential of the redox probe, and the electron/charge transfer resistance ($R_{et}$ or $R_{ct}$) is calculated from the faradaic impedance spectrum obtained at different frequencies usually in the form of Nyquist plot. Changes in the mass of the interfacial electrode/solution cause changes in $R_{ct}$, which are related to the analyte concentration in solution (Lisdat and Schafer, 2008).

#### *5.5.1.4 Chemical-sensitive Field Effect Transistor*

They are classical metal-oxide-semiconductor field-effect transistors (MOSFETs), where the charge on the gate is regulated by a chemical interaction between the analyte and the active coating of the gate, leading to changes in the source-drain current. Ion selective field-effect transistors (ISFETs) are composed of an ion-selective membrane applied to the insulating gate. The potential of the gate is dependent on the electrical charge of the interface, and it is influenced by pH changes in its close vicinity. The immobilization of enzymes on the gate surface, whose activity is accompanied by a change in pH, turned those devices into enzyme FET biosensors (Dzyadvych et al., 2006). Not only enzymes but also antibodies (immunological FET) or DNA have been immobilized onto the gate of ISFETs or MOSFETs devices.

### 5.5.2 Optical Biosensors

They are based on changes in the optical properties of the system as a result of the interaction of the analyte and the biorecognition layer. A breakthrough in the development of optical biosensors was the implementation of optical fibers in the 60s and 70s as waveguides, because they permit remote and in vivo sensing (medical applications). The probe containing the biological component is called optode or optrode from the term "optical electrode," so that the recognition element is immobilized at one of its end and the detection system in the other end. Changes in optical properties propagate through the optical fiber to the detection system, usually a phototube or a photomultiplier. There are varieties of optical fibers configurations available for any optical technique and currently most optical biosensors are based on this kind of transducers. Optical biosensors can be classified according with the sensing principles on which they are based.

#### *5.5.2.1 Absorbance*

They are based on the changes in the intensity of the light due to the absorptivity of the analyte itself or other species after the reaction with an indicator. Since absorption of light from a monochromatic source follows the Lambert-Beer's law, there is a linear relationship between the absorbance and the concentration of the absorbing species (sometimes the analyte) that can be directly related to the concentration of the analyte.

#### *5.5.2.2 Fluorescence*

The light emitted by a molecule previously irradiated is measured. When the analyte is not fluorescent by itself, it can be labeled with a fluorophore. An alternative and widely extended approach takes advantage of the interaction between the analyte and another molecule causing a variation in the emission of fluorescence (quenching or energy transfer). The quencher species can be another fluorophore or an acceptor that absorbs the excitation or the emitted light. Quantum dots have attracted great attention as fluorescent molecules due to their photostability, tunable color by modifying the size and material and high quantum yields (Wolfbeis., 2005).

#### *5.5.2.3 Chemo/Electro/Bioluminescence*

Luminescence is the light produced by an excited species returning to the ground state. If this reaction is catalyzed by an enzyme or takes place in a microorganism, the process is called bioluminiscence. A similar phenomenon called electrochemiluminescence (ECL) (Richter., 2004) occurs when a potential is applied to an electrode, and the resulting oxidized or reduced species participate in the reaction yielding the excited species. The instrumentation is clearly reduced in comparison to other optical techniques because neither a monochromator nor light source is required.

#### *5.5.2.4 Evanescent Wave Biosensors*

They exploit the total internal reflection of light at a surface–solution interface to produce an electromagnetic field extending a short distance into solution, which is a surface-sensitive physical phenomenon. One of the most popular techniques within this group is SPR, which responds with high sensitivity to changes in the dielectric constant of the adjacent medium, and consequently, to the refractive index. This feature makes it very suitable for detecting the formation of affinity complexes such as antigen-antibody or hybridization event between complementary DNA strands. This technique is based on the transfer of energy from photons to a cloud of electrons (plasmons) of a metal surface when the energy of the former matches exactly the quantum energy level of the plasmons. Resonant mirror (RM), ellipsometry, and interferometry are also used in biosensing but their contribution is limited. The exponential decay of evanescent wave implies a penetration depth of only a few nanometers, which is a very interesting feature to discriminate between adsorbed and bulk solution species with no need of separation (Daghestani and Day, 2010). Figure 5.2 illustrates the schematic of a SPR and the method of detecting the formation or dissociation of an affinity complex.

### 5.5.3 Mass-sensitive Biosensors

Piezoelectric biosensors are a type of mechanical biosensors that use the piezoelectric effect, i.e., the production of electricity/acoustic waves caused by mechanical stress or pressure (Pohanka, M., 2017). Piezoelectric materials typically include quartz, lithium tantalite, and lead zirconate titanate. The biosensing principle relies on applying an alternating current or radio frequency excitation to electrodes patterned on a piezoelectric material, which generates an acoustic wave that propagates in the direction perpendicular to the surface of the material. Such propagation takes place either into the bulk medium [bulk acoustic wave (BAW)] or along the surface of the material [surface acoustic wave (SAW)] (Fu et al., 2017). The use of this technique for biosensing is owed to the fact that wave oscillation can be affected by biomolecular events occurring at the electrode surface. There is a linear relationship between changes in resonance frequency and mass accumulation. Therefore, such frequency shifts are measured and related to the mass load, serving as a "nanogravimetric" system. QCM are the most commonly used BAW devices for biosensing and are made of a bulk piezoelectric material, i.e., a quartz crystal sandwiched between two metallic electrodes, typically gold. Biorecognition elements are commonly immobilized onto the gold surface.

### 5.5.4 Thermometric Biosensors

Thermometric biosensors or thermistors are capable of measuring the variation in temperature of the biocatalytic reaction, which is directly related to the concentration of the

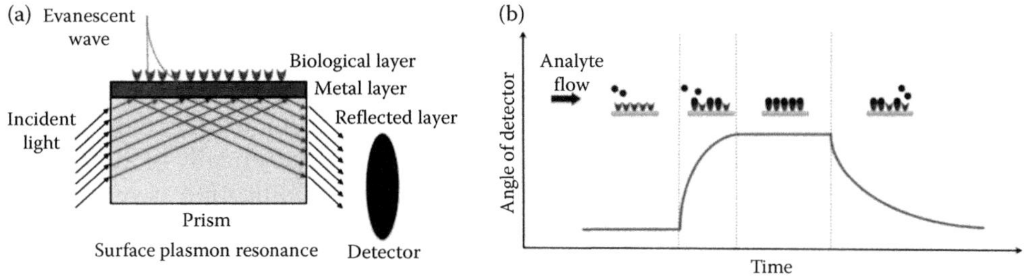


FIGURE 5.2 (a) Schematic of a surface plasmon resonance (SPR) biosensor (Kretchmann configuration). Light reflected from a prism induces an evanescent field in both the metal and dielectric (biological) layer, with the field being greater in the latter. Light is then reflected out of the prism and a detector records the angle at which resonance is satisfied. (b) Detection of binding events for SPR and RM. As analyte begins to flow over the sensing layer and binds to substrate, the angle of reflectivity that satisfies the resonance condition will change accordingly until it reaches saturation and all the binding sites have been occupied. The dissociation of analyte from the substrate causes the angle of the detector to return to baseline once all the analyte has been completely removed. [Reproduced from Daghestani and Day, 2010 (open access)].

analyte. For analytical purposes, almost all thermistors make use of enzymatic reactions as biochemically selective heat generators (enzyme thermistors). They present the advantages of working in flow injection systems with no electrochemical, optical or by-product interferences. Differential measurements improve sensitivity by using two-reaction columns, one of them with an immobilized enzyme and the other as a reference with no enzyme. The temperature probe is encased in an aluminum block to avoid ambient temperature fluctuations.

### 5.5.5 Nanomechanic Biosensors

Microcantilevers can transduce a number of different phenomena, such as changes of mass, temperature, heat, or stress, into bending (static mode) or a change in resonant frequency (dynamic mode), which can be monitored. Adsorption of molecules, when they are restricted to one of the cantilever surfaces, produces differential surface stress that bends the cantilever. At the same time, the resonant frequency of the cantilever also varies due to mass loading. The bending and the changes in resonant frequency can be monitored by several techniques, with optical beam deflection, piezoresistivity, piezoelectricity, interferometry, capacitance, and electron tunneling among the most important ones (Carrascosa et al., 2006). Microcantilevers are typically made of silicon/silicon nitride or polymer materials, with dimensions ranging from tens to hundred of μm long, some tens of μm wide and hundreds of nm thick. High-throughput platforms using arrays of cantilevers have been developed for simultaneous measurement and read-out of hundreds of samples. Figure 5.3 illustrate a schematic representation of the microcantilever-based biosensor and a sequential readout of microcantilever arrays.

## 5.6 BIOSENSORS AS PLATFORMS FOR GENETICALLY MODIFIED ORGANISM DETECTION

In order to reveal the presence of genetically modified organisms (GMOs) in food, two classical approaches can be used in the development of biosensors based on the detection of two kinds of macromolecules, DNA or protein. The most common detection approach relies on the knowledge that part of the genetic information in genetically modified plants differs from that of the wild type line. Thus, the genetic modification is by definition detectable at the DNA level. The second approach involves the detection of the new protein(s) encoded by the inserted trait gene via immunoassays. However, given their, generally, lesser stability, proteins are not considered suitable for GMO detection in a wide range of products (e.g., processed food/feed) (Holst-Jensen et al., 2012). Therefore, most of the papers available in the literature nowadays have focused on DNA detection for GMO monitoring.

According to the DNA targets present in GMOs, DNA-based methods can be categorized into different levels of specificity (Figure 5.4) (Holst-Jensen):

a. *Screening methods*, which are the least specific methods because the targets include common DNA elements in GMOs, such as promoters and terminators that are present in many different events. Sometimes, marker genes are also used as screening targets, such as the nptII gene.

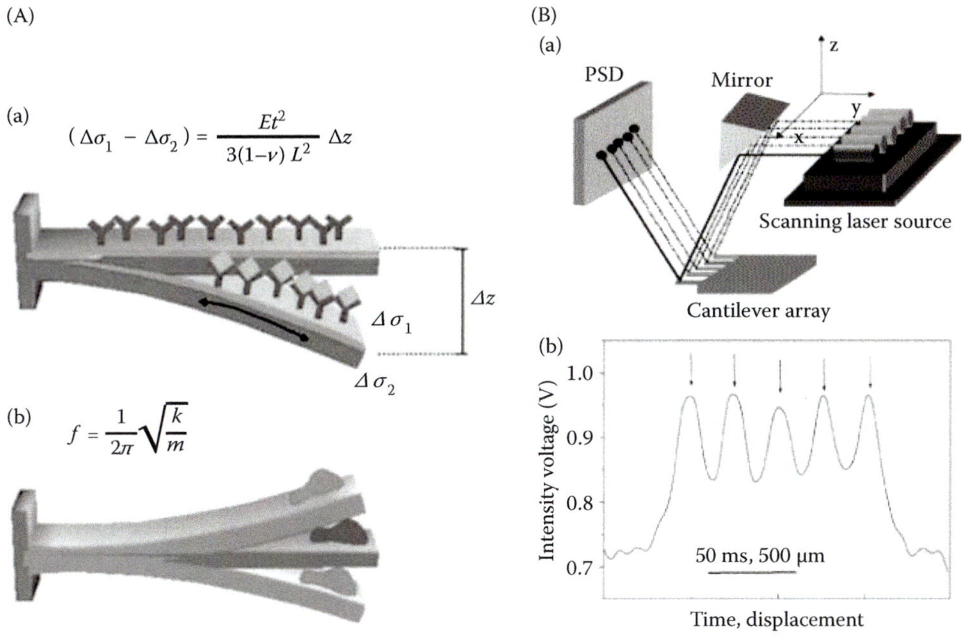


FIGURE 5.3 (A) Schematic representation of the microcantilever-based biosensor working principles, (a) static mode and, (b) dynamic mode. [Reproduced from Alvarez y Lechuga., 2010, with permission from Royal Society of Chemistry]. (B) (a) Schematic depiction of the technique for sequential readout of microcantilever arrays. (b) Experimental measurement of the total intensity of the position-sensitive optical detector as function of the laser beam position and time. Intensity maxima correspond with the laser beam positions, in which each cantilever is illuminated. The experiment was performed with an array composed of five silicon cantilevers with a length of 400 µm, a width of 100 µm, and thickness of about 1 µm. [Reproduced from Alvarez y Tamayo, 2005, with permission from Elsevier].

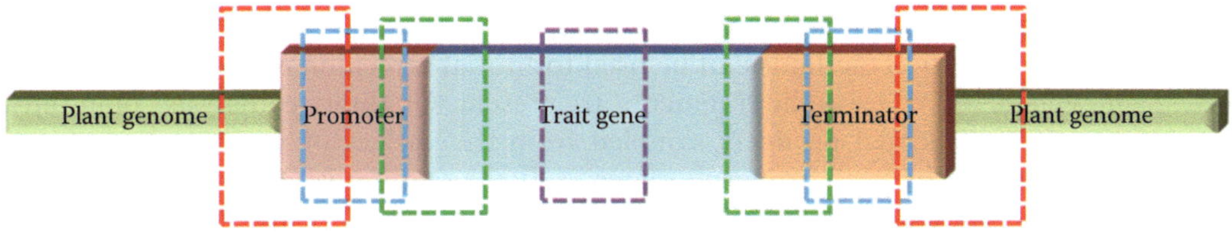


FIGURE 5.4 Levels of specificity of GMO methods based on the targeted DNA region: screening (blue dashed square), gene-specific (purple square), construct-specific (green), and event-specific (red) [Adapted from Holst-Jensen et al., 2012 with permission from Elsevier].

b. *Gene-specific methods*, which detect a part of the trait gene associated with the specific genetic modification. Examples are the Bt or the CP4 5-enolpyruvylshikimate-3-phosphate synthase (EPSPS) genes. If a positive signal is obtained, the presence of GM-related sequences is highly probable, but it is not possible to identify the specific GM crop because the trait gene can be used in different transformation events. Both screening and gene-specific methods are based on DNA sequences present in nature so the risk of obtaining false positives increases significantly.

c. *Construct-specific methods*, which target the junction between two DNA elements, such as the promoter-trait gene or trait gene-terminator. As these methods target DNA sequences that are not present in nature, their presence ensures that the sample contain a GMO. However, different GMOs may share the same constructs. Such is the case for two distinct GMO maize, MON809 and MON810, which have the same promoter-trait gene junction.
d. *Event-specific methods*, which provide the highest level of specificity because the target is the unique junction, characteristic of each event, found at the integration locus between the inserted DNA construct and the recipient genome. Although, stacked events cannot be distinguished with these methods.

While in enzymatic biosensors the sample-to-measurement process is usually short and ideally no pretreatment is required, this is not the case for DNA biosensors. DNA brings an entirely different scenario: samples must be processed to isolate genomic DNA from cell components and other matrix-derived interfering species (e.g., carbohydrates and phenols, usually present in food samples). Figure 5.5 shows a schematic diagram of this process. The genetic material must be extracted from a sample in the form of supercoiled genomic DNA of great size. The target sequence represents a small fragment of this complex genomic structure. Hybridization directly using genomic DNA is unlikely to be efficient on the electrode surface due to steric effects. Moreover, in the case of processed food samples, DNA is extracted in ultralow quantities. Hence, target size restriction and amplification are necessary to reach detectable levels of the analyte, both of which can be accomplished via PCR. In some cases, if the biosensor surface is not specific enough against physical adsorption or other types of nonspecific interactions that could lead to high background currents, then amplified DNA must be purified post-PCR. However, to this day surface chemistries have been extensively optimized to surpass this problem. Finally, detection of the amplicons takes place. The whole process can take approximately from one to three days, depending on the protocol for sensor fabrication, which can involve overnight procedures and/or lingered nanoparticle synthesis/bioconjugations in the case of nanoparticle-labeled strategies.

Qualitative detection methods can be used for initial screening of food products, to investigate whether GMO specific fragments are present. Qualitative analysis could thus be performed on packaged products sampled from the shelves of supermarkets, from stocks at the supply chain or from raw material. If the qualitative analysis provides an indication of the presence of GMOs, a subsequent quantitative test might give a decisive answer concerning the labeling requirement (Querci et al., 2006).

The steps involved in the design of a genosensor are: (i) transducer selection, (ii) target-sequence selection, (iii) selection of a convenient probe-immobilization strategy; and (iv) evaluation of labeling marks and detection methods. (Lucarelli et al., 2004).

Although several transducers have been used in biosensors and genosensors, as far as we know, only DNA biosensors with optical, piezoelectric, and electrochemical transduction have been successfully developed for the detection of GMO sequences, as was recently reviewed by Arugula and Simonian (2016). However, electroanalytical techniques provide important advantages, such as relative simplicity, low cost of equipment, and automatic on-line and portable options.

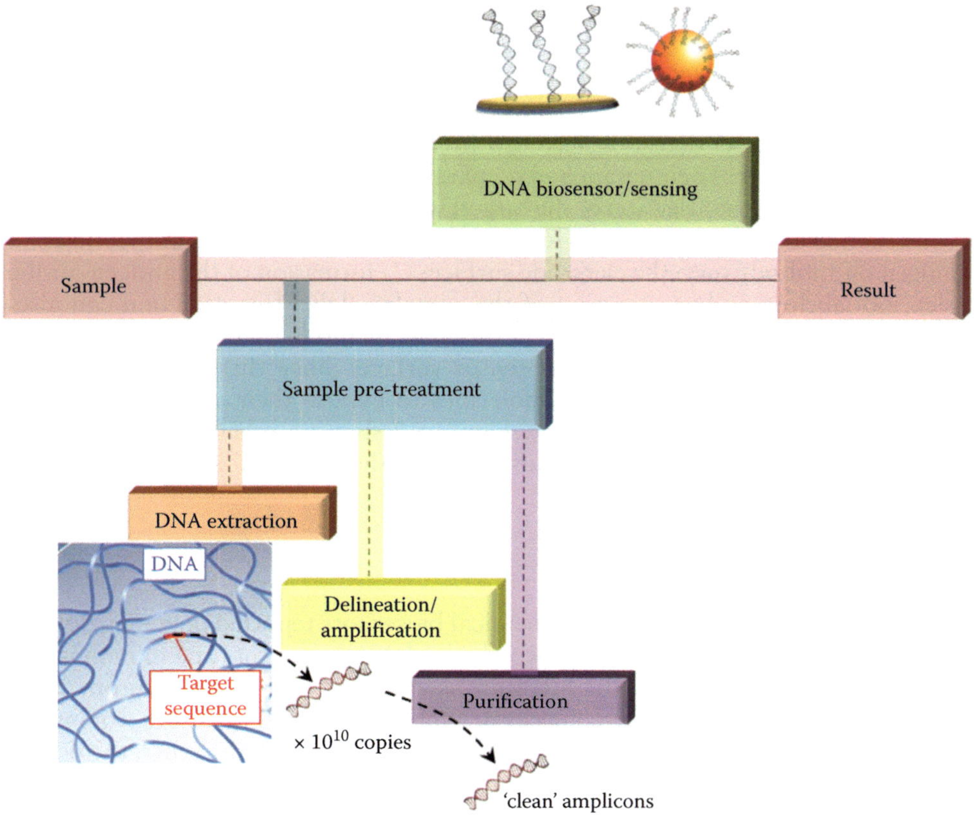


FIGURE 5.5 Analytical overview of DNA detection with electrochemical biosensors/sensing platforms from the sample to the final result.

In GMO detection, the selection of the target sequence is relatively easy. It depends on the aim of the assay (i.e., screening, qualitative or quantitative). The nucleic acid sequences of authorized or pre-evaluated transformed plants are well characterized and described in open-access databases (http://www.gmo-compass.org/eng/gmo/db/, http://gmo-crl.jrc.ec.europa.eu/gmomethods/, and http://gmdd.shgmo.org/). The taxon-specific or reference genes have also been described in official PCR methods, which are necessary for the relative quantification of GMOs and for species identification.

The probe immobilization step plays a major role in determining the performance of a DNA biosensor. Control of the surface chemistry and coverage is crucial for the analytical performance of DNA biosensors. The key features of DNA-modified surfaces are DNA density and hybridization accessibility (Kasry et al., 2009). Moreover, the immobilization chemistry should be sufficiently specific for probe binding and offer efficient surface blockage in order to avoid unspecific adsorption by other molecular species (e.g., proteins, short oligonucleotides, genomic DNA, etc.).

Two kinds of formats can be used for the detection of the target DNA sequence: direct or indirect, also called sandwich assay. The direct assay consists of a capture probe complementary to the analyte sequence, this assay requires the labeling of one of the two DNA involved sequences, the analyte or the capture probe. The most common is the sandwich assay, which involves two probes, a capture probe partially complementary to the target and anchored to the electrode, and a labeled signaling probe that hybridizes with the rest of the target. The steps involved in the design of electrochemical genosensors are illustrated in Figure 5.6.

Although DNA is the most frequently used target in GMO detection, the use of immunosensors in GMO detection has also been described and will also be discussed throughout this chapter. Their design and preparation hold similarities with DNA biosensors, except regarding the selection of the target, which in this case is a protein or peptide. The construction of an immunosensor involves the following stages: (1) immobilization of the antigen or antibody onto the electrode surface; (2) formation of the antigen-antibody complex; (3) labeling and/or detection of the complex (label-free detection can also be done). Antibodies can be immobilized via different methods that can yield oriented or randomly-distributed antibodies on the sensor surface. Since these glycoproteins only have one binding site, orienting these molecules to expose their antigen-binding fraction can improve biosensor performance. Figure 5.7 shows a schematic diagram of the oriented (A) and not oriented (B) immunosensors (Malvano et al., 2016).

### 5.6.1 Electrochemical Biosensors

Considering the high amount of electrochemical biosensors reported up to date for GMO monitoring, we have divided them into two blocks: DNA biosensors and immunosensors. In the case of DNA biosensors, the literature is extensive and varied. On one hand, a subclassification was thus considered necessary for this type of biosensors, comprehending electrode modification and immobilization strategies, and on the other, the detection

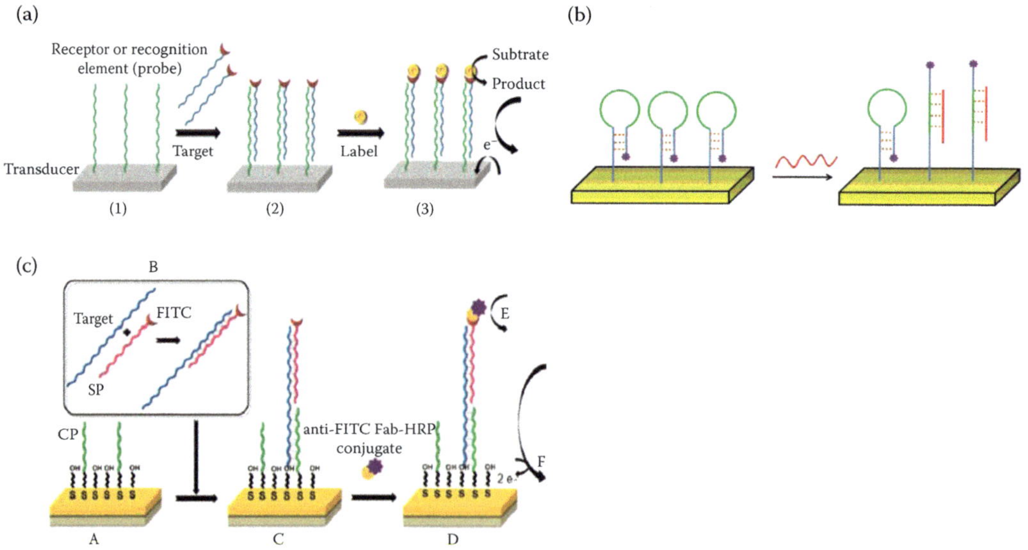


FIGURE 5.6 Steps in the design of genosensors: (a) direct assay with labeled target [Reproduced from Manzanares-Palenzuela et al., 2015a, with permission from Elsevier], (b) direct assay with labeled hairpin capture probe. [Reproduced from Pursey et al., 2017 (open access)] and (c) sandwich assay. [Adapted from Martín-Fernández et al., 2014, with permission from Elsevier].

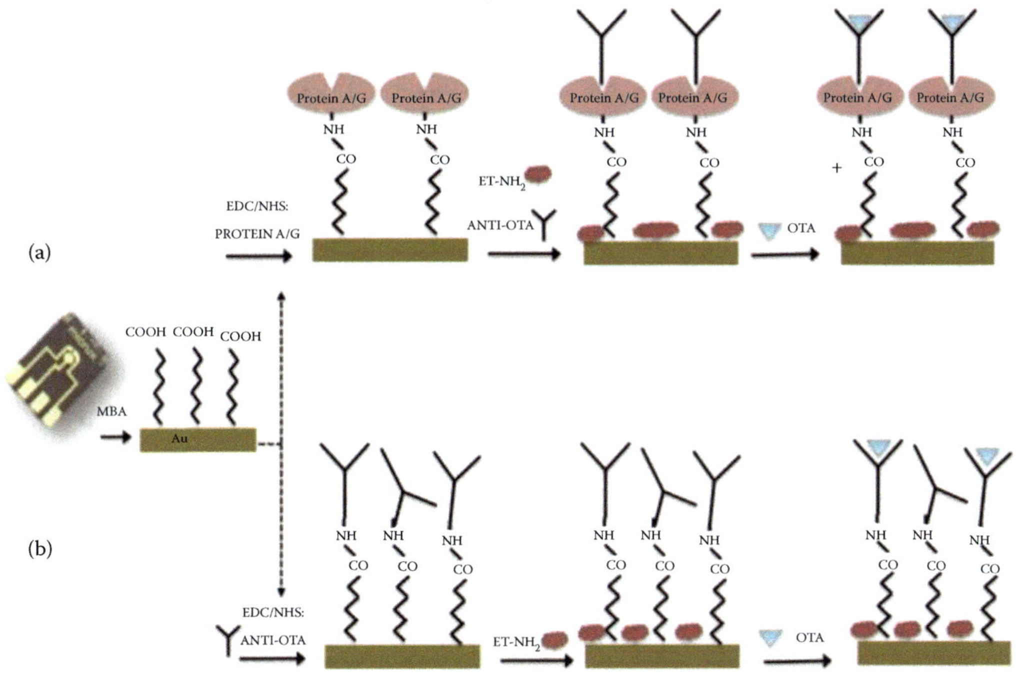


FIGURE 5.7 Schematic diagram of the oriented (a) and not oriented (b) immunosensors. [Reproduced from Malvano et al., 2016, with permission from Elsevier].

strategies. All according to the level of specificity (screening, gene-specific, and event-specific biosensors) for a more comprehensive reading.

#### *5.6.1.1 DNA Biosensors*

Half of the reported DNA sensors are screening methods, i.e., methods with the least specificity level in GMO testing. In some cases, gene-specific methods have been anchored to screening assays with the goal of reducing false positive results. Some authors have reported the simultaneous determination of nitric oxide synthase (NOS) and phosphinothricin acetyltransferase (PAT) gene fragments using genosensors (Yang et al., 2007a; Yang et al., 2008; Jiang et al., 2008; Yang et al., 2009). Fewer works were based on event-specific biosensors (Duwensee et al., 2009; Mix et al., 2012; Liao et al., 2013, Sun et al., 2013; Sun et al., 2014, Manzanares-Palenzuela et al., 2015b, ). Moreover, most GMO genosensors have been applied to the analysis of powdered plant tissues, whereas only a few articles assessed the analysis of commercial food and feed products (Manzanares-Palenzuela et al., 2017).

*5.6.1.1.1 Electrode Modification and Immobilization Strategies* Gold and carbon electrodes are among the most popular electrode materials employed in the development of DNA sensors. The reason gold is widely used is most likely to be the spontaneous and robust self-assembly of thiols and other sulfur-containing compounds onto gold surfaces, which can be used to covalently immobilize thiolated DNA (Lucarelli et al., 2004). Yet, conventional gold electrodes require tedious and time-consuming mechanical and chemical procedures to regenerate a new bare surface. The availability of disposable printed, photolithographed, and screen-printed gold electrodes (Carpini et al., 2004; Lucarelli et al.,

2005) has greatly facilitated genosensing protocols. On the other hand, glassy paste electrodes (GPE) and carbon paste electrodes (CPE), respectively), also widespread materials used in the design of genosensors, are advantageous because they have a wide potential window, they are chemically inert and can be modified with a wide variety of surface chemistries and procedures. In contrast to the relatively complicated modifications of solid substrates, carbon pastes can be easily modified to obtain sensors with predefined properties. Glassy carbon combines glassy and ceramic properties with those of graphite, conferring the electrodes high temperature and chemical resistance. Screen-printed carbon electrodes (SPCE) are also commercially available, eliminating the need of surface regeneration and allowing portable on-field analysis.

Other materials have been incorporated in the design of GMO genosensors in recent years, such as conductive polymers and carbon nanotubes (CNTs), due to their high electrical conductivity and long-term stability. In addition, CNTs show very good mechanical strength (Balasubramanian and Burghard, 2005). The ability of CNTs-modified electrodes to promote electron-transfer reactions has been reported in connection with many important biomolecules. The use of multi-wall carbon nanotubes (MWCNTs)-doped polypyrrole (PPy) on gold interdigitated electrodes for 35S detection have been reported (Lien et al., 2010). The combination of Ppy and CNTs enhances charge density, electrical conductivity, and electrocatalytic activity compared to both individually.

Taking into account the number of GMO events authorized worldwide nowadays, one of the most important challenges in the field of GMO testing is the development of multiplex analysis. In this sense, electrode arrays provide a great platform for a complete and fast analysis. These types of multiplex sensors have been reported in the literature and will be discussed in the following sections.

5.6.1.1.1.1. Screening biosensors Most of the reported works have been focused on the detection of the 35S promoter, which represents the main inserted fragment in transgenic constructs and therefore the model target for GMO screening.

Thiol-based self-assembled monolayers (SAMs) are the most common approach with gold electrodes. In order to control the density of the immobilized thiol capture probe on the electrode surface, in such a way that unspecific adsorptions of nucleotide bases can be prevented without hindering the access of the target sequence, a second thiol component, usually mercaptohexanol (MCH) is added to the surface.

There are several examples of this type of designs. Carpini et al. (2004) proposed it for the detection of 35S using a mixed monolayer of a 25-mer thiolated DNA probe and MCH. Wang et al. (2009) reported a similar strategy for the detection of a specific fragment of nptII (253-mer), amplified from genomic DNA of transgenic plants by PCR and used as target sequence for sandwich hybridization with the immobilized capture probe and a biotinylated signaling probe. Another SAM-based approach involves the immobilization of the target sequence instead of the capture probe and a subsequent step of hybridization with a DNA probe. An example of this approach was proposed by Sun et al (2007), aimed at detecting NOS fragments. In this case, the formation of a SAM with mercaptoethanol onto a gold electrode surface is proposed. The covalent linkage of DNA onto the SAM/Au was achieved via phosphate ester linkage between the 5′-phosphate group of the target DNA sequence (20-mer) and the hydroxyl group of mercaptoethanol.

Carbodiimide coupling has also been widely used for DNA immobilization. There are three different types of covalent coupling activated by carbodiimide (a) hydroxyl, (b) amino-terminated SAMs coupled to the 5′-phosphate end of DNA and (c) carboxyl-terminated SAMs coupled to the 3′-hydroxy end of the nucleic acid.

Amino-terminated SAMs for immobilizing 5′-phosphate capture probes were developed for the detection of 35S and NOS. 21-mer ssDNA probes were immobilized on cysteamine SAM-modified gold electrode surfaces by covalent binding in the presence of 1-ethyl-3(3′-dimethylaminopropyl)-carbodiimide (EDC) and *N*-hydroxysulfosuccinimide (NHS) as activators (Tichoniuk et al., 2008).

Another kind of carbodiimide coupling was used by Zhu et al. (2008) for the detection of NOS sequences. After a mercaptoacetic acid SAM was formed on the electrode surface, covalent immobilization of the DNA probe was done through the carboxylate ester formed between the 3′-hydroxy end of the DNA and the carboxylic group of mercaptoacetic acid, using NHS and EDC.

Zhan et al. (2017) developed a biosensor for the detection of 35S based on a molecular beacon end-labeled *in situ* with an electroactive copper crown cycle. First, the modified hairpin-structured capture probe, thiolated on one end, was immobilized onto the gold disk surface *via* SAM chemistry (without spacer thiols as backfillers). Second, the "crown cycle," namely 4′- aminobenzo-18-crown (AbC), was covalently grafted on the 5′-carboxylic acid end of the capture probe through carbodiimide coupling. The AbC-probe modified electrode was then incubated in $Cu(NO_3)_2$ to achieve the assembly of electroactive $Cu^{2+}$, coordinated within the AbC molecule. Hybridization with the target sequence resulted in a drop of the electrochemical signal of the AbC-$Cu^{2+}$ label recorded by differential pulse voltammetry (DPV), given that the hairpin "opens up" to hybridize with its complementary sequence pushing the electroactive molecule further away from the electrode surface.

Compared to the works described with gold electrodes, genosensors using carbon electrodes exhibit a wide variety of immobilization strategies, such as electrodeposition, adsorption onto polymer films, polymer-carbon nanotubes surfaces, etc. This versatility, along with the low chemical reactivity and wide potential window, results in the extended use of carbon electrodes as transduction platforms.

Kerman et al. (2006) used direct immobilization of a 25-mer capture probe, complementary to a 35S fragment, onto a glassy carbon electrode surface by adsorption.

Ligaj et al. described a DNA sensor for the detection of nptII gene (Ligaj et al., 2003). A 92-mer fragment of nptII gene and a capture probe of 21-mer were used. The DNA probe was immobilized on a carbon paste electrode surface by electrodeposition.

Meric et al (2004) described a genosensor based on disposable SPCE for NOS detection based on the immobilization of a 25-mer DNA probe and hybridization with the target, both under held potential.

Although it is easy to immobilize DNA probes by adsorption, the immobilized oligonucleotides could be attached on multiple sites, resulting in a lower reactivity for hybridization and a decrease in the specificity of the recognition layer. In addition, some of the probes could leave the support during the assay.

Covalent immobilization of DNA exhibits some advantages, especially when nucleic acid chains are intentionally bound to the electrode surface only by one end, which ensures structural flexibility and increases hybridization efficiency without DNA leakage. To achieve this with glassy carbon surfaces, most papers have reported the use of a connector for one-site covalent immobilization.

Xu et al. reported a DNA sensor for detection of 35S (20-mer) (Xu et al., 2006) comparing two immobilization strategies for the immobilization of a 20-mer DNA probe: 1) directly on a bare GCE and 2) introducing an ethylenediamine onto an electrochemically oxidized GCE (EDA/GCE). EDA was employed as a connector to introduce amino groups on the GCE for one-site covalent immobilization of probes in the presence of EDC and NHS. Results obtained with CV measurements showed that ssDNA immobilized on the EDA/GCE hybridized with the target more effectively than that immobilized via adsorption directly on the bare GCE. This connector seemed to increase DNA mobility and improved the approachability of the complementary DNA.

More recent approaches involve the use of hybrid material based on nanoparticles and polymers for DNA immobilization. These complex matrices enhance the electron transfer process and increase the active surface. An overall improvement in sensitivity is often obtained.

A regenerable electrochemical DNA biosensor based on a new type of acrylic microspheres and gold nanoparticles (AuNPs) composite coated onto a screen-printed electrode (SPE) has been successfully developed by Ulianas et al., 2014 for specific determination of the 35S promoter gene in soybean. DNA probe was immobilized onto acrylic microspheres via covalent bonding. The presence of modified genes in soybean was detected via hybridization of cauliflower mosaic virus (CaMV) 35S gene-modified DNA with the immobilized DNA probe, which was monitored by DPV using anthraquinone-2-sulfonic acid monohydrate sodium salt as redox indicator during hybridization event.

Xie et al. proposed a DNA electrochemical biosensor fabricated with cetyltrimethylammonium bromide modified-semicondutive PbSe nanoparticles and chitosan composite films (nanoPbSe-chitosan) on the electrode. Chitosan has good biocompatibility and affinity toward DNA, allowing the adsorption of the capture probe in the modified electrode (Xie et al., 2008).

In another report, a Pt-nanoparticles-based platform was electrochemically formed onto a GCE surface. The capture probe (19-mer) for 35S detection was immobilized on the nanoPt/GCE surface by adsorption (Mao-Qing et al., 2008).

Yang et al (2012a) reported a sensor for the quantitative determination the less common promoter, the PEP gene, by EIS detection. Polytyramine films were electropolymerized on a GCE surface, followed by electrodeposition of Au-Pt nanoparticles. Immobilization of $NH_2$-modified capture probe (20-mer) on the electrode was done due to the affinity of amino groups toward Au-Pt nanoparticles. Potential-controlled hybridization was carried out. As it was shown by CV results, the combination of Au and Pt nanoparticles produced an increased $[Fe(CN)_6]^{3-/4-}$ redox activity compared to polytyramine alone and both metals alone. This confirms a conductivity synergistic effect with these nanoaggregates.

Wang et al. (2016) reported the use of gold nanoparticles-decorated multiwalled carbon nanotube-reduced graphene oxide nanoribbon (Au NPs/MWCNT-rGONR) composites for 35S detection using EIS. The nanocomposite was dropcasted onto the bare GCE surface, followed by probe immobilization *via* electrostatic interaction.

Aghili et al. (2017) recently proposed the use of exfoliated graphene oxide (EGO) and gold nano-urchins (GNU) for the modification of the SPCE, as well as the use of hematoxylin as electroactive intercalator. The working electrode was modified by dropcasting EGO, followed by GNU. A thiolated capture probe was immobilized *via* thiol-gold chemistry, followed by backfilling with MCH.

5.6.1.1.1.2. Gene-specific biosensors Frequently, gene-specific methods are anchored to screening assays with the goal of reducing false positive results. For example, a given sample could be positive for the presence of 35S, however this does not ensure that the sample contains GMOs. If a gene-specific test performed on the same sample gives a positive result for a trait gene such as PAT, then the conclusion from both methods indicate that the sample is very likely to contain a GMO. Most genosensors based on gene-specific detection use PAT gene (herbicide resistance) as target and include a screening procedure consisting on PCR amplification and detection of NOS gene. Another commonly inserted gene in genetically engineered food is the Bt gene obtained from *Bacillus thuringiensis*.

Ren et al. (2005) reported a DNA sensor for the detection of specific sequences related to the bar gene in transgenic corn and CP4 EPSPS gene from transgenic Roundup Ready soybean. The electrode was prepared by mixing graphite powder, paraffin, and stearic acid to produce a homogeneous paste, resulting in a negatively charged surface, followed by electrodeposition of Al (III) cations. DNA capture probe was immobilized by adsorption in the aluminum film owed to the electrostatic attraction between the positively charged ion film and the negatively charged phosphate backbone of DNA.

Ligaj et al. (2006) also used stearic acid-modified CPE for qualitative bar gene detection. In this case, only the outer carbon paste layer (0.5 mm) was modified with stearic acid with the aim of preventing a decrease of the conductivity. Ethylenediamine was used as linker for immobilization of the capture probe, by reacting with the carboxyl groups of the stearic acid-modified electrode surface. A mixture of the DNA probe (21-mer) and the activators EDC and NHS was added to form a covalent bond between the ethylendiamine and the phosphate end of DNA.

Ma et al. (2008) designed a genosensor for PAT detection based on a Nano-$SiO_2$/*p*-aminothiophenol (PATP) film, fabricated by self-assembly and electrodeposition. A feature of $SiO_2$-nanoparticles is their negative charge, which could electrostatically attract the amino group of PATP, firmly immobilized onto the Au surface. This nanomaterial seemed to enhance electron transfer and also increased surface area. The capture probe (20-mer) was immobilized in the modified electrode by potential-controlled adsorption due to the expected affinity between $SiO_2$ and the phosphate groups at the 5′ end of DNA.

Different sensors for the determination of PAT gene based on modified electrodes with different combinations of nanomaterials and polymers have been reported. In the first propose (Yang et al., 2007b), 2,6-pyridinedicarboxylic acid (PDC) was electrodeposited into a GCE surface followed by the adsorption of gold nanoparticles on the PDC/GCE. The capture probe was adsorbed on the modified surface by the interaction of gold nanoparticles with DNA. The incorporation of PDC improved the electrochemical properties.

A similar approach was later reported using the same polymer in combination with carbon nanotubes (Yang et al., 2007a). The proposed sensor was based on the modification of a GCE surface with a copolymer film consisted on carboxyl-group-functionalized SWNTs and PDC. The resulting surface, being rich in oxygen-containing groups, was an ideal platform for the electrodeposition of zirconia films ($ZrO_2$). The strong affinity of $ZrO_2$ for phosphate groups made it possible to attach DNA strands through their phosphate 5′ ends. With the aim of obtaining a positively charged surface, appropriate for DNA immobilization cationic polyelectrolyte, poly(diallyldimethyl ammonium clorhide) was used instead of $ZrO_2$ (Yang et al., 2008). Zhang et al., 2008 reported a modification of this film based on $ZrO_2$/gold nanoparticles.

In another work, polyaniline (PANI) nanoparticles were combined with chitosan and gold nanoparticles as DNA immobilization matrix (Feng et al., 2008), and, 5′-amino-functionalized capture probe (20-mer) was adsorbed into the modified electrode, hybridization was carried out by electrodepositing the target, followed by electrochemical readout using EIS for PAT gene detection.

Single-walled carbon nanotubes (SWCNT), functionalized with carboxylic groups were used to modify the surface of the CPE followed by the electropolymerization of poly-L-lysine films (p-Lys). A 20-mer capture probe was immobilized by potential-controlled adsorption via electrostatic affinity between the amino groups of p-Lys and the phosphate skeleton of the DNA molecule. Hybridization was carried out also by controlled potential (Jiang et al., 2008).

In recent years, polyaniline hybrid materials (i.e., the product of combining this polymer with other kinds of nanomaterials) have been used as immobilization systems onto different transducers for sensor development due to the high sensitivity of the resulting devices.

Yang et al., 2009 proposed the modification of a carbon paste electrode with MWNT/PANI composite dispersed in chitosan for quantification of PAT gene. This approach was based on the synergistic effect between PANI and MWNT nanocomposites in chitosan film, which results in a highly enhanced conductivity and an increase of the surface area that consequently increases the load of the DNA probes.

Chitosan was changed by gold nanoparticles (Zhou et al., 2009) in a CPE modified with polyaniline nanofibers (nano-PANI). This nano-PANI/CPE served as interface for the immobilization of a gold nanoparticles and carbon nanotubes hybrid (nanogold-CNT). The immobilization of the DNA probe onto the nanogold-CNT/nano-PANI/CPE surface was performed by potential-controlled adsorption followed by the hybridization with the target at constant potential.

Another approach involved the electrodeposition of L-tyrosine on the electrode surface, followed by the addition of PANI-$ZrO_2$ nanoparticles (Yang et al., 2012a). The resulting PANI-nano$ZrO_2$ composite exhibited an interconnected dendritic structure, which provided high specific surface area for the electron transfer and for the immobilization of the capture probe.

5.6.1.1.1.3. Event-specific biosensors The highest specificity is obtained when the target DNA is the unique junction between the inserted transgenic construct and the plant genome and it is targeted by event-specific methods.

A genosensor based on partially reduced graphene oxide (p-RGO) modified carbon ionic liquid electrode (CILE) was reported by Sun et al. (2013) for the detection of transgenic soybean A2704–12. Graphene has been extensively investigated in recent years owing to its unique planar sheet structure. Due to its wide potential window, large surface area, good electrocatalytic activity, and relatively inertness, graphene-based electrodes have been widely reported. On the other hand, ionic liquids (Ils) have also shown great electrochemical advantages. The good solvating properties, high conductivity, non-volatility, low toxicity, large electrochemical window, good electrochemical stability and biocompatibility, make Ils suitable for biosensing applications. The CILE was prepared by mixing graphite powder and 1-butylpyridinium hexafluorophosphate to form a homogeneous carbon paste. Graphene oxide was added onto the freshly prepared CILE surface and subsequently electroreduced at constant potential. Due to the partial reduction of graphene oxide, unreduced oxygen groups remained on the electrode surface, which were activated with EDC and NHS in order to link the amino-modified capture probes via covalent binding. Hybridization with the synthetic target sequence (21-mer), related to the A2704-12 soybean, was carried out at room temperature and the electrochemical measurements were performed by DPV, using MB as indicator. Authors reported a larger signal of MB for dsDNA than that of ssDNA-modified electrode, ascribing this effect to the intercalation model.

Fátima-Barroso et al. (2015) reported a genosensor for the event-specific detection of MON810 transgenic maize using nanostructured 3D gold electrodes and ternary monolayers containing a dithiol (1,6-hexanedithiol), monothiol (MCH) and thiolated capture probe. A sandwich-type hybridization was carried out using a FITC-labeled signaling probe. An anti-FITC-peroxidase conjugate was used to perform the electrochemical read-out via the chronoamperometric measurement of TMB reduction.

More event-specific biosensors have been reported, but, considering that the novelty of the design has to do with the detection method rather than the immobilization system, they will be included in the detection section.

*5.6.1.1.2 Detection Methods*

5.6.1.1.2.1. Screening biosensors Detection can be direct or indirect. Direct electrochemical detection involves the oxidation of oligonucleotides or impedimetric measurements. A wide variety of indirect methods are available that can (i) detect changes in interfacial properties, (ii) use markers non-covalently attached to the DNA strands but via electrostatic attraction, affinity binding (streptavidin-biotin) or intercalation, and (iii) use markers covalently attached.

Carpini et al. (2004) proposed the use of an enzymatic conjugate as label, streptavidin-alkaline phosphatase, to mark the biotinylated target-capture probe duplex. This was followed by the addition of α-naphthyl phosphate as enzymatic substrate. The product of the enzyme-substrate reaction is an electroactive molecule, detected in this work by means of DPV.

In order to eliminate the need of biotinylated primers in PCR amplification, a genosensor based on sandwich hybridization was proposed later by the same group (Lucarelli et al., 2005). The amplification of the signal was mediated by the addition of alkaline phosphatase-streptavidin conjugate binding to the biotynilated signaling probe. The enzyme transforms 5-bromo-4-chloro-3-indolyl phosphate/nitro blue tetrazolium mixture in an insoluble and insulating product which precipitates on the sensing interface. EIS was used in the presence of $[Fe(CN)_6]^{3-/4-}$. This technique allows the study of the surface properties of a modified electrode measuring changes in charge transfer resistance (i.e., $R_{ct}$ values). An increase in the $R_{ct}$ value was observed after hybridization due to the precipitation of the insulating enzymatic product onto the surface (Figure 5.8).

Wang et al. (2009) proposed a similar assay, but changing the enzyme to catalase, and the detection system to square wave voltammetry (SWV), which is a faster and equally sensitive technique. After hybridization, the biotinylated signaling probe was labeled with streptavidin, followed by the linking of biotinylated catalase. Then, the biosensor was incubated in a mixture of aniline/$H_2O_2$ in an acidic medium, triggering the accumulation of protonated aniline molecules around the double-stranded DNA (dsDNA) owed to the electrostatic interaction between aniline and the negatively charged phosphate groups

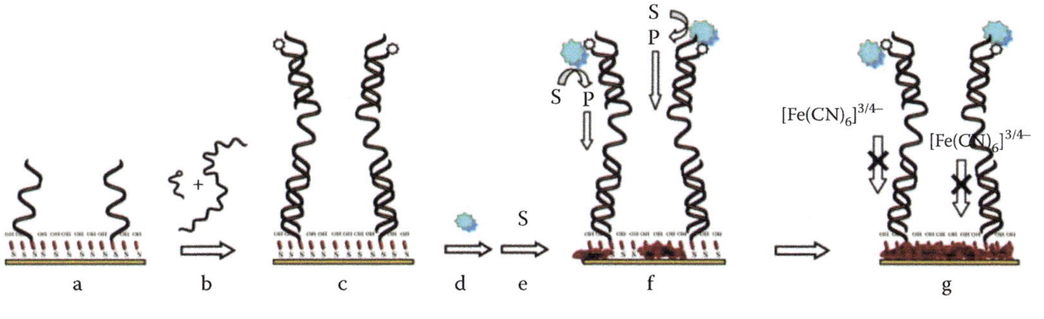


FIGURE 5.8 Schematic representation of the described genosensor. [Reproduced from Lucarelli et al., 2005, with permission from Elsevier].

of DNA, followed by the polymerization of aniline to polyaniline (PANI), resulting in a PANI/DNA complex. The presence of this complex was detected by SWV.

The Phenothiazine dye methylene blue (MB) was reported to be an effective electrochemical marker of DNA hybridization due to its differential affinity to ss- and ds-DNA, specifically to guanine bases, and easy electrochemical detection.

Tichoniuk et al. (2008) proposed a direct hybridization format and SWV detection of the double helix with MB. Quantification was based on an increase of the electrochemical signal when ssDNA is present on the electrode surface and a decrease when hybridization (dsDNA) occurs. This is attributed to lower MB binding to dsDNA because of the lower accessibility of MB to the guanine bases, which are packed between the bulky double DNA helix (Tichoniuk et al., 2008). Similar results were obtained by Xu et al., who found a decrease of the peak height in DPV, directly proportional to the target concentration was observed after MB intercalation. The genosensor was regenerated by the application of a high ionic strength buffer and the device could be reused for up to three days (Xu et al., 2006).

MB was also used as electrochemical indicator in a different work where cyclic voltammetry (CV) was chosen as the measurement technique (Zhu et al., 2008). In contrast to other works, a higher electrochemical signal was obtained with dsDNA compared to ssDNA. MB presents two types of binding models: surface electrostatic attraction on ssDNA and intercalation of MB on the dsDNA molecules, inside the double helix. The increase in the peak current of MB with dsDNA observed in this work was explained by the intercalation model that may be favored when a high concentration of MB is used.

Another intercalator that acts like MB, giving a signal decrease when dsDNA is formed, is methylene violet. It was used as hybridization indicator by Xie et al. (2008). With this approach, a 18-mer specific sequence of the 35S promoter was sensitively detected by DPV.

Kerman et al. (2006) studied the interaction between oligonucleotide probes and a cobalt-based coordination complex, $[Co(NH_3)_6]^{3+}$. After the hybridization process, this indicator molecule was added and then DPV was recorded. Since this complex lacks aromatic and planar ligands that can intercalate with DNA, it only interacts with the negatively charged phosphate backbone electrostatically. It is therefore a sequence-neutral binder. This, coupled with the fact that it is electrochemically active, makes it suitable as hybridization indicator. The hybridization process with 139-mer amplicons from an asymmetric PCR increased the negative charge on the electrode surface, thus generating an accumulation of $[Co(NH_3)_6]^{3+}$ ions; i.e., an increase in the response was observed when the duplex was formed. The device was suitable for qualitative detection of 35S from Roundup Ready soybean (reference material).

Another strategy for 35S detection was reported by Mao-Qing, et al (2008), in which, the hybridization event was monitored by SWV using $[Co(phen)_3]^{+3}$ (phen = 1,10-phenanthroline) as electroactive hybridization indicator. Current increased when the double helix was present, showing that this ion had more affinity for the duplex than for the ssDNA. The sensor could be reused up to eight times without signal change after exposing dsDNA/nanoPt/GCE to boiling and ice water baths successively.

Aghili et al. (2017) have reported recently the use of hematoxylin, which intercalates into the dsDNA structure, for 35S detection. Hematoxylin was detected by means of DPV.

Another alternative method with suitable performance in the detection of DNA is the use of metallic nanoparticles attached to the DNA probe. Sun et al (2007), reported an approach aimed at detecting NOS fragments based on the immobilization of the target sequence to the electrode surface, instead of the capture probe, and a subsequent step of hybridization with a 5′-amino functionalized 20-mer ssDNA probe labeled with mercaptoacetic acid-modified CdS nanoparticles. CdS nanoparticles attached on the hybrids were completely dissolved by immersing the Au electrode in a $HNO_3$ solution. The resulting solution was transferred to a $Hg^{+2}$-containing buffer in order to form a mercury film on the surface of a GCE in situ, to obtain the electrochemical readout of $Cd^{2+}$ by differential pulse anodic stripping voltammetry (DPASV). Figure 5.9 illustrates this process. The anodic stripping current of $Cd^{2+}$ had a linear relationship with the logarithmic value of the target concentration. The same group reported the detection of 35S using mercaptoacetic acid for SAM preparation and PbS nanoparticles for labeling (Sun W. et al., 2008). The current of $Pb^{2+}$ also showed a semilogarithmic relationship with the target concentration.

Li et al. (2016) reported a photoelectrochemical (PEC) biosensor for the detection of 35S. Chitosan was dropped onto the surface of indium tin oxide (ITO) slides, followed by the addition of gold nanoparticles-reduced graphene oxide, which acted as "nanocarriers" for the immobilization of a thiolated probe. After hybridization of the probe with the target sequence, a signaling-probe complex, alleged "nanocomplex," was incorporated as labeling mark. This labeling complex consisted of $SiO_2$ nanoparticles, covalently coated with 5 nm CdTe quantum dots, which carried multiple probe strands at the surface. PEC detection was carried out at in a buffer containing ascorbic acid, which served as a sacrificial electron donor during the photocurrent measurement. White light, with a spectral range of 200–2500 nm, was used as excitation light and was switched on and off every 20 s. The applied potential was 0.2 V (Figure 5.10).

5.6.1.1.2.2. Gene-specific biosensors The work of Ren et al. (2005) involved the detection of specific sequences related to the bar gene in transgenic corn and CP4 EPSPS gene from transgenic Roundup Ready soybean, in which the hybridization events were monitored by DPV using MB as hybridization indicator. Later, Ligaj et al. (2006) made use of the complex 2,2′-(bipyridil)cobalt (III) as hybridization indicator, detecting it by SWV. This indicator generated higher voltammetric peaks after intercalation with dsDNA, compared to ssDNA.

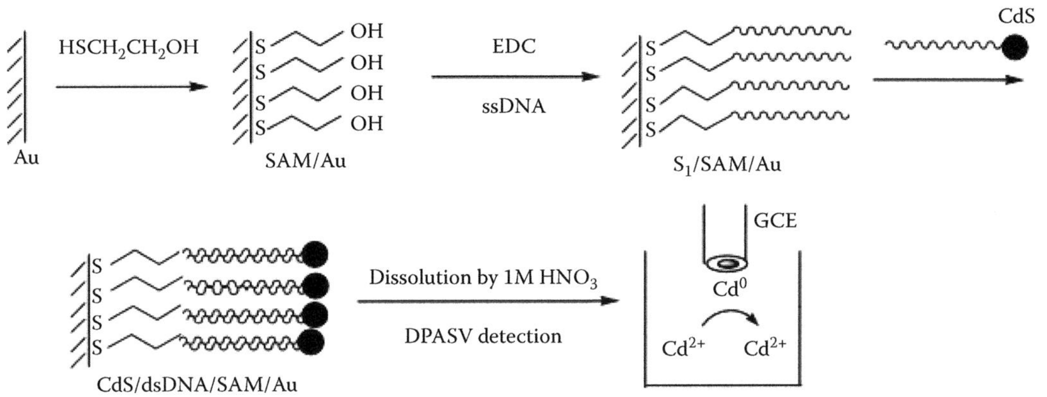


FIGURE 5.9 Schematic representation of electrochemical DNA detection with CdS nanoparticle labels. [Reproduced from Sun et al., 2007, with permission from Springer].

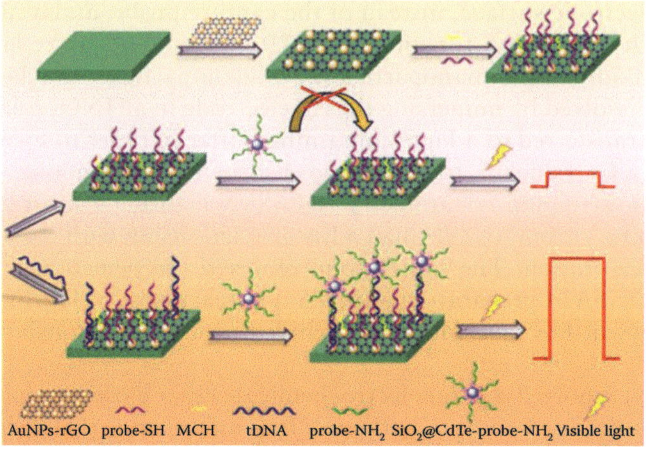


FIGURE 5.10 Schematic illustration of the fabrication procedure of the PEC biosensor and detection of the 35S promotor. [Reproduced from Li et al., 2016, with permission from Elsevier].

Jiang et al. (2011) presented a highly sensitive strategy for the detection of a 30-mer Bt fragment based on solid-state voltammetry. The authors proposed a sandwich hybridization format, with biotinylated Ag nanoparticles signaling probe. The modified electrode was incubated with streptavidin and more biotinylated Ag nanoparticles were added in order to form aggregates. Measurements were based on a solid-state Ag/AgCl process, in which the Ag from the aggregates was oxidized to $Ag^+$ and the electrogenerated $Ag^+$ formed insoluble AgCl on the electrode surface in the presence of $Cl^-$ ions. The solid AgCl on the electrode was then reduced to Ag (Figure 5.11).

5.6.1.1.2.3. Event-specific biosensors Dinh Tam (2015) reported two types of biosensors, both based on SWCNTs and both label-free. One used EIS as detection technique and the other was based on a FET. For the electrochemical sensor, platinum interdigitated microelectrodes were fabricated and modified with drop-casted SWCNT dispersed in ethylendiamine to form an amine-functionalized layer suitable for immobilization of EDC-activated DNA. The FET device was fabricated by sputtering ~10 nm of Ti and ~200 nm of Pt on an ~100 nm thick $SiO_2$ layer thermally grown on top of a silicon wafer. SWCNTs were added on the device and DNA was immobilized by electrostatic force.

The EIS-based system showed an increase in $R_{ct}$ upon hybridization, whereas the FET device depicted a decrease in the drain current. The authors suggested that the presence of the DNA duplex at the surface of SWCNTs in the FET device could affect the electronic properties of the nanotubes, possibly decreasing the conductivity by increasing the band gap of the nanomaterial.

Manzanares-Palenzuela et al. (2016b) reported the design of a nanostructured phthalocyanine-based biosensor for the label-free detection of an event-specific sequence related to Roundup-Ready soybean. FTO electrodes were silanized with amine-terminated silane onto which layer-by-layer films consisting of copper phthalocyanine tetrasulfonate and poly(allyl)amine hydrochloride were sequentially deposited by simple charge-based adsorption. One to five bilayers were constructed and the last layer being positively charged was suitable for electrostatic interaction with the capture probe. Hybridization

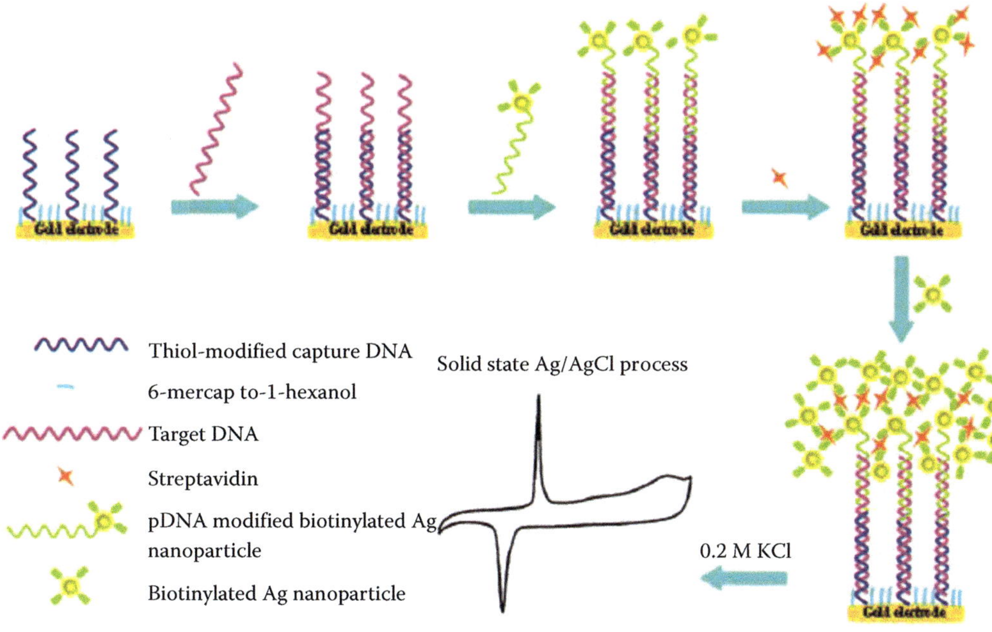


FIGURE 5.11 Schematic image of the DNA sensing strategy. [Reproduced from Jiang et al., 2011, with permission from Elsevier].

with the target sequence took place and the process was monitored by means of EIS. The biosensor was able to differentiate the target from a non-complementary sequence by a decrease in the impedance signal after specific hybridization.

5.6.1.1.2.4. Multiplex detection methods An interesting contribution published in 2009 proposed an event-specific genosensor for detecting a transgenic variety of maize (MON810) (Duwensee et al., 2009) and its application in maize flour samples (Mix et al., 2012). The genosensor relied on a direct assay, where the capture probe was immobilized by mixed SAMs with MCH onto gold electrodes. The complex $OsO_4$(bipy) was utilized as an electrochemically reversible redox probe covalently bound to DNA. It reacts only with the pyrimidine bases of ssDNA. The reaction involves the oxidation of the C=C double bond in the pyrimidine ring giving a diester of osmic (VI) acid.

With the aim of protecting the target from excessive binding of thymine or cytosine residues with [$OsO_4$(bipy)] the target sequence hybridizes partially (80 per cent) with a protective strand. Then a solution of the osmium-complex is added and only unprotected pyrimidine bases are able to react with [$OsO_4$(bipy)]. After the protective strand-target complex labeled with [$OsO_4$(bipy)] is formed, the excess of the osmium complex is removed by dialysis. The electrode is then dipped in the solution containing the osmium-labeled hybrid. In this step, the capture probe (immobilized on the Au surface) displaces the protective strands and hybridizes with the target. The protective strands were designed with 3–5 mismatches to ease this displacement by the immobilized probe. SWV was used to detect the DNA-osmium complex, based on the fact that each pyrimidine [$OsO_4$(bipy)] bond delivers two electrons during the voltammetric scan.

Four different targets, two from wild type maize and two from genetically modified maize were simultaneously labeled and detected using four working electrodes, each modified with a specific capture probe. As positive control for the detection of natural maize, two probes were designed: one for the synthase gene Iib (SSIIb) and the other for the invertase gene (ivrp) of maize. To identify the genetic modification, two probes were designed: one for detecting the trait gene CryIa/b and the other one designed to detect the event-specific junction between the maize DNA and the inserted transgene in MON810.

The application of the previous device to detect MON810 in maize flour samples employed an asymmetric PCR, that is, a PCR that preferentially amplifies one DNA strand in a double stranded DNA template using a great excess of one of the primers. Results showed that it was possible to discriminate between maize and GM maize in real samples from 0.6 per cent of GMO content. No significant detection of MON810 was possible when only 0.5 per cent of transgenic maize was present in the sample, most likely due to insufficient amplification of the template DNA (Mix et al., 2012).

Liao et al. (2013) reported a genosensor that provides a multiplex GMO analysis in a gold 16-array format. The proposed device implemented a biomolecular computational assay based on the logic gates principle. This consists on logic operations from dual or multiple inputs to produce a single logic output. Exploiting this principle, GMO-related target sequences were used as inputs and the output was the electrochemical signal obtained if hybridization of the targets with specific probes occurred.

A monolayer-modified Au electrode surface was prepared with a thiolated capture probe and 3-mercaptopropionic acid. Target DNA was incubated with two signaling probes (functionalized with fluorescein isothiocianate, FITC, and biotin) and loaded onto the DNA capture probe of Au surfaces. A mixture of anti-FITC-peroxidase and avidin-glucose oxidase was added followed by the addition of a mixture of their substrates, i.e., glucose and tetra- methylbenzidine (TMB). Only when all the probes (capture and signaling probes) recognized the target, an enzymatic cascade reaction occurred in which Gox catalyzed the oxidation of glucose to produce $H_2O_2$, which was subsequently reduced by HRP along with the resulting TMBox (Figure 5.12). The latter was finally detected by chronoamperometry. If one of the probes does not hybridize with target because target lacks its complementary sequence, there is no signal (Figure 5.13).

Different target sequences were designed corresponding to different GM events. Each sequence was composed by fragments of three GMO regions: a promoter (35S or Glb1), a trait gene (CP4 EPSPS, PAT, and cordapaA) and an endogenous gene (soybean: lectin gene, maize: SSIIb gene). A specific probe recognized each region: the capture probe was complementary to the promoter region and the FITC-labeled and biotinylated signaling probes were complementary to the trait and endogenous genes, respectively. According to the authors, the number of oligonucleotide bases separating the target sequences, especially trait genes from endogenous genes, may play a role in the efficiency of the cascade enzymatic reaction, which requires further attention to meet sequence diversity in various GMOs.

A relationship between the output current and the concentration (0–5 per cent) of GM genes was found. Additionally, this device was capable to integrate screening and event-specific methods, and a multiplex detection toward different GM events in one analysis. Considering DNA amplification is not included in this method, it is important to mention that a high amount of starting material is required to carry out the analysis with the aim of assessing the labeling regulation in Taiwan (set at 5 per cent of GMO).

Manzanares-Palenzuela et al. (2015b), aimed at the detection and quantification of Roundup Ready Soybean in real samples, reported the development of a multiplex magnetoassay comprising the immmobilization of biotinylated capture probes onto the surface of commercial streptavidin-coated magnetic beads. Subsequently, a sandwich

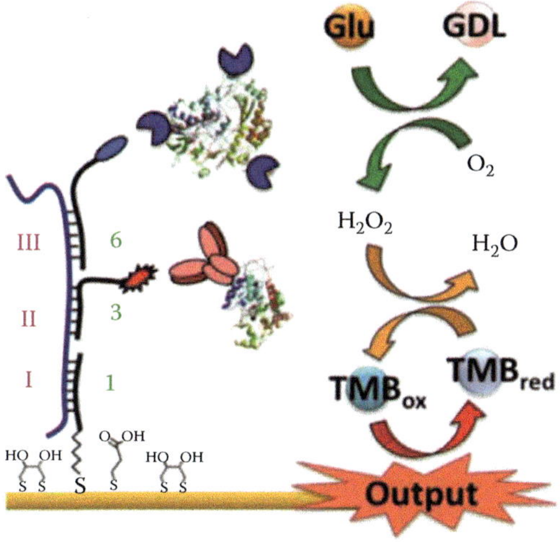


FIGURE 5.12 Envisioned configuration of biomolecular detection of GMO on the chip, wherein the computing relies on three hybridization reactions, two affinity recognition events, and biocatalytic cascade reactions in connection to a resulting output displayed in terms of the electrochemical transformation of oxidized TMB ($TMB_{ox}$) to reduced TMB ($TMB_{red}$). Right: schematic representations of the various substances involved in the gate. [Reproduced from Liao et al., 2013, with permission from Elsevier].

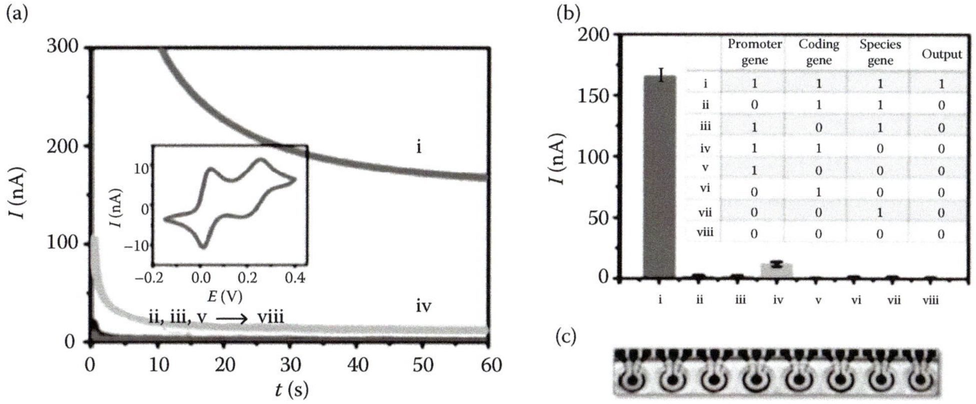


FIGURE 5.13 (a) Chronoamperometric transients of the bioanalytical system in the presence of eight combinations of inputs (promoter gene, coding gene and species gene). Inset: cyclic voltammogram of the substrate solution (0.1 mg/ML TMB and 250 mM glucose) recorder over a bare gold electrode chip. (b) Bar chart of the magnitudes of responses of the combinations (i–viii) generated from the system for GMO analysis at 60 s. Inset: corresponding truth table drawn from the combinations of input signals. (c) Visualized output interpretations displayed in an array corresponding to the combinations of input signals (i–viii). Blue color representing the oxidized form of TMB, indicates the simultaneous presence of promoter, coding, and species genes. [Reproduced from Liao et al., 2013, with permission from Elsevier].

hybridization was carried out with FITC- and digoxigenin-labeled signaling probes to subsequently perform a bi-labeling step using anti-FITC and anti-digoxigenin alkaline phosphatase and peroxidase conjugates, respectively, for the event-specific and taxon-specific targets, respectively. DPV and chronoamperometry were the techniques used to measure the enzymatic substrates α-naphthyl phosphate and TMB for alkaline phosphatase and peroxidase, respectively (Figure 5.14).

#### 5.6.1.2 Immunosensors

To the best of our knowledge, there are only three reports on electrochemical immunosensors for GMO detection. Volpe et al. (2006) reported an immunomagnetic sandwich assay for the detection of the transgenic protein Cry1Ab in corn flours. Commercial magnetic beads are precoated with monoclonal antibody specific for the Fc region of all mouse IgG.

Cry1Ab was sandwiched between the mouse monoclonal anti-Cry1Ab antibodies coated on the surface of IgG-magnetic beads and rabbit polyclonal anti-Cry1Ab antibodies (Pab). The sandwich complex was then revealed using anti-rabbit IgG labeled with the enzyme alkaline phosphatase. After immunological reactions, the beads were localized onto the surface of a magnetized screen-printed electrode using α-naphthyl phosphate

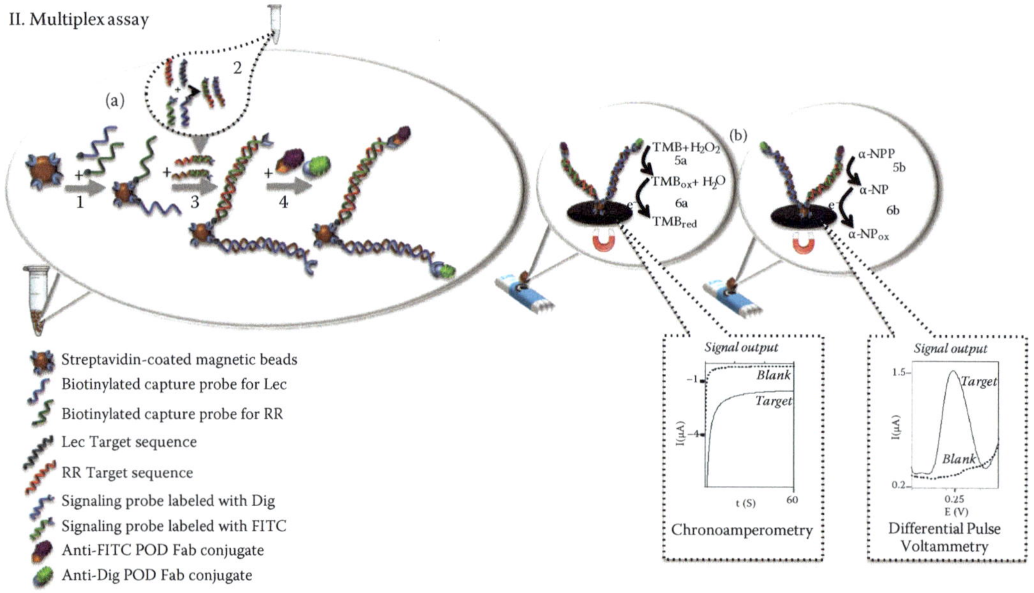


FIGURE 5.14 Scheme of the (I) single assays and (II) multiplex assay divided into two steps, recognition (a) and measurement (b): (1) attachment of capture probe(s) to the surface of magnetic beads; (2) homogeneous hybridization between a labeled-probe and target sequence; (3) heterogeneous hybridization with capture probe bound to the beads; (4) addition of the Fab-enzyme conjugate; (5a–6b) enzymatic reactions occurring after adding the enzymatic substrate (TMB/α-NPP); (6a) chronoamperometric measurement of TMB reduction at the electrode surface; (6b) voltammetric measurement of naphthol oxidation current at the electrode surface. Only showed part II. [Reproduced from Manzanares-Palenzuela et al., 2015b, with permission from Elsevier].

as enzymatic substrate, which was converted to the electroactive molecule α-naphthol detected by means of DPV.

Freitas et al. (2016) have recently reported another approach to detect the same protein. They propose a label-free fashion EIS detection system using ITO electrodes. The electrode surface was silanized to form an amine-terminated monolayer that could be later used to covalently immobilize specific polyclonal antibodies *via* carbodiimide coupling. The protein interaction with the Pab recognition platform was directly monitored and measured by CV and electrochemical impedance spectroscopy using commercially Cry1Ab protein.

Zhu et al., 2015 describe an electrochemical immunoassay for the Cry1Ab toxin. It is making use of a nanobody (a heavy-chain-only antibody) (Figure 5.15). Single variable domain called the variable domain of heavy-chain-only antibody (VHH) or Nanobody® derived from the heavy chain antibody present in camels, llamas, alpacas, and sharks has gained much more focus. VHH is the smallest available, functional, and intact antigen-binding fragment. Compared to the conventional antibody, nanobody (Nb) showed more excellent stability and it can recognize more inaccessible and cryptic sites. Moreover, it can be functionally modified with enzyme, isotope, toxin, fluorescein and so on for diversified applications. A biotinylated primary nanobody and a HRP-conjugated secondary nanobody were applied in a sandwich immunoassay where horseradish peroxidase (HRP) was used to produce polyaniline (PANI) from aniline. PANI can be easily detected by DPV, which makes the assay fairly selective.

### 5.6.2 Optical Biosensors

Optical biosensors have also been reported for GMO detection due the high selectivity of the technology that involves the interaction between the selective biomolecule binding layer and the transducer.

As with electrochemical biosensors, most of the optical biosensors developed to be applied in the detection of GMOs are based on the measurement of DNA, while protein-based biosensors are uncommon. The majority of the described optical DNA biosensors

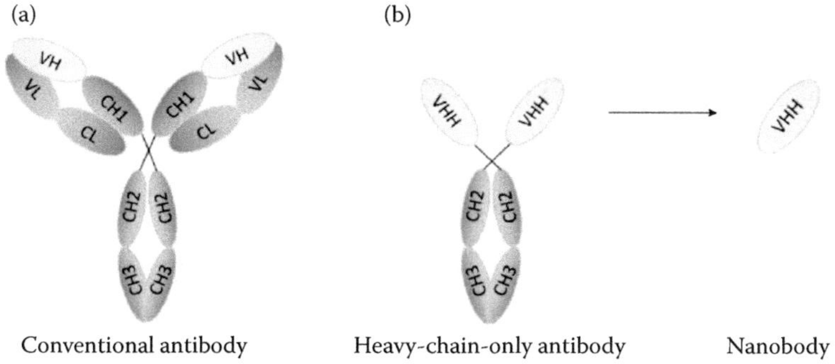


FIGURE 5.15 Nanobody and the amino acid sequences of Nanobodies deduced from their DNA sequences. a Nanobody was isolated from the heavy-chain only antibody. b Framework regions 1–4 (FW 1–4) and complementarity-determining regions 1–3 (CDR 1–3) are shown. According to the diversity of CDR3, these Nanobodies were classified into four families. Only showed part II. [Reproduced from Zhu et al., 2015, with permission from Springer].

are based on screening methods, the least specific level, as detect common DNA elements in GMOs, such as promoter 35S and terminator NOS. There is also optical-based devices which detect a part of the train gene associated with the specific genetic modification (i.e., "gene-specific methods"). As an example, detection of Cry1Ab genes has been reported, among others.

SPR is the optical technique more used in GMO detection, but surface-enhanced Raman scattering (SERS) spectroscopy and electroluminescence have also been applied. Visual detection is another strategy to confirm the presence of GMO.

Most of the systems have been applied to the detection of synthetic oligonucleotides, with high sensitivity, the analysis of certified reference materials have been also reported.

Because of the special characteristics and requirements of the detection systems used in optical biosensors, unlike in case of electrochemical biosensors, we consider more appropriate to group them not according to the nature of the target, but depending on the detection system.

#### *5.6.2.1 SPR Biosensors*

The recent development of SPR-based biosensor technologies for biospecific interaction analysis (BIA) enables the monitoring of a variety of molecular reactions in real time. The biomolecular interactions occur at the surface of a flow cell of a sensor chip between a ligand immobilized on the surface and an injected analyte.

Many of the SPR biosensors for analysis of GMOs use SA chip sensors, whose surface consists of a carboxymethylated dextran matrix pre-immobilized with streptavidin to immobilize biotinylated probes, or a CM5 chip sensor in which the surface has a carboxymethylated dextran matrix coating on a gold film. Between them is the one reported by Mariotti et al. aimed of detecting 35S and NOS. The gold sensor chip was modified with carboxylated dextran and thiol to immobilize streptavidin and the biotinylated oligonucleotide respectively. The hybridization with the target oligonucleotides was performed injecting the oligonucleotide solution in a hybridization buffer at the SPR flow cell and maintained 10 min. The system was tested with 2 per cent transgenic soya flour certificated material. After PCR amplification, a pretreatment of the double DNA strand of PCR products was necessary, previous to sensing. The procedure consisted on a denaturation step with alkaline agents followed by physical separation of the two strands with magnetic particles coated with immobilized streptavidin. The resulting single-stranded target sequence was able to hybridize with the immobilized probe on the surface, avoiding the reannealing phenomenon (Mariotti et al., 2002).

SPR-based BIA was used to detect genetically modified Roundup Ready soybean gene sequences. First, single-stranded biotinylated oligonucleotides containing soybean lectin and Roundup Ready gene sequences were immobilized on SA sensor chips, and the efficiency of hybridization to oligonucleotide probes differing in length was determined. Second, biotinylated PCR products from non-transgenic soybeans (genomes carrying only the lectin gene), as well as from genetically modified Roundup Ready soybean, were immobilized and the oligonucleotide probes injected. Furthermore, the sensor chips carrying either lectin and Roundup Ready soybean PCR products or 21-mer oligonucleotide as probes were used, and both non-purified and purified asymmetric PCR products injected (Figure 5.16). The results obtained show that 13 and 15 mer oligonucleotides are suitable probes to detect genetically modified Roundup Ready soybean gene sequences (either target oligonucleotides or PCR products) under standard BIA experimental conditions. By contrast, when 11 mer DNA probes were employed, no efficient hybridization was obtained. All the SPR-based formats were found to be useful for detection of

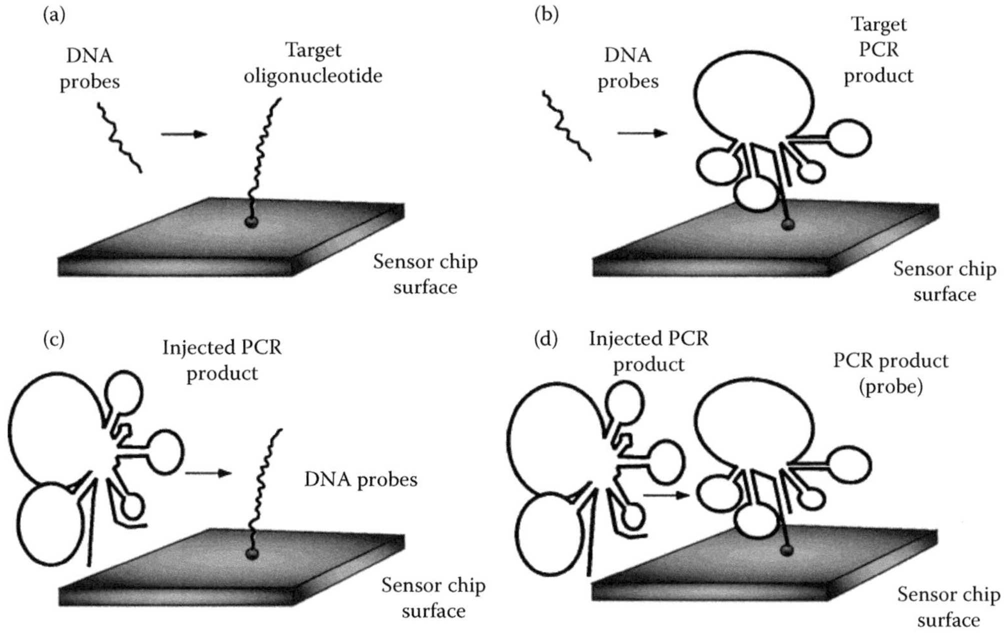


FIGURE 5.16 Experimental strategies and formats for GMO detection using SPR-based BIA and sensor chips carrying lectin or Roundup Ready oligonucleotides or PCR products. [Reproduced from Feriotto et al., 2002, with permission from ACS publications].

Roundup Ready gene sequences, suggesting that these procedures are useful for the real-time monitoring of hybridization between target single-stranded PCR products (Feriotto et al., 2002). In other work biotinylated multiplex PCR products from non-transgenic and transgenic maize (Bt-176 sequence) were immobilized in the SA sensor chip coated. The device allows discrimination between samples containing 0.5 and 2 per cent Bt-176 maize. However, authors stated that further work was needed to apply this method to processed samples, suggesting the incorporation of suitable internal standards (Feriotto et al., 2003).

Giakoumaki et al. developed an optical biosensor based on SPR (BiacoreX™) for detection of 35S in PCR-amplified products of soybean powder, maize samples, and pBI121 plasmid. The dextran sensor chip was modified with streptavidin to anchor the biotinylated DNA probe. The sensor could be regenerated after denaturation of the duplex with HCl, allowing the sensor to be a "multi-use" device (Giakoumaki et al., 2003).

Wang et al. reported a DNA biosensor based on SPR transduction coupled with PCR. The gold sensor chip was covered with a thiol-funtionalized probe and then treated with a blocking thiol solution (MCH) (Wang et al., 2004a).They implemented a non-conventional denaturation method of the PCR-derived double-stranded DNA. It consisted on the use of high temperature and small oligonucleotides that were designed to be complementary to a part of the strand near the probe-hybridization region, but positioned in a way that they do not overlap the probe-complementary portion of the target in order to prevent reannealing of the DNA sister strands (Figure 5.17). This method proved to be efficient in producing a distinguishable signal between blank and target.

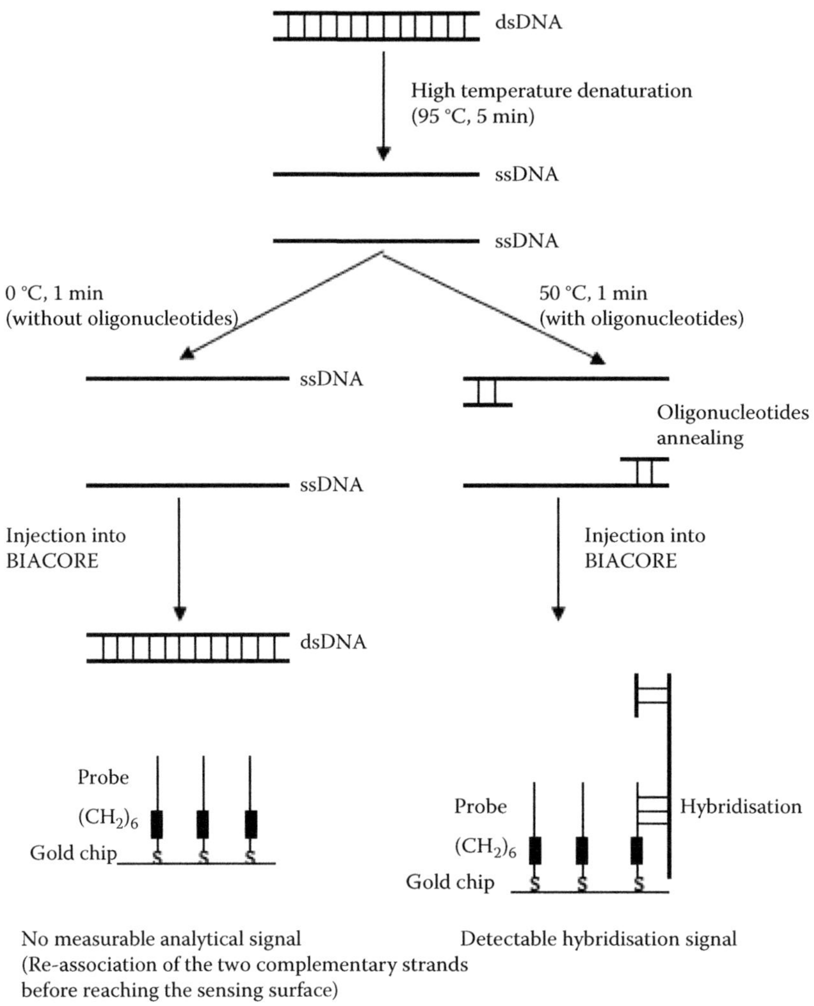


FIGURE 5.17 Treatments to dissociate the dsDNA PCR samples. Left: high temperature denaturation (95°C for 5 min, 1 min in ice). Right: high temperature denaturation with oligonucleotides (95°C for 5 min, 1 min incubation with oligonucleotides at 50°C). After the treatments, the sample is injected into the instrument for the interaction with the immobilized probe. [Reproduced from Wang et al., 2004a, with permission from Elsevier].

DNA samples extracted from plant were tested after amplification by PCR. The probe corresponded to a region of the 35S promoter. The sensor could be regenerated more than 100 times after an acidic or alkaline treatment.

A comparison between later devices, BIACORE X™ (bench instrument) and a dextran-modified sensor chip or a bare gold sensor chip, and the SPR device SPREETA™ (portable instrument) and a bare gold, for 35S detection was carried out by the same group (Wang et al., 2004b). The performances of the BIACORE SPR-based DNA sensors resulting from direct coupling of thiol-derivatized DNA probes onto the gold chip were described and compared with the immobilization method based of biotinylated oligonucleotide probes onto a streptavidin coated dextran sensor surface. In this case, chemical denaturation and high temperature denaturation were carried out. In the detection of PCR-amplified samples, and when chemical denaturation method was applied, a positive signal was obtained with GMO maize samples, but PCR blanks also resulted in high signal. If high temperature denaturation was used, negligible responses with PCR blanks were obtained. Similar results were obtained in PCR samples detection with SPREETA. Authors concluded that considering the advantages of the thiol derivatized probe/blocking thiol immobilization method (high reproducibility and stability, good sensitivity, specificity, and lifetime of sensor chip), it appears to be an efficient immobilization technique useful for DNA-based biosensor.

Zhao et al described both, protein and DNA-based devices for detection of transgenic Cry1Ac cotton (Gossypium spp.) (Zhao et al., 2013). In the immunosensor, monoclonal anti-Cry1Ac antibodies were immobilized on the surface of a CM5 sensor chip. The SPR sensor response to solutions containing Cry1Ac was significantly greater than to solutions without Cry1Ac. In the case of genosensing, transgenic DNA Bt cotton variety Nucotn33B expressing the Cry1Ac protein was detected. 25-mer biotinylated oligonucleotide probe was immobilized on a SA sensor chip and PCR products of Cry1Ac were detected.

Two Fourier transform-SPR immunosensors were developed for detection of the Bacillus thuringiensis Cry1Ab protein (Ming et al., 2015). Sensor chips were modified by a first layer of 1,6-hexanedithiol, a second layer of Au/Ag alloy nanoparticles, and a third layer of 3-mercaptopropionic (sensor 1), and extra layer of protein A was applied to one of them (sensor 2). Cry1Ab monoclonal antibody was immobilized on the later layer (Cry1Ab monoclonal antibody-MPA-Au/Ag alloy nanoparticles/HDT). Au/Ag alloy nanoparticles were introduced for increasing sensitivity. Although sensor 2 is able to immobilize fewer monoclonal antibodies, protein A is interesting because of the primary binding site for protein A is on the Fc fragment, leaving the Fab fragment exposed to Cry1Ab proteins. As a result, sensor 2 could increase the detection sensitivity, extend the detection range, and slightly decrease the detection limit compared with sensor 1.

#### *5.6.2.2 SERS Biosensors*

Surface-enhanced Raman scattering (SERS) spectroscopy also has been used for optical biosensor developed in GMO detection. This technique involves the interaction of light, molecules, and metal nanostructures to enhance Raman signals that can resolve the structures down to single-molecule level. The enhancement occurs due to the resonant interaction between optical fields and surface plasmons in the metal. The principle relies on the incident light excited surface plasmons that radiate a dipolar field, which together leads to redistribution of the electric field around the metal clusters. This effect can cause enhanced excitation intensity from the molecule adsorbed on the metal surface and shift the frequency between incident and excited laser light.

A SERS-barcoded nanosensor was used to detect Bacillus thuringiensis (Bt) gene in transformed rice, the gene of rice sucrose phosphate synthase (SPS) was used as interior reference gene (Chen et al., 2012). The SERS-barcoded nanoparticles were fabricated with a golden core for optical enhancement, a layer of Raman reporter molecules absorbed onto the surface of gold core for spectroscopic barcoding, and a silica shell for protection and functionalization. After conjugated with specific oligonucleotides, the SERS-barcoded tags were ready for barcoding target gene. The capture DNA of Bt and SPS were immobilized at each corresponding testing zone of glass substrate. The fixed fragments were barcoded with SERS tags by hybridization to complementary sequences. Finally, the testing results were decoded by reading the SERS spectra at the detection

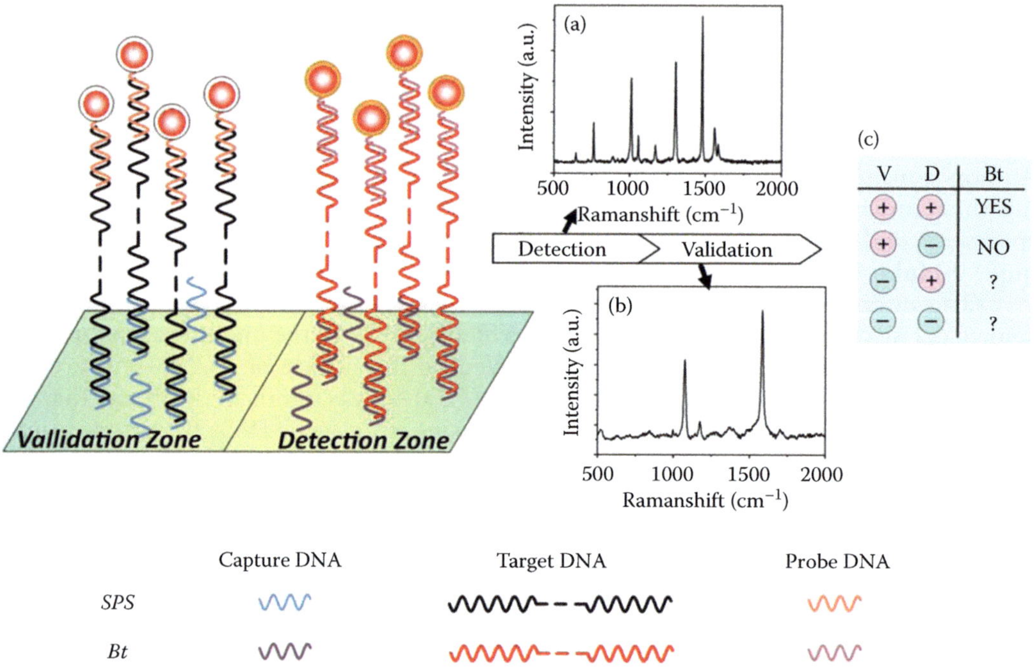


FIGURE 5.18 Schematic illustration of Bt gene detection procedure using SERS-barcoded nanotags. (a) Representative SERS spectrum of Bt; (b) representative SERS spectrum of SPS; (c) table of detection results and results determination. [Reproduced from Chen et al., 2012, with permission from Elsevier].

zone and verified testing effectiveness at the validation zone. Simultaneously, through analyzing the Raman intensity, the amount of transgenic fragments in samples was estimated. Figure 5.18 shows a schematic illustration of the biosensor working principle.

The same technology was applied to detect the 35S sequence of Bt-176 maize sample (Guven et al., 2012). The capture probe was immobilized on spherical magnetic gold nanospheres funcionalized with mercapto-undecanoic acid by covalent bond with the amino group of the probe. On the other hand, a SAM was formed on gold nanorods using 5,5′-dithiobis (2-nitrobenzoic acid) (DTNB). These rod shaped nanoparticles were used as Raman label. A second probe specific for 35S target was immobilized on the activated nanorod surface. Both captures probes (DNT labeled gold nanorod-probe and gold coated magnetic nanosphere-probe) were hybridized with target DNA to form a sandwich structure in solution (Figure 5.19). Quantification of the target concentration was performed via SERS spectra of DTNB on the nanorods.

### *5.6.2.3 Chemiluminescence Biosensors*

Electrochemiluminescence (ECL) is an electrochemical process in which molecules undergo electrontransfer reactions at an electrode surface, leading to a singlet excited photon emission state. The process is controlled by the applied potential, allowing precise control over the emission, so photon collection efficiency can be optimized. Although many labels can be used, the majority of ECL biosensors employ the tris (2,2′-bipyridine) ruthenium(II) complex, $Ru(bpy)_3^{2+}$. $Ru(bpy)_3^{2+}$ is oxidized at the electrode surface in the present of a co-reactant system as a tertiary amine, after the oxidation the complex

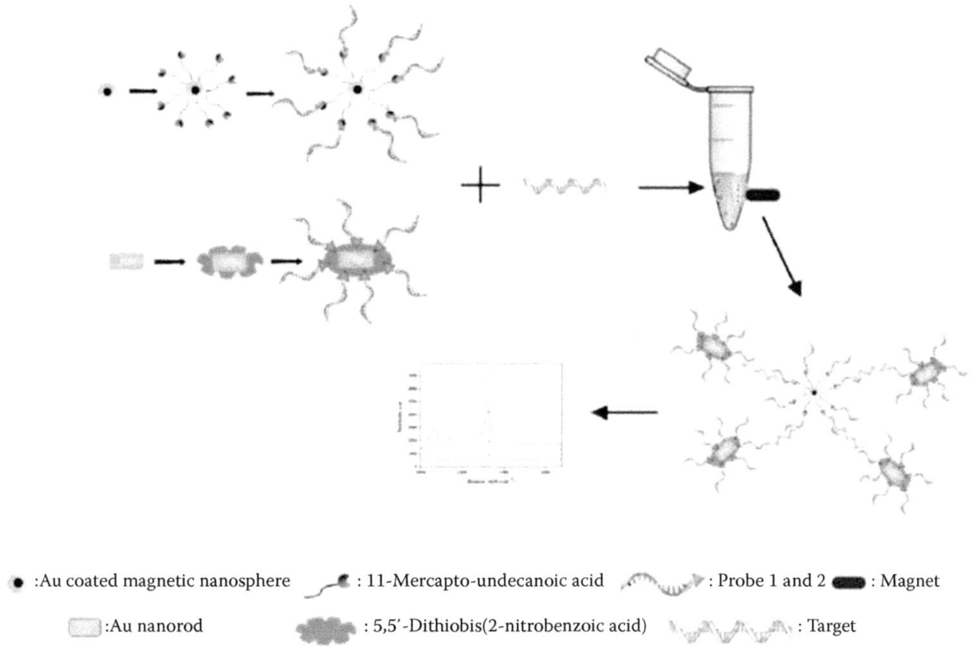


FIGURE 5.19 Schematic illustration of MS-SERS based sandwich assay for the target oligonucleotide. [Reproduced from Guven et al., 2012, with permission from Royal Society of Chemistry].

receive an electron from the radical intermediate of the amine (also formed at the electrode surface) to produce an excited state. This label was extensively used in association with a tertiary amine (generally tri- propylamine, TPA) in the so-called co-reactant system, in which $Ru(bpy)_3^{2+}$ is oxidized at the electrode surface and then receives an electron from the radical intermediate of the co-reactant (also formed at the electrode surface) to produce an excited state. Under these conditions, one molecule of the $Ru(bpy)_3^{2+}$ label can produce many photons.

Zhu et al. (2010) reported an ECL-based optical DNA sensor for 35S and NOS detection. Biotinylated probes were immobilized onto streptavidin-coated magnetic beads and placed in a platinum working electrode. GMO target DNA and ruthenium (II) tris–bipyridal (TBR)-probe were added to the electrochemical detection cell. The GMO target DNA was hybridized with the immobilized biotin-functionalized probe and with the TBR-probe to form a sandwich complex, at 50°C. Hybridization with TBR reacted with tripropylamine (TPA) resulted in emission of light for electroluminescence detection. A voltage of 1.25 V was applied to start the reaction between TBR and TPA. A linear range was obtained from 5 nM to 5 μM for 35S detection. The sensor was able to differentiate between the non-GM tobacco and GM tobacco.

Jang et al., 2011 propose a miniaturized chemiluminometric immunosensor array for quantitative detection of traces of genetically modified products. Different capture antibodies were immobilized on predetermined regions of a glass slide solid matrix, and a sandwich-type immunoassays were developed. Photodiodes were located at the bottom of the glass slides in an aligned arrangement to the immobilized antibody sites such that the light signal resulting from the immunoassays could be detected in situ (Figure 5.20).

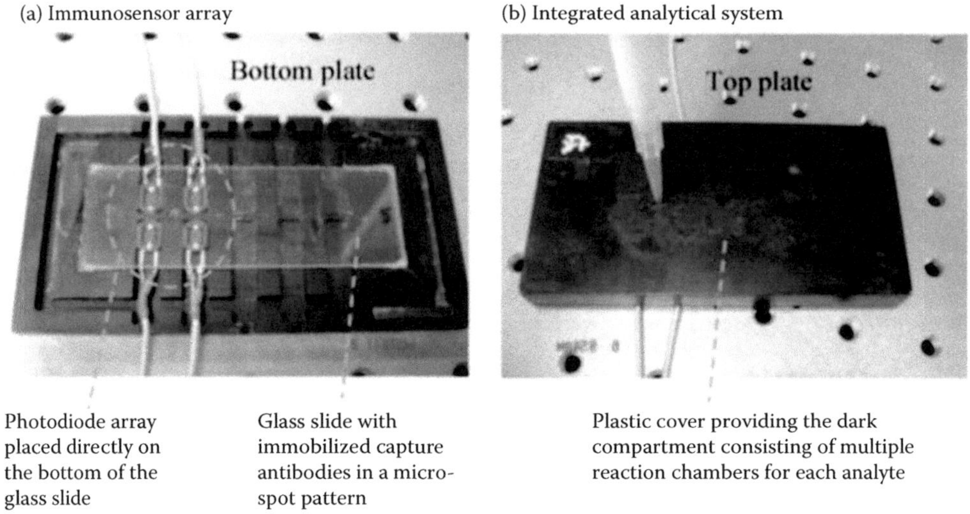


FIGURE 5.20 Development of a photodiode-embedded immunosensor array for chemiluminometric detection. The sensor consisted of a glass slide where the immune reactions occurred and photodiodes, which were on the bottom and aligned to each reaction site for the detection of chemiluminometric signals. The sensor array was placed on the black bottom plate (a) and covered with a top plate to ensure complete darkness within the sensor (b). The top plate also contained a port so reagents could be supplied to the reaction chamber. [Reproduced from Jang et al., 2011, with permission from Elsevier].

Three capture antibodies specific to recombinant marker proteins expressed in GMOs were used: EPSPS, neomycin phosphotransferase II (NPTII), and PAT.

#### 5.6.2.4 Visual Biosensors

Visual detection has also been applied as detection method in DNA sensors for GMO. Kalogianni et al., (2006) reported a dry-reagent dipstick configuration for visual detection of 35S promoter and NOS terminator sequences. Oligonucleotide-conjugated gold nanoparticles were used as probes to hybridize with biotinylated PCR product. The hybrids were captured by the immobilized streptavidin at the test zone of the sensor giving a characteristic red line due to the accumulation of the nanoparticles. Soybean powder certified reference material with 0.1 per cent GMO content was also clearly detectable for 35S and NOS sequences.

Bai et al., 2007 reported custom-designed optical silicon thin-film biosensor chips to detect GMOs. In the first step, the aldehyde-capture probes were covalently immobilization onto the hydrazine-derivatized biosensor chip surface. Then, the hybridization of biotinylated PCR amplicon target with capture probes was carried out. And finally, the anti-biotin IgG HRP conjugated was added and TMB, used as the enzymatic substrate, was converted into a precipitated product by HRP to increase the thin-film thickness. Differing amounts of precipitates resulted in differing colors ranging from purple to light blue. Five DNA targets were amplified from a maize Bt11 sample corresponding to Ivr1, CaMV 35S promoter, NOS terminator, BAR (pat), and CryIAb. In 2010, the same procedure was reported for detecting six GM maize lines (Bt11, Bt176, GA21, MON810, NK603, and T25) (Bai et al., 2010).

### 5.6.3 Piezoelectric Biosensors

These kind of sensors enable the selective and label-free detection of biological events in real time. QCM are the most commonly used BAW devices for biosensing, and are made of a bulk piezoelectric material, i.e., a quartz crystal sandwiched between two metallic electrodes, typically gold. Biorecognition elements are commonly immobilized onto the gold surface. In fact, piezoelectric sensors have also been developed for GMOs detection because of the increase in mass that occurring in the hybridization and antigen/antibody reactions, which results in a decrease in the resonance frequency. QCM devices are capable of detecting nanogram changes in mass.

There are several reports involving GMO detection with QCM that target screening and gene-specific sequences, most commonly promoter 35S and terminator NOS DNA fragments, but also the Cry1Ab, CTP4, and EPSPS genes, using different immobilization procedures. Most of the biosensors reported use synthethic oligonucleotide for optimization and flours, seeds, or processed food as the target raw material.

Mascini's group was probably one of the pioneers in GMO-biosensing research and probably the first (Minunni et al., 2001) to propose a piezoelectric method for GMO screening in food matrices. They did it so in a time when the field of GMO detection was in early stages. In this work, the quartz crystal was housed inside a methacrylate cell such that only one side of the crystal was in contact with the solution in the cell well. The frequency variations were continuously recorded using a quartz crystal analyzer. The gold on the quartz was modified with 11-mercaptoundecanol and carboxylated dextran to immobilize streptavidin and then the biotinylated capture probe. This oligonucleotide was 25-nt long, complementary to a 25-nt synthetic target sequence and partly complementary with lengthier target sequences (195 and 180-nt of 35S and NOS fragments, respectively) that had been PCR-amplified from a plasmid and from certified reference material (soybean powder, Roundup Ready®). The authors tried to detect amplified and non-amplified (genomic and plasmidic) DNA.

The frequency shift is usually negative upon biomolecular interactions because wave oscillation is slowed down by the mass load put onto the piezoelectric system. The reusability of the sensor surface was also evaluated, and the results suggested that it could be reused for up to 10 measurement cycles, after regenerating the surface with an acidic treatment.

As regards to the PCR-amplified plasmidic and genomic DNA, the authors reported that the amplification was carried out in three different laboratories to test the reproducibility of the PCR reaction. The amount of amplified DNA was considerably different from the three laboratories, which they attributed to the PCR reaction as being highly variable by nature. Amplified DNA was diluted and the measured signal was found to be independent of the dilution factor, meaning that the system failed to quantify. The sensor was considered as semi-quantitative. Interestingly, no quantitative method existed at this point.

As to the non-PCR attempt, the authors revealed that even though the sensor was able to obtain a measurable frequency shift with non-amplified DNA, they were unable to distinguish between the transgenic and non-transgenic varieties of soybean. The possibility of unspecific adsorptions of the big-sized genomic and plasmidic DNAs without specific recognition by the probe was argued as being the plausible cause of this behavior.

In a later work (Mannelli et al., 2003), the capture probe was immobilized onto the gold surface using two different chemistries and GMO detection was accomplished in complex samples (e.g., supermarket products). In addition to the thiol-dextran chemistry for biotin-streptavidin recognition used in the previous work, it was tested here another surface functionalization using the classical mixed SAM approach with thiolated probes and a short blocking thiol (MCH) (Figure 5.21). Both immobilization procedures exhibited similar analytical performances, but the SAM strategy was considered to be faster and more practical than the thiol-dextran one.

The authors were concerned with the double-stranded nature of the PCR amplicons, which would harness hybridization on the sensor surface. Thus, several approaches were evaluated to denature the DNA: elevated temperature, magnetic separation of the strands, and enzymatic digestion of one strand. PCR was performed with 5′-biotinylated and 5′-phosphorylated primers for the magnetic and enzymatic strategies, respectively. In the first approach, streptavidin-coated paramagnetic particles were used for strand separation and, in the second approach, lambda exonucleases were used to digest one strand of the duplex DNA from the 5′-phosphorylated end. None of these strategies exhibited satisfactory results as the authors found that the thermal treatment was more convenient in terms of cost, time, and simplicity of the experimental procedure. The analysis of diluted PCR-amplified DNA obtained from real samples such as a drink, snack bar, and soybean crackers revealed a frequency shift corresponding to the lower region of the calibration plot of synthetic DNA, thus, a measurable signal was obtained. Nevertheless, the authors stated the following: "At the moment it is impossible to use this system in a quantitative manner and to compare the measurements with the law normative" and they further explained that this might be due to the fact that the samples were submitted to PCR amplification up to the plateau phase.

Further on, Minunni et al. (2005) succeeded at developing a PCR-free system based on QCM for GMO detection. To accomplish such task, genomic DNA extracted directly from genetically engineered tobacco leaves was enzymatically digested to yield

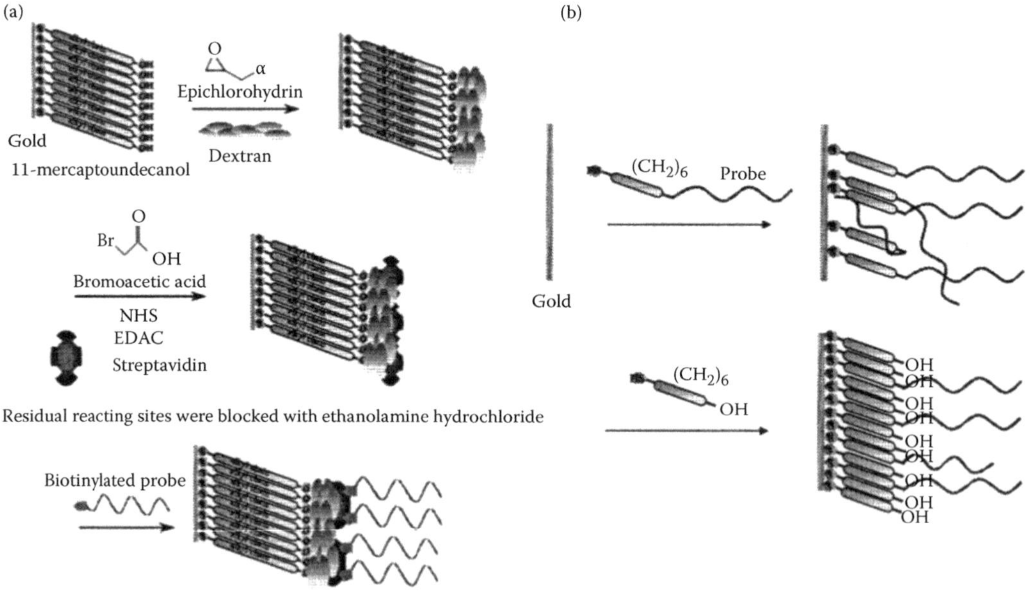


FIGURE 5.21 Immobilization procedure. (a) Thiol-dextran immobilization procedure; (b) thiol-derivatized probe/blocking thiol immobilization procedure. [Reproduced from Mannelli et al., 2003, with permission from Elsevier].

shorter fragments. The digestion was designed to preserve the target sequence within these shorter, digested fragments. They tested different procedures to denature double-stranded genomic DNA: thermal and chemical (formamide buffer) treatments and the use of a thermal procedure combined with blocking-oligonucleotides designed to hybridize to the region near the target sequence and near the sister strand, in order to prevent them from reannealing. The latter resulted in the highest signal-to-blank ratios in the detection of 35S from transgenic tobacco. This work was a relevant contribution to the field, given that PCR-free detection of single-copy genes had not been achieved with biosensors at this point.

In 2009, the group reported a biosensing approach to detect transgenes in a Roundup Ready® soybean processing line (Bogani et al., 2009). The work relied on the previously reported thiol-dextran-streptavidin immobilization procedure and thermal denaturation. The rest of experimental conditions remained unchanged as to their 2003 report. In this work, the authors employed PCR to amplify CTP4 and 35S target sequences from samples of diverse complexity i.e., unprocessed, crushed, and expanded seeds, and soy and protein flours. The results showed that this method was suitable for the discrimination of genetically modified soybean in these samples, which were chosen to represent the different stages of the soybean industrial production chain.

Passamano and Pighini (2006) have also made important contributions to the field of QCM-based GMO detection. They reported a QCM system for the detection of a 200-bp fragment of the Cry1Ab gene using a streptavidin-modified gold surface and biotynilated 200-nt probes. PCR amplification was carried out in certified reference material containing different levels of genetically modified maize and the system exhibited a linear relationship between the analytical response and the percentage of genetically modified MON 810 maize flour from 0.1 to 5 per cent. A biscuit sample was prepared in the laboratory with known GMO amount and was quantitatively analyzed using this system. The result was seemingly in concordance with the theoretical GMO percentage or added amount. Although only one sample was submitted to quantitative analysis, this level of accuracy with a quantitative determination had not been accomplished by previous works.

Stobiecka et al. (2007) developed a DNA biosensor for the determination of Roundup® soybean through the detection of the EPSPS gene inserted within the transgenic cassette. The electrodes were modified by avidin after a succinimidyl-based functionalization. 21-nt biotinylinated probes were immobilized onto the avidin-coated gold electrodes (Figure 5.22). A synthetic target sequence of the same length was used as the capture probe to optimize and characterize the system in terms of analytical performance. The number and density of DNA molecules immobilized on the QCM electrode surface were calculated from frequency changes according to Sauerbrey's equation.

DNA samples extracted from animal feed containing 30 per cent of transgenic soybean and amplified by PCR (169-bp) were also detected, as well as non-amplified genomic DNA from this sample. Regarding PCR-amplified samples, amplicon purification was required, followed by thermal denaturation of the double-stranded DNA. The authors spectrophotometrically determined the DNA target concentration post-PCR. The experimental approach taken here intended to simulate the content of a real sample where not only genomic DNA is present, but also there is the possibility of having a nonspecific PCR-amplified fragment in relatively elevated amounts. So the authors amplified a similarly long sequence and mixed both in different ratios. They found that this nonspecific product actually decreased the signal significantly, but did not eliminate it completely. The detection limit for the EPSPS target was in the nanomolar range with relatively high coefficient of variation (~30 per

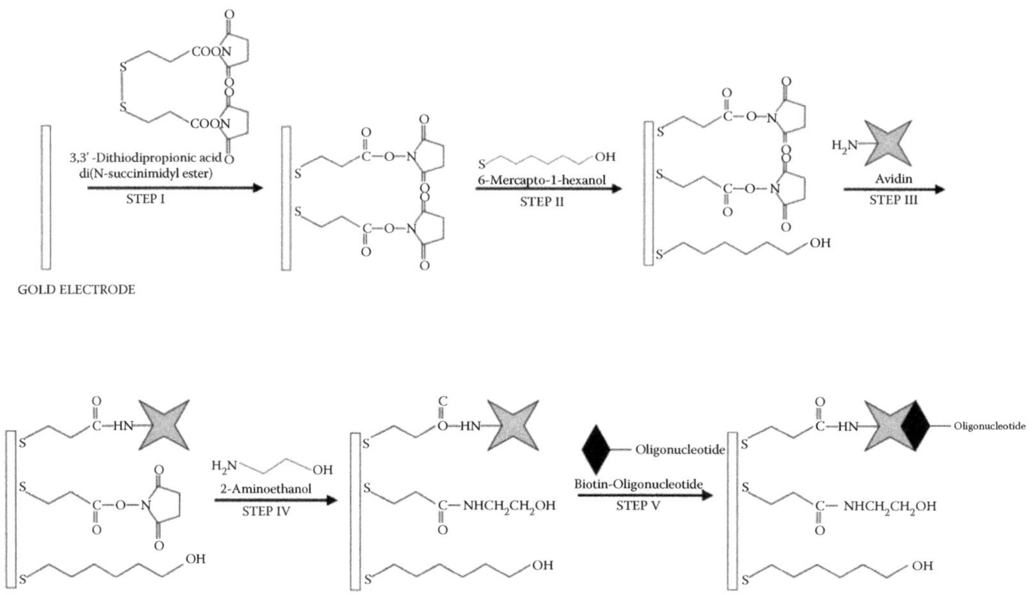


FIGURE 5.22 Steps of modification of the gold piezoelectrode. [Reproduced from Stobiecka et al., 2007, (open access)].

cent). In spite of these unfavorable results, this work reported highly encouraging data regarding the detection of non-amplified genomic DNA from the same feed: the sensor was able to detect from 3.6 µg of genomic DNA ($4.7 \times 10^6$ numbers of genome copies contained EPSPS gene). Although it is important to point out that the negative control, genomic DNA extracted from unmodified soybean, generated a small frequency shift, which the authors attributed to the possible direct adsorption of DNA onto the gold electrode surface without hybridization to the probe or weak, nonspecific interactions between the probe and partially complementary sequences present in very long genomic DNA.

Karamollaoglua et al. (2009) described a QCM biosensor for the detection of 35S using AT-cut Ti/Au polished piezoelectric quartz crystals (24.4 mm) with gold electrodes evaporated on both sides. The quartz crystal was held inside a methacrylate QCM flow-cell. The performance of different immobilization procedures, i.e., chemisorption based on thiol–gold interaction (SAM) with thiolated capture probes and blocking MCH, and covalent attachment based on functionalization of ethylenediamine (EDA)-polymerized surface using amined probes, were investigated. Capture probes were the same sequences used in the previous work by Mannelli (Mannelli et al., 2003). The EDA-based immobilization was carried out by treating the quartz substrate in a glow-discharge system generating a radio-frequency for EDA plasma polymerization. The primary amine groups created on the crystal surface after EDA plasma-polymerization were further converted to aldehyde groups by treating the surfaces with glutaraldehyde. The authors intended to covalently bind one aldehyde group of glutaraldehyde to the amine group of the EDA-derivatized surface, while the other aldehyde group would remain available for immobilization of the amino-functionalized probe. Results pointed out that a mildly enhanced signal (higher frequency decrease) was observed after hybridization of the synthetic target sequence and the thiolated probe. Moreover, the thiol-modified surfaces were more stable and could be regenerated up to five times after acidic treatment, compared to only three times using the EDA-based system. Interestingly, according to Sauerbrey's equation, which was employed in this work to determine the extent by which the surface was covered by the DNA probes, both thiolated and aminated probes resulted in similar values. Yet, the thiol-gold chemistry was chosen for biosensor construction. No calibration plot was included in this work, yet a decreasing trend in frequency changes was observed as the target concentration was increased, resulting in a bell-shaped plot. It seemed that 500 nM was the slowest target concentration tested with this system, and the authors obtained a similar frequency shift than the one observed by Mannelli et al. at lower levels.

Detection of "real" target DNA was done with PCR-amplified fragments and direct genomic DNA (PCR-free attempt) after enzymatic digestion or sonication to decrease steric effects. Heat denaturation was carried out in all cases. A plasmid was used as DNA source for PCR and genomic DNA extracted from transgenic tobacco plants was used for the PCR-free tryout. The same decreasing-signal with increasing-concentration behavior was obtained with the PCR-amplified samples, which the authors attributed to the fact that an increased number of target sequences might cause steric hindrance and the efficiency of denaturation might be reduced leading to the regeneration of the double-stranded configuration unable to hydridize at the sensor surface.

As to the PCR-free experiments, the system was evaluated using both genomic DNAs from wild type tobacco plants (as control) and transgenic tobacco plants. Both wild-type and transgenic DNA produced a signal increase with increasing analyte concentration using either enzymatically digested DNA or sonicated DNA. The authors concluded that the concentration range of the genome DNA was far below the linear ranges of the sensor, which could explain why the responses of both wild-type and transgenic systems did not correlate to the expected behavior.

Lien et al. (2010) reported a piezoelectric biosensor for the detection of 35S as well (same probes and sequences as previous works). The immobilization chemistry described here was based on the electrochemical deposition of polypyrrole films with MWCNTs, simultaneously mixed with oligonucleotides end-functionalized with pyrrole groups. The MWCNT-doped polypyrrole system depicted remarkable sensitivity with the QCM system, down to the detection of 4 pM of synthetic target sequence.

The saturation was reached at a concentration of 300 pM of target. In order to validate the transduction effect as being specific to the analyte, on one hand, a non-complementary sequence was tested and, on the other hand, the modified electrode was evaluated without the probe. Both experiments did not result in any frequency variation but only a slight destabilization of the quartz, which demonstrated that the resonance frequency variation was uniquely due to hybridization.

The biosensors described above have demonstrated the potential of QCM as a micro-weighing device as being suitable for GMO detection given the advantages of regeneration of the surface which enables the reuse of the quartz and also the label-free condition of the method. Yet, according to Ferreira et al. (2009), although the use of QCM as a transducer in biosensor development has exploited mainly the direct relationship between mass and frequency, as described by the Sauerbrey equation, this approach is biased because viscoelastic effects are not taken into consideration. This is particularly important when biomolecules are used due to complex biological media and buffers often required for bioconjugation. In addition, biomolecules commonly lead to considerable alterations of the viscoelastic properties near the sensor surface, which renders the signal from the sensor unsuitable to be interpreted under the ideal conditions that allow the use of the Sauerbrey equation. Moreover, variations in resonant frequency are also affected by changes in the roughness of the sensor surface, the solution permittivity and conductivity, as well as by the presence of charged species near the sensor surface. All of which might explain why this type of technique is more rarely reported than, for example, electrochemical and optical methods for GMO biosensing.

Considering that is important to know the kinetics of DNA degradation and amplificability in all the food processing chain, Bogani et al developed a systematic approach for tracing the transgenes along the whole food processing chain (Bogani et al., 2009). Roundup Ready soybean was specifically analyzed in eight types of processed materials—seeds, crushed seeds, expander, crude flour, protein flour, crude oil, degummed oil, and lecithin—all derived from the same initial source and produced during the manufacturing process. Biotinylated probe was immobilized into a gold sensor surface modified with thiol/dextran/streptavidin. Hybridization with PCR products amplified DNA containing 35S, extracted from the processing chain products was performed. In this way, it was possible study the traceability of the same targets in different materials, undergoing to different degree of processing, starting from the same source.

## 5.7 FINAL REMARKS

Compliance with GMO labeling thresholds must be guaranteed throughout the production chain, for which GMO quantification is ultimately required. This is a highly demanding analytical task that is, at present, solely fulfilled by qPCR methods, which are not utterly available in resource-limited environments and are often inadequate for decentralized and on-field analysis. Inmunosensors and, especially DNA-based biosensors, represent viable alternatives for this end. But there are still fundamental limitations in the field that we have summarized in two fundamental standpoints:

- From a technological perspective, methods that combined nanostructured or material-modified surfaces generally provided the highest sensitivities. However, the fabrication of these sensors often appeared to be time-consuming and laborious owed to multiple-step synthesis procedures and lingered electrode modifications. In this sense, the development of simpler and genuinely easy-to-execute protocols remains a challenge.
- From an analytical standpoint, the inability to quantify a specific protein or DNA sequences derived from "real" samples is a critical drawback. Scarce "real-sample" application and lack of quantitative analysis regarding taxon-specific-to-event-specific ratios stand out as two of the most important gaps of this technology. In addition, most reported GMO sensors have been focused on screening purposes, while very few attained event-specific detection.

We consider the second drawback to be the most crucial: if the actual analytical purpose is rarely achieved, which is to trace down specific genetic modifications in real foodstuffs (e.g., supermarket products), then the technological limitations regarding sensor fabrication can be overlooked. In this sense, the first aspect to consider is that a GMO genosensor is designed to detect a specific fragment contained within a genomic DNA extract, in which the ratio between the target and interfering species will often be very low. Although some genes are present in high copy numbers in the genome of some species, analysts generally deal with single-copy genes when working with GM plants, making amplification necessary. So far, PCR has been the most frequent amplification process coupled to genosensing. However, other amplification strategies, such as isothermal amplification, could be coupled to biosensors, but this type of amplification is not of widespread used in the field of GMO sensors (Ahmed et al., 2009). An enormous breakthrough in the field would be provided by non-PCR genosensors, meaning that these would surpass the need to incorporate an amplification step prior to electrochemical readout. This is a major challenge yet to be conquered in the GMO biosensing field.

Another aspect to be considered is that GMO content should be determined in relation to a taxon-specific gene and not simply as an absolute estimation of marker sequences. In this sense, it is important to highlight that the ultrasensitive genosensors reported so far, which show promising potential for application due to their prominent analytical performances, suffer from a major limitation related to the lack of true quantitative capacity. This fact seriously limits the applicability of the methods up to now reported that remain restricted to simple identification or quantitation of transgenic events in an absolute fashion that is not acceptable to establish compliance with legislation, which requires the GMO content to be expressed in percentage.

Other considerations to keep in mind when designing a GMO (DNA-based) biosensor are: on one hand, small DNA fragments should be targeted in order to ensure the detection GMOs in highly processed foods. On the other hand, DNA extraction, which is a crucial step in the analysis, must result in high quality and in sufficient DNA quantities from a variety of samples. Moreover, the amplification step must also be carefully optimized to obtain close-to-linear responses with the sensor. Overall, all the necessary steps that come before the sensing step must be thoroughly evaluated to obtain accurate results. Ideally, all of these steps would be integrated in a single platform but this envisioned sensing technology is yet to be accomplished.

Most recently, other challenges have become crucial in the field of GMO detection, affecting both PCR and biosensor technologies. These are the detection of unauthorized GMOs and the development of high-throughput multitarget techniques. Although some biosensors have been described for the simultaneous detection of different GMO sequences (Duwensee et al., 2009; Liao et al., 2013, Mix et al., 2012), it has not yet been possible to develop a multiplex quantitative sensor with analytical characteristics comparable to those of quantitative PCR. Until now, what has been achieved so far in terms of simultaneous determination is an electrochemical magnetoassay for the detection of a specific event of transgenic soybean (Manzanares et al., 2015b y 2016a), being necessary to perform the amplification and electrochemical measurement separately. One important goal to achieve yet would be to provide a multiplex device enabling simultaneous determination of at least two different DNA sequences (reference gene and inserted gene), in which all phases of the assay, extraction, amplification, and measurement, occur simultaneously. In this sense, the development of DNA biosensors with multiple electroactive markers that allow the detection of different transgenic events is a very promising aspect hardly explored to date.

The interest in DNA biosensors for GMO detection has been growing due to their possibility for automation and microfabrication based on simple and portable detection systems. Electrochemical microarray-based systems for multiplex DNA detection have become the most interesting kind of approach given that several construct elements can be co-detected, thus allowing high-throughput GMO diagnostics (Michelini et al., 2008). Optical platforms based on fast, visual results are also attractive at the consumer level.

Although a remarkable advance in biosensor technology for GMO testing has been reached, there is still much to explore and to achieve in the field, for which a great load of research is invested each year given the increasing interest in enforcing food control regulations and in guarantying transparency regarding food composition to the growingly aware consumers.

## REFERENCES


Aghili, Z., Nasirizadeh, N., Divsalar, A., Shoeibi, S., Yaghmaei, P. 2017. A nanobiosensor composed of exfoliated graphene oxide and gold nano-urchins, for detection of GMO products. *Biosensors and Bioelectronics*, 95:72–80.

Ahmed MU, Saito M, Hossain MM, Rao SR, Furui S, Hino A, Takamura Y, Takagi M, Tamiya E. 2009. Electrochemical genosensor for the rapid detection of GMO using loop-mediated isothermal amplification. Analyst, 134(5):966–72.

Alvarez, M., Tamayo, J. 2005. Optical sequential readout of microcantilever arrays for biological detection. *Sensors and Actuators B:Chemical*, 106:687–690.

Alvarez, M., Lechuga, L.M. 2010. Microcantilever-based platforms as biosensing tools. *Analyst*, 135:827–836.

Arugula, M.A., Simonian. A.L. 2016. Biosensors for detection of genetically modified organisms in food and feed. In *Genetically Modified Organisms in Food. Production, Safety, Regulation and Public Health*. 1st Edition Ross Watson, R., Preedy, V.R. (Eds.), pp. 97–110. Copyright © 2016 Elsevier.

Bai, S., Zhang, J., Li, S., Chen, H., Terzaghi, W., Zhang, X., Chi, X., Tian, J., Luo, H., Huang, W., Chen, Y., Zhang, Y. 2010. Detection of six genetically modified maize lines using optical thin-film biosensor chips. *Journal of Agriculture and Food Chemistry*, 58:8490–8494.

Bai, S.-L., Zhong, X., Ma, L., Zheng, W., Fan, L.-M., Wei, N., Deng, X.W., 2007. A simple and reliable assay for detecting specific nucleotide sequences in plants using optical thin-film biosensor chips. *Plant Journal for Cell and Molecular Biology*, 49:354–366.

Balasubramanian, K., Burghard, M. 2005. Chemically functionalized carbon nanotubes. *Small*, 1:180–192.

Bogani, P., Minunni, M., Spiriti, M.M., Zavaglia, M., Tombelli, S., Buiatti, M., Mascini, M. 2009. Transgenes monitoring in an industrial soybean processing chain by DNA-based conventional approaches and biosensors. *Food Chemistry*, 113:658–664.

Carpini, G., Lucarelli, F., Marrazza, G., Mascini, M. 2004. Oligonucleotide-modified screen-printed gold electrodes for enzyme-amplified sensing of nucleic acids. *Biosensors and Bioelectronics*, 20:167–175.

Carrascosa, L.G., Moreno, M., Álvarez, M., Lechuga, L.M. 2006. Nanomechanical biosensors: A new sensing tool. *TrAC Trends in Analytical Chemistry*, 25:196–206.

Chen, K., Han, H., Luo, Z., Wang, Y., Wang, X. 2012. A practicable detection system for genetically modified rice by SERS-barcoded nanosensors. *Biosensors and Bioelectronics*, 34:118–124.

Daghestani, H.N., Day, W. 2010. Theory and applications of surface plasmon resonance, resonant mirror, resonant waveguide grating, and dual polarization interferometry biosensors. *Sensors*, 10:9630–9646.

Dinh Tam., P. 2015. Genetically modified organism (GMO) detection by biosensor based on SWCNT material. *Current Applied Physics*, 15:397–401.

Duwensee, H., Mix, M., Broer, I., Flechsig, G-U. 2009. Electrochemical detection modified maize gene sequences by multiplexed labeling with osmium tetroxide bipyridine. *Electrochemistry Communications*, 11:1487–1491.

Dzyadvych, S.V., Soldatkin, A.P., El'skaya, A.V, Martelet, C., Jaffrezic-Renault, N. 2006. Enzyme biosensors based on ion-selective field-effect transistors. *Analytica Chimica Acta*, 568:248–258.

Ellington, AD., Szostak, J.W. 1990. In vitro selection of RNA molecules that bind specifi ligands. *Nature*, 346:818–822.
Fátima Barroso, M.F., Freitas, M., Oliveira, M.B., de-los-Santos-Álvarez, N., Lobo-Castañón, M.J., Delerue-Matos, C. 2015. 3D-nanostructured Au electrodes for the event-specific detection of MON810 transgenic maize. *Talanta*, 134:158–164.
Feng, Y., Yang, T., Zhang, W., Jiang, C., Jiao, K. 2008. Enhanced sensitivity for deoxyribonucleic acid electrochemical impedance sensor: Gold nanoparticle/polyaniline nanotube membranes. *Analytical Chimica Acta*, 616:144–151.
Ferreira, G.N.M., da-Silva, A.C., Tome, B. 2009. Acoustic wave biosensors: Physical models and biological applications of quartz crystal microbalance. *Trends in Biotechnology*, 27:689–697.
Feriotto, G., Borgatti, M., Mischiati, C., Bianchi, N., Gambari, R., 2002. Biosensor technology and surface plasmon resonance for real-time detection of genetically modified roundup ready soybean gene sequences. *Journal of Agricultural Food Chemistry*, 50:955–962.
Feriotto, G., Gardenghi, S., Bianchi, N., Gambari, R. 2003. Quantitation of Bt-176 maize genomic sequences by surface plasmon resonance-based biospecific interaction analysis of multiplex polymerase chain reaction (PCR). *Journal of Agricultural Food Chemistry*, 51:4640–4646.
Freitas, M., Correr, W., Cancino-Bernardi, J., Fátima Barroso, M., Delerue-Matos, C., Zucolotto, V. 2016. Impedimetric immunosensors for the detection of Cry1Ab protein from genetically modified maize seeds. *Sensors and Actuators B: Chemical*, 237:702–709.
Fu, Y.Q., Luo, J.K. Nguyen, N.T. Walton, A.J. Flewitt, A.J., Zu, X.T., Li, Y., McHale, G., Matthews, A., Iborra, E., Du, H., Milne, W.I. 2017. Advances in piezoelectric thin films for acoustic biosensors, acoustofluidics and lab-on-chip applications. *Progress in Materials Science*, 89:31–91.
Giakoumaki, E., Minunni, M., Tombelli, S., Tothill, I.E., Mascini, M., Bogani, P., Buiatti, M. 2003. Combination of amplification and post-amplification strategies to improve optical DNA sensing. *Biosensors and Bioelectronics*, 19:337–344.
Grieshaber, D., MacKenzie, R., Voros, J., Reimhult, E. 2008. Electrochemical biosensors-sensor principles and archittectures. *Sensors*, 8:1400–1458.
Guven, B., Hall Boyaci, I., Tamer, U., Alik, P.C. 2012. A rapid method for detection of genetically modified organisms based on magnetic separation and surface-enhanced Raman scattering. *Analyst*, 137:202–208.
Holst-Jensen, A., Bertheau, Y., Loose, M., Grohmann, L., Hamels, S., Hougs, L., Morisset, D., Pecoraro, S., Pla, M., Van den Bulcke, M., Wulff., D. 2012. Detecting un-authorized genetically modified organisms (GMOs) and derived materials. *Biotechnology Advances*, 30:1318–1335.
Jang, H.-J., Cho, I.-H., Kim, H.-S., Jeon, J.-W., Hwang, S.-Y., Paek, S.-H., 2011. Development of a chemiluminometric immunosensor array for on-site monitoring of genetically modified organisms. *Sensors and Actuators B Chemical*, 155:598–605.
Jarata, J. 1989. *Principles of Chemical Sensors*. Plenum Press, New York.
Jiang, C., Yang, T., Jiao, K., Gao, H. 2008. A DNA electrochemical sensor with and its application for the highly sensitive EIS detection of PAT gene fragment and PCR amplification of NOS gene. *Electrochimica Acta*, 53:2917–2924.
Jiang, X., Chen, K., Han, H. 2011. Ultrasensitive electrochemical detection of *Bacillus thuringensis* transgenic sequence base don *in situ* Ag nanoparticles aggregates induced by biotin-streptavidin system. *Biosensors and Bioelectronics*, 28:464–468.

Kalogianni, D.P., Koraki, T., Christopoulos, T.K., Ioannou, P.C., 2006. Nanoparticle-based DNA biosensor for visual detection of genetically modified organisms. *Biosensors and Bioelectronics*, 21:1069–1076.

Karamollaoglua, I., Avni-Öktema, H., Mutlub, M. 2009. QCM-based DNA biosensor for detection of genetically modified organisms (GMOs). *Biochemical Engineering Journal*, 44:142–150.

Kasry, A., Borri, P., Davies, P. R., Harwood, A., Thomas, N., Lofas, S., Dale, T. 2009. Comparison of methods for generating planar DNA-modified surfaces for hybridization studies. *ACS Applied Materials and Interfaces*, 1:1793–1798.

Kerman, K., Vestergaard, M., Nagatani, N., Takamura, Y., Tamiya, E. 2006. Electrochemical genosensor based on peptide nucleic acid-mediated PCR and asymmetric PCR techniques: Electrostatic interactions with a metal cation. *Analytical Chemistry*, 78:2182–2189.

Li, Y., Sun, L., Liu, Q., Han, E., Hao, N., Zhang, L., Wang, S., Cai, J., Wang, K. 2016. Photoelectrochemical CaMV35S biosensor for discriminating transgenic from non-transgenic soybean based on $SiO_2$@CdTe quantum dots core-shell nanoparticles as signal indicators. *Talanta*, 161:211–218.

Liao, W.C., Chuang, M.C., Ho, J.A. 2013. Electrochemical sensor for multiplex screening of genetically modified DNA: Identification of biotech crops by logic-based biomolecular analysis. *Biosensors and Bioelectronics*, 50:414–420.

Lien, T.T.N., Lam, T.D., An, V.T.H., Hoang, T.V., Quang, D.T., Khieu, D.Q., Tsukahara, T., Hoon Lee, Y., Kim, J.S. 2010. Multi-wall carbon nanotubes (MWCNTs)-doped polypyrrole DNA biosensor for label-free detection of genetically modified organisms by QCM and EIS. *Talanta*, 80:1164–1169.

Ligaj, M., Oczkowski, T., Jasnowska1, J., Musiał, G.W., Filipiak, M. 2003. Electrochemical genosensors for detection of L. monocytogenes and genetically-modified components in food. *Polysh Journal of Food and Nutrition Sciences*, 12/53:61–63.

Ligaj, M., Jasnowska, J., Musiał, W.G., Filipiak, M. 2006. Covalent attachment of single-stranded DNA to carbon paste electrode modified by activated carboxyl groups. *Electrochimica Acta*, 51:5193–5198.

Lisdat, F., Schafer, D. 2008. The use of electrochemical impedance spectroscopy for biosensing. *Analytical and Bioanalytical Chemistry*, 391:1555–1567.

Lucarelli, F., Marrazza, G., Turner, A.P.F., Mascini, M. 2004. Carbon and gold electrodes as electrochemical transducers for DNA hybridisation sensors. *Biosensors and Bioelectronics*, 19:515–530.

Lucarelli, F., Marrazza, G., Mascini, M. 2005. Enzyme-based impedimetric detection of PCR products using oligonucleotide-modified screen-printed gold electrodes. *Biosensors and Bioelectronics*, 20:2001–2009.

Ma, Y., Jiao, K., Yang, T., Sun, D. 2008. Sensitive PAT gene sequence detection by nano-$SiO_2$/p-aminothiophenol self-assembled films in DNA electrochemical biosensor based on impedance measurement. *Sensors and Actuators B: Chemical*, 131:565–571.

Malvano, F., Albanese, D., Pilloton, R., Di Matteo, M. 2016. A highly sensitive impedimetric label free immunosensor for Ochratoxin measurement in cocoa beans. *Food Chemistry*, 212:688–694.

Mannelli, I., Minunni, M., Tombelli, S., Mascini, M. 2003. Quartz crystal microbalance (QCM) affinity biosensor for genetically modified organisms (GMOs) detection. *Biosensors and Bioelectronics*, 18:129–140.

Manzanares-Palenzuela, C.L., Martín-Fernandez, B., Sánchez-Paniagua, M., López-Ruiz, B. 2015a. Electrochemical genosensors as innovative tools for detection of genetically modified organisms. *Trends of Analytical Chemistry*, 66:19–31.

Manzanares-Palenzuela, C.L., Santos-Alvarez, N., Lobo-Castañon, M.J., López-Ruiz, B. 2015b. Multiplex electrochemical DNA platform for femtomolar-level quantification of genetically modified soybean. *Biosensors and Bioelectronics*, 68:259–265.

Manzanares-Palenzuela, C.L., Mafra, I., Costa, J., Barroso, M.F., de-los-Santos-Álvarez, N., Delerue-Matos, C., Oliveira, M.B., Lobo-Castañón, M.J., López-Ruiz, B. 2016a. Electrochemical magnetoassay coupled to PCR as a quantitative approach to detect the soybean transgenic event GTS40-3-2 in foods. *Sensors and Actuators B: Chemical*, 222: 1050–1057.

Manzanares-Palenzuela, C.L., Fernandes, E.G.R., Lobo-Castañon, M.J., López-Ruiz, B., Zucolotto, V. 2016b. Impedance sensing of DNA hybridization onto nanostructured phthalocyanine-modified electrodes. *Electrochimica Acta*, 21:86–95.

Manzanares-Palenzuela, C.L., Martín-Clemente, J.P., Lobo-Castañon, M.J., López-Ruiz, B. 2017. Electrochemical detection of magnetically-entrapped DNA sequences from complex samples by multiplexed enzymatic labelling: Application to a transgenic food/feed quantitative survey. *Talanta*, 164:261–267.

Mao-Qing, W., Xiao-Yan, D., Li-Yan, L., Qian, S, Xian-Chen, J. 2008. DNA biosensor prepared by electrodeposited Pt-nanoparticles for the detection of specific deoxyribonucleic acid sequence in genetically modified soybean. *Chinese Journal of Analytical Chemistry*, 36:890–894.

Mariotti, E., Minunni, M., Mascini, M., 2002. Surface plasmon resonance biosensor for genetically modified organisms detection. *Analytica Chimica Acta*, 453:165–172.

Martín-Fernández, B., Miranda-Ordieres, A.J., Lobo-Castañón, M.J., Frutos Cabanillas, G., de-los-Santos-Álvarez, N., López-Ruiz, B. 2014. Strongly structured DNA sequences as targets for genosensing: Sensing phase design and coupling to PCR amplification for a highly specific 33-mer gliadin DNA fragment. *Biosensors and Bioelectronic*, 60:244–251.

Meric, B., Kerman, K., Marrazza, G., Palchetti, I., Mascini, M, Ozsoz, M. 2004. Disposable genosensor, a new tool for the detection of NOS-terminator, a genetic element present in GMOs. *Food Control*, 15:621–626.

Michelini E, Simoni P, Cevenini L, Mezzanotte L. 2008. Roda ANew trends in bioanalytical tools for the detection of genetically modified organisms: an update. *Anal Bioanal Chem*, 392(3):355–67

Ming, H., Wang, M., Yin, H., 2015. Detection of *Bacillus thuringiensis* Cry1Ab protein based on surface plasmon resonance immunosensor. *Analytical Biochemistry*, 468:59–65.

Minunni, M., Tombelli, S., Pratesi, S., Mascini, M., Piati, P., Bogani, P., Buiatti, M. 2001. A piezoelectric affinity biosensor for genetically modified organisms (GMOs) detection. *Analytical Letters*, 34:825–840.

Minunni, M., Tombelli, S., Fonti, J., Spiriti, M.M., Mascini, M., Bogani, P., Buiatti, M. 2005. Detection of fragmented genomic DNA by PCR-free piezoelectric sensing using a denaturation approach. *Journal of the American Chemical Society*, 127:7966–7967.

Mix, M., Rüger, J., Krüger, S., Broer, I., Flechsig, G.U. 2012. Electrochemical detection of 0.6% genetically modified maíz MON810 in real flour samples. *Electrochemistry Communications*, 22:137–140.

Navani, N.K., Li, Y.F. 2006. Nucleic acid aptamers and enzymes as sensors. *Current Opinion in Chemical Biology*, 10:272–281.

Patris, S., Kauffmann, J.M. 2016. Antibodies as target for affinity biosensors. *Trends in Analytical Chemistry*, 79:239–246.

Pohanka, M. 2017. The piezoelectric biosensors: Principles and applications, a review. *International Journal of Electrochemistry*, 12:496–506.

Querci, M., Guy, V., Jermini, M. 2006. Overview, general introduction on genetically modified organisms (GMOs), EU legislation joint research centre (European Commision).

Passamano, M., Pighini, M. 2006. QCM DNA-sensor for GMOs detection. *Sensors and Actuators B*, 118:177–181.

Pursey, J., Chen, Y., Stulz, E., Park, M.K., Kongsuphol, P. 2017. Microfluidic electrochemical multiplex detection of bladder cancer DNA markers. *Sensors and Actuators B:Chemical*, 251:34–39.

Ren, Y, Jiao, K., Xu, G., Sun, W., Gao, H. 2005. An electrochemical DNA sensor based on electrodepositing aluminum ion films on stearic acid-modified carbon paste electrode and its application for the detection of specific sequences related to bar gene and CP4 epsps gene. *Electroanalysis*, 17:2182–2189.

Richter, M.M. 2004. Electrochemiluminescence (ECL). *Chemical Reviews*, 104:3003–3036.

Sanchez-Paniagua Lopez, M., Lopez-Ruiz. B. 2011. Inhibition biosensor, based on calcium phosphate materials for detection of benzoic acid in aqueous and organic media. *Electroanalysis*, 23:264–271.

Sánchez-Paniagua López, M., Redondo Gómez, E., López Ruiz, B. 2017. Electrochemical enzyme biosensors based on calcium phosphate materials for tyramine detection in food samples. *Talanta*, 175:209–216.

Sassolas, A., Blum, L.J., Leca-Bovier, B.D. 2012. Immobilization strategies to developed enzymatic biosensors. *Biotechnology Advances*, 30:489–511.

Smuc, T., Ahn, I-Y., Ulrich, H. 2013. Nucleic acid aptamers as high affinity ligands in biotechnology and biosensorics. *Journal of Pharmaceutical and Biomedical Analysis*, 81–82:210–217.

Stobiecka, M, Ciesśla, J.M., Janowska, B., Tudek, B., Radecka, H. 2007. Piezoelectric sensor for determination of genetically modified soybean roundup ready® in samples not amplified by PCR. *Sensors*, 7:1462–1479.

Sun, W., Zhong, J., Zhang, B., Jiao, K. 2007. Application of cadmium sulphide nanoparticles as oligonucleotide labels for the electrochemical detection of NOS terminator gene sequences. *Analytical Bioanalytical Chemistry*, 389:2179–2184.

Sun, W., Zhang, Y., Hu, A., Lu, Y., Shi, F., Lei, B., Sun, Z. 2013. Graphene oxide modified carbon ionic liquid electrode for the detection of transgenic soybean A2704-12 gene sequence. *Electroanalysis*, 25:1417–1424.

Sun, W., Lu, Y., Wu, Y., Zhang, Y., Wang, P., Y. Chen. 2014. Electrochemical sensor for transgenic maize MON810 sequence with electrostatic adsorption DNA on electrochemical reduced graphene modified electrode. *Sensors and Actuators B: Chemical*, 202:160–166.

Tichoniuk, M., Ligaj, M., Filipiak, M. 2008. Application of DNA hybridization biosensor as a screening method for the detection of genetically modified food components. *Sensors*, 8:2118–2135.

Ulianas, A., Heng, L.Y., Ahmad, M., Lau, H.Y., Ishak, Z., Ling, T.L. 2014. A regenerable screen-printed DNA biosensor based on acrylic microsphere–gold nanoparticle composite for genetically modified soybean determination. *Sensors and Actuators B: Chemical*, 190:694–701.

Volpe, G., Ammid, N.H., Moscone, D., Occhigrossi, L., Palleschi, G. 2006. Development of an immunomagnetic electrochemical sensor for detection of BT-CRY1AB/CRY1AC proteins in genetically modified corn samples. *Analytical Letters*, 39:1599–1609.

Wang, J. 1998. DNA biosensors based on peptide nucleic acid (PNA) recognition layers. A review. *Biosensensors and Bioelectronics*, 13:757–762.

Wang, R., Minunni, M., Tombelli, S., Mascini, M., 2004a. A new approach for the detection of DNA sequences in amplified nucleic acids by a surface plasmon resonance biosensor. *Biosensors and Bioelectronics*, 20:598–605.

Wang, R., Tombelli, S., Minunni, M., Spiriti, M.M., Mascini, M., 2004b. Immobilisation of DNA probes for the development of SPR-based sensing. *Biosensors and Bioelectronics*, 20:967–974.

Wang, J., Qinling, S., Tian, N., Chen, L., Ziqin, X. Zheng, J. 2009. Electrochemical detection of the neomycin phosphotransferase gene (NPT-II) in transgenic plants with a novel DNA biosensor. *Journal of Applied Electrochemistry*, 39: 935–945.

Wang, S., Liu, Q., Li, H., Li, Y., Hao, N., Q, J., Zhu, W., Wang, K. 2016. Fabrication of label-free electrochemical impedimetric DNA biosensor for detection of genetically modified soybean by recognizing CaMV 35S promoter. *Journal of Electroanalytical Chemistry*, 782:19–25.

Wei Sun*, Jianghua Zhong, Peng Qin, Kui Jiao. 2008. Electrochemical biosensor for the detection of cauliflower mosaic virus 35 S gene sequences using lead sulfide nanoparticles as oligonucleotide labels. Analytical Biochemistry, 377:115–119

Wolfbeis, O.S. 2005. Materials for fluorescence-based optical chemical sensors. *Journal of Material Chemistry*, 15:2657–2669.

Xie, J-K., Jiao, K., Liu, H., Wang, Q-X., Liu, S-F., Fu, X. 2008. DNA electrochemical sensor base don PbSe nanoparticle for the sensitive detection of CaMV35S gene sequence. *Chinese Journal of Analytical Chemistry*, 36:874–878.

Xu, G., Jiao, K., Fan, J., sun, W. 2006. Electrochemical detection of specific gene related to CaMV35S using methylene blue and ethylenediamine-modified glassy carbon electrode. *Acta Chimica Slovenica*, 53:486–491.

Yang, J, Jiao, K, Yang, T. 2007a. A DNA electrochemical sensor prepared by electrodepositing zirconia on composite films of single-walled carbon nanotubes and poly(2,6-pyridinedicarboxylic acid), and its application to detection of the PAT gene fragment. *Analytical and Bioanalytical Chemistry*, 389:913–921.

Yang, J, Yang, T, Feng, Y, Jiao, K. 2007b. A DNA electrochemical sensor based on nanogold-modified poly-2,6-pyridinedicarboxylic acid film and detection of PAT gene fragment. *Analytical Biochemistry*, 365:24–30.

Yang, T., Zhang, W., Du, M., Jiao, K. 2008. A PDDA/poly(2,6-pyridinedicarboxylic acid)-CNTs composite film DNA electrochemical sensor and its application for the detection of specific sequences related to PAT gene and NOS gene. *Talanta*, 75:P987–994.

Yang, T., Zhou, N., Zhang, Y., Zhang, W., Jiao, K., Li., G. 2009. Synergistically improved sensitivity for the detection of specific DNA sequences using polyaniline nanofibers and multi-walled carbon nanotubes composites. *Biosensors and Bioelectronics*, 24:2165–2170.

Yang, T., Zhou, N., Li, Q., Guan, Q., Zhang, Q., Jiao, K. 2012a. Highly sensitive electrochemical impedance sensing of PEP gene based on integrated Au-Pt alloy nanoparticles and polytyramine. *Colloids and surfaces B: Biointerfaces*, 97:150–154.

Zhan, F., Liao, X., Gao, F., Qiu, W., Wang, Q. 2017. Electroactive crown ester-Cu2+ complex with in-situ modification at molecular beacon probe serving as a facile electrochemical DNA biosensor for the detection of CaMV 35s. *Biosensors and Bioelectronics*, 92:589–595.

Zhang, W., Yang, T., Jiang, C., Jiao, K. 2008. DNA hybridization and phosphinothricin acetyltransferase gene sequence detection based on zirconia/nanogold film modified electrode. *Applied Surface Science*, 254:4750–4756.

Zhao, Z., Chen, Y., Xu, W., Ma, M. 2013. Surface plasmon resonance detection of transgenic Cry1Ac cotton (gossypium spp.) *Journal of Agricultural and Food Chemistry*, 61:2964–2969.

Zhou, N., Yang, T., Jiang, C., Du, M., Jiao, K. 2009. Highly sensitive electrochemical impedance spectroscopic detection of DNA hybridization based on Aunano–CNT/PANnano films. *Talanta*, 77:1021–1026.

Zhu, L., Zhao, R., Wnag, K., Xiang, H., Shang, Z., Sun, W. 2008. Electrochemical behaviours of methylene blue on DNA modified electrode and its application to the detection of PCR product from NOS sequence. *Sensors*, 8:5649–5660.

Zhu, D., Liu, J., Tang, Y., Xing, D., 2010. A reusable DNA biosensor for the detection of genetically modified organism using magnetic bead-based electrochemiluminescence. *Sensors and Actuators B Chemical*, 149:221–225.

Zhu, M., Li, M., Li, G., Zhou, Z., Liu, H., Lei, H. 2015. Nanobody-based electrochemical immunoassay for bacillus thuringiensis Cry1Ab toxin by detecting the enzymatic formation of polyaniline, *Microchimica Acta*, 182:2451–2459.

# CHAPTER 6

# The Application of Nucleic Acid Microarrays for the Detection of Genetically Modified Organisms

*Stuart J. Lucas*
Sabanci University Nanotechnology Research and Application Center (SUNUM)

CONTENTS



## 6.1 INTRODUCTION

The use of genetically modified organisms (GMOs) to address the challenges faced by global agriculture continues to be a highly contentious issue. GMO crops, and to a lesser extent animals, are presented by their proponents as the best opportunity to provide food security for a growing world population. However, sceptics are equally insistent that GMOs present risks to health and the environment, resulting in widespread public distrust of the technology (see Lucas, Türkeç, and Karlik 2016 for a recent review of the issues).

In response to these concerns, many national and international authorities have enacted regulations controlling the transport and use of GMOs and their products, such as the Cartagena Protocol on Biosafety (Secretariat of the Convention on Biological Diversity 2003). These regulations in turn create a need for methods that provide accurate monitoring of GMO presence, both in the field and in food production chains.

An ideal GMO detection method should:

i. be comprehensive enough to detect most, if not all, existing GMOs
ii. be specific enough to distinguish between different GM events with >95 per cent accuracy
iii. be sensitive enough to detect and quantify GMOs at concentrations down to 0.9 per cent (based on EU regulations)
iv. be labor- and cost-effective enough for routine monitoring
v. be robust and fast enough to be reproduced in multiple laboratories without extensive specialist training (Von Götz 2010)

While real-time polymerase chain reaction (PCR) assays remain the most widely used technology for GMO monitoring, they are limited to detecting one or a few genetic elements in each assay. In spite of the controversy surrounding them, the planted area and variety of GMO crops on the market is increasing steadily. Between 2008 and 2014, the number of different GM events approved for commercial use somewhere in the world more than doubled from 42 to 102, and based on those currently in the development pipeline, this figure could double again by 2020 (Figure 6.1.) Moreover, these figures do not take into account "stacked" GMOs, in which two or more GM events are combined in a single plant by conventional crossbreeding. If these are considered as separate varieties, by the end of 2016, 210 different GMOs had been approved for use in at least one country.

Testing for such a large number of different GM crops by single or multiplex real-time PCR is rapidly becoming prohibitively expensive. Therefore, methods that allow high-throughput screening of numerous specific DNA sequences are urgently required for GMO monitoring. One approach that has generated considerable research interest is microarray technology.

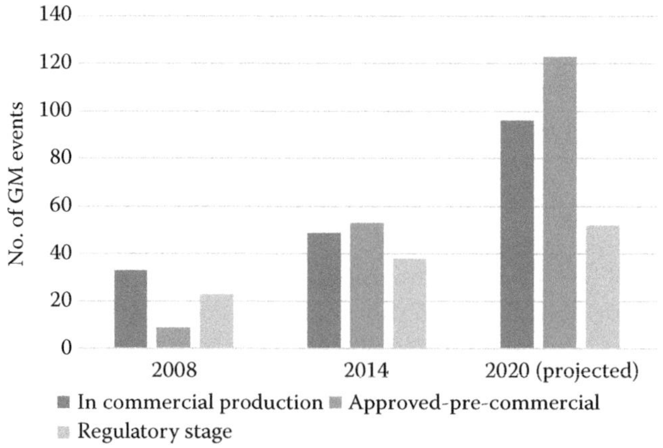


FIGURE 6.1 Bar chart showing the expansion in the number of distinct GM events in production in at least one country from 2008 to 2014, and projected growth by 2020. (Parisi, Tillie, and Rodríguez-Cerezo 2016.)

## 6.2 NUCLEIC ACID MICROARRAY TECHNOLOGY

Microarrays provide a platform on which anywhere from a few to tens of thousands of specific biomolecules can be detected simultaneously. As a result, significant research effort has been put into developing microarray-based methods for GMO detection, to overcome the multiplexing limitations of real-time PCR. While protein microarrays are attracting interest for some biotechnological applications (Sutandy et al. 2013), to date the GMO field has focused exclusively on the detection on the detection of transgenic DNA, which is much more likely to survive crop and food processing. In this chapter, the essential features of microarrays used for DNA detection will be reviewed, the different GMO-specific microarrays that have been developed will be compared, and the prospects for the use of this technology in the future will be discussed.

### 6.2.1 Essential Features

The basic principle of nucleic acid microarrays is simple, and relies on the capacity of DNA/RNA strands to bind those with matching complementary sequences with high specificity. A microarray experiment consists of four main steps, as summarized in Figure 6.2.

First, the array itself is constructed by immobilizing probes (specific sequences of single-stranded DNA) on a solid support, in an ordered 2D pattern. Various methods can be used to generate ssDNA probes, such as reverse transcription; however, as microarray technology has matured, synthetic oligonucleotides have become the probes of choice, as they are much easier to produce consistently in large numbers.

Second, the genomic DNA from the sample of interest must be processed to produce short (<1000 nt) targets that can bind to the probes on the array. This typically involves fragmentation and/or PCR amplification to generate smaller segments from high molecular weight DNA, which may be followed by synthesis of the targets by DNA or RNA polymerase starting from an oligonucleotide primer. The targets are also labeled, usually by incorporation of a fluorophore or biotin.

During the third step, hybridization, the labeled targets are incubated with the microarray, which is subsequently washed to remove unbound targets. Hybridization conditions must be optimized to minimize non-specific binding and ensure a good signal:noise ratio.

Finally, the targets bound to the washed and dried microarray are visualized by colorimetric or fluorimetric methods. The locations of the spots on the resulting image indicate which target sequences were present in the sample; in some applications, their intensity can also be used to quantify the concentration of the targets in the original sample.

In the GMO detection field, a variety of approaches have been applied for each of these steps, as detailed in the following sections.

### 6.2.2 A Brief History of GMO Microarrays

The first use of a hybridization approach to detect DNA from different GMOs was reported by Blais and colleagues in 2002 (Blais, Phillippe, and Vary 2002), who immobilized PCR products from two transgene elements, P35S (the cauliflower mosaic virus 35S promoter) and tNOS (the *Agrobacterium tumefaciens* nopaline synthase terminator), and two plant-specific genes (maize invertase and soybean lectin) onto strips of polyester

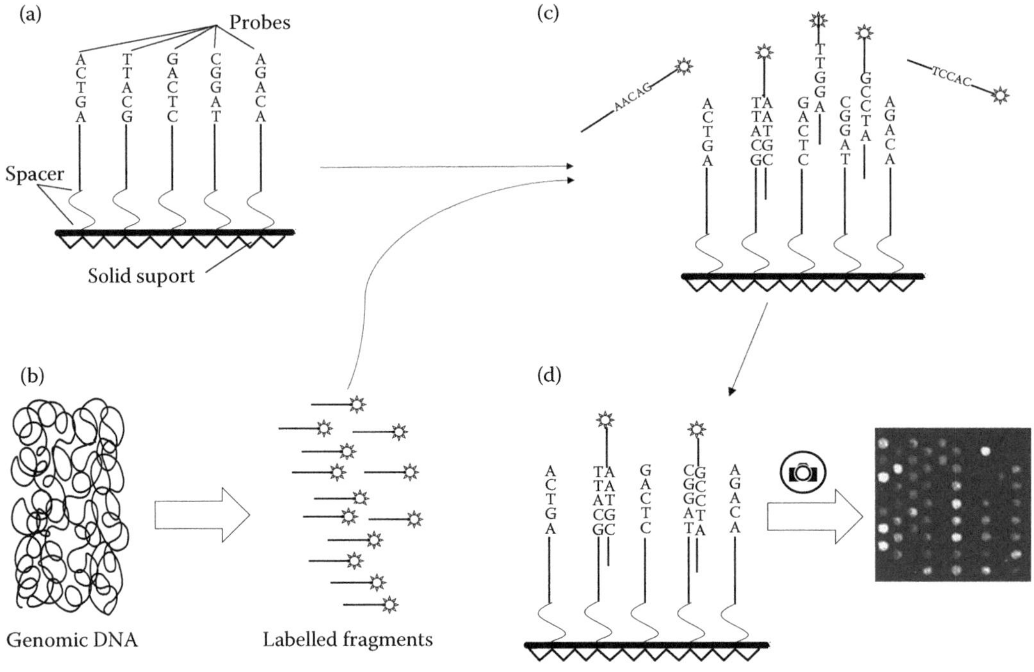


FIGURE 6.2 Schematic of the essential elements of a DNA microarray experiment. (a) *Microarray synthesis.* Oligonucleotide probes of known sequences are immobilized in specific locations on a solid support. (b) *Sample processing.* Genomic DNA is either fragmented, or target regions amplified, and a tag attached to produce labeled target fragments. (c) *Hybridization.* The labeled targets are incubated with the array to allow targets to bind to their complementary probes. Unbound targets are washed away. (d) *Visualization.* After drying, the array is imaged, for example, using a microarray scanner. Brightness of spots on the image corresponds to the amount of target bound to each probe.

cloth. They also designed a multiplex PCR to amplify the same four elements from isolated maize and soya DNA. Digoxigenin-11-dUTP was included in the multiplex PCR to label the targets; after hybridization, these were detected colorimetrically using antibody-horseradish peroxidase (HRP) conjugate specific for digoxigenin. By this method, the four genetic elements could be detected simultaneously and specifically, so that GM and non-GM soya and maize flour could be distinguished from each other.

Although DNA hybridization technology was still in its infancy, this study provided a proof of concept for its use in GMO detection, and included all of the essential features of a microarray experiment. In studies published over the following years, these core elements remained largely unchanged, although many novel technical improvements have been made (Table 6.1). The cloth support was rapidly replaced by nitrocellulose membrane (Su et al. 2003; Rudi, Rud, and Holck 2003). The comprehensive work by Rudi et al. also identified many key considerations for a useful diagnostic microarray, including sensitivity, a linear dose-response to enable quantification of the DNA targets, and the use of reference GMO materials to calibrate the assay (Rudi, Rud, and Holck 2003).

The introduction in 2003 of legislation by the European Union requiring all food and feed products containing ≥0.9 per cent GMO material to be labeled as such

TABLE 6.1 Summary of Reported GMO Microarray Detection Methods

| References | Microarray Type | Target Amplification/Labeling | Visualization/ Detection |
|---|---|---|---|
| Blais, Phillippe, and Vary (2002) | PCR products on cloth strips | Multiplex PCR with 11-DIG-dUTP | Anti-DIG-HRP conjugate |
| Rudi, Rud, and Holck (2003) | Oligonucleotides on nitrocellulose | 2-step multiplex PCR; fluorescein-ddCTP labeling | Fluorescence/ Anti-fluorescein-HRP conjugate |
| Su et al. (2003) | Oligonucleotides on nitrocellulose | Multiplex PCR with biotinylated primers | Streptavidin-alkaline phosphatase |
| Germini et al. (2004); Germini et al. (2005) | PNAs on glass slides | Multiplex PCR; asymmetric PCR with 5′-Cy5-primers | Fluorescence array scanner |
| Bordoni et al. (2005); Bordoni et al. (2004) | Oligonucleotides on glass slides | Multiplex PCR; ligation detection with Cy3-oligos | Fluorescence array scanner |
| Xu et al. (2005) | Oligonucleotides on glass slides | Asymmetric multiplex PCR with 5′-Cy3 primers | Fluorescence array scanner |
| Xu et al. (2006); Xu et al. (2007) | Oligonucleotides on glass slides | Multiplex PCR incorporating Cy5-dCTP | Fluorescence array scanner |
| Leimanis et al. (2006); Leimanis et al. (2008); Hamels et al. (2009) | Oligonucleotides on glass slides (DualChip GMO) | Multiplex PCR (4 sets) incorporating biotinylated dATP & dCTP | Streptavidin-gold nanoparticles, SilverQuant system |
| Morisset et al. (2008); Dobnik, Morisset, and Gruden (2010) | Oligonucleotides on glass slides | Multiplex NASBA; ligation to dendrimers harboring Oyster-550 dye | Fluorescence array scanner |
| Prins et al. (2008); Prins et al. (2010) | Oligonucleotides on glass slides | Multiplex Padlock Probe Ligation; asymmetric PCR with 5′-Cy5-primers | Fluorescence array scanner |
| Tengs et al. (2007); Tengs et al. (2010) | Affymetrix/Agilent HD arrays | Whole genome fragmentation/labeling | Fluorescence array scanner |
| Schmidt et al. (2008) | Oligonucleotides on glass slides | Multiplex PCR; Cy3-ULS | Fluorescence array scanner |
| Kim et al. (2010) | Oligonucleotides on glass slides | Multiplex PCR (4 sets) with 5′-Cy3 primers | Fluorescence array scanner |
| Shao et al. (2014) | Oligonucleotides on glass slides | Microwell PCR; universal PCR with 5′-Cy3 primers | Fluorescence array scanner |
| Turkec et al. (2016) | Agilent Custom CGH array | Whole genome fragmentation/labeling | Fluorescence array scanner |
| Liu et al. (2016) | Oligonucleotides on glass slides | Multiplex PCR; ligation detection with Cy3-oligos | Fluorescence array scanner |

(European Commission 2003a; European Commission 2003b) prompted a rapid acceleration in the development of GMO detection methods. At the same time, the availability of automated microarray printers enabled researchers to produce custom microarrays in a highly reproducible fashion by spotting the probes onto functionalized glass slides (Germini et al. 2004; Xu et al. 2005). Probes produced from peptide nucleic acids, pseudo-DNA strands in which the sugar-phosphate backbone is replaced by *N*-aminoethylglycine, were tested as an alternative to DNA oligonucleotides (Germini et al. 2004). Furthermore, it was demonstrated that inclusion of a short spacer between the probe and the glass support improved the microarray signal, presumably by reducing steric hindrances to hybridization (Bordoni et al. 2005; Germini et al. 2005).

By 2006, biotechnology companies were beginning to market oligonucleotide microarrays for a variety of applications. Accordingly, the first commercial microarray-based GMO detection kits were developed by Leimanis and colleagues (Leimanis et al. 2006, 2008) and produced by Eppendorf Array Technologies (Namur, Belgium) as "DualChip GMO." This system had a number of novel features that illustrate important issues for transferring a microarray suitable for research to a marketable product. The target GM elements were amplified in optimized multiplex PCR reactions; in order to include elements specific for all GMOs that were approved in the EU at the time, as well as plant-specific genes, the DualChip GMO kit used four different PCR mixes with 2–4 primer pairs in each. The PCR procedure incorporated biotin labeling and dUTP instead of dTTP; this allows uracil-*N*-glycosylase treatment to be included before amplification, which will degrade any contaminating PCR products from previous reactions—an important consideration for a diagnostic laboratory.

The pooled PCR products were then hybridized to the microarray chip, which was spotted with probes for 15 GM and plant elements, plus hybridization controls. As antibody and fluorescence-based detection methods are relatively expensive, these chips instead used streptavidin-linked gold nanoparticles to bind the biotinylated PCR products. The gold nanoparticles act as a catalyst for reduction of silver ions, allowing the microarrays to be visualized with EAT's SilverQuant reagents and scanner. Finally, analysis software was provided to give the user an immediate interpretation of the microarray results, and the procedure was validated in 11 laboratories (Hamels et al. 2009).

The DualChip kit remains the only microarray-based GMO detection kit to have been commercialized, and it is no longer on the market. One major limitation was that, although the microarray could in principle be expanded to include probes for many more GM elements, the requirement for multiplex PCR to amplify and label the targets before hybridization imposed a major limiting factor. Most multiplex PCRs, even after extensive optimization, can only reliably amplify 2–5 targets at once, although one study reported a 10-plex PCR allowing microarray detection of GM canola (Schmidt et al. 2008). In any case, as the number and diversity of GMOs on the market has increased, using multiplex PCR in screening methods has become increasingly impractical.

In order to address this problem, a number of non-PCR methods have been proposed for multiplex target amplification prior to microarray analysis, such as NASBA (Morisset et al. 2008) and Padlock Probe Ligation (Prins et al. 2008); these approaches will be discussed in detail in the next section. Most recently, Shao et al. designed a microwell chip to carry out 91 individual PCRs simultaneously, before hybridizing the pooled products with a GMO microarray (Shao et al. 2014).

All of the approaches mentioned above used relatively low-density microarrays that can be printed in a laboratory equipped with a microarray spotter, with fewer than 100 different probes. The production of high-density microarrays with thousands of probes requires highly specialized technology, and is currently only offered by three companies: Affymetrix, Agilent, and Illumina. However, the use of a large excess of probes is extremely powerful; by including probes encompassing all known GM transformation vector sequences, even unknown GMOs can be detected and identified (Tengs et al. 2007; Tengs et al. 2010). Also, high-density arrays may be sensitive enough directly to detect the presence of GMO DNA in mixed samples without PCR amplification (Turkec et al. 2016). These high-density arrays have not yet been applied to routine GMO screening due to the high cost of the individual arrays, and the complexity of data analysis.

The large majority of GMO microarrays described to date have been designed to detection of the most widespread GMO crops, soybean and maize. However, more recent studies have included microarrays specifically for the detection of GM canola (Schmidt et al. 2008) and rice (Liu et al. 2016).

### 6.2.3 Hybridization Biosensors

In contrast to standard DNA microarray technology, where the underlying membrane or glass slide simply provides a solid support for the probes, another alternative is offered by electrochemical biosensors. In these systems, the DNA probe is immobilized on a matrix such as a quartz crystal microbalance (QCM) or a gold electrode; on hybridization of the target, the change in mass generates an electrical signal in the matrix, removing the need for an additional visualization step. A small number of reports have explored the potential of this technology for GMO detection. Mannelli et al. (Mannelli et al. 2002) immobilized ssDNA probes for P35S and tNOS on a QCM chip, and showed that PCR-amplified DNA targets could be bound and then washed off, meaning that the chip could be re-used up to 20 times. In a similar QCM chip carrying a 200nt probe derived from the *cry1Ab* gene, it was shown that DNA from bt176 maize could be detected across a range of 0.1–5 per cent GMO, with a linear relationship between GMO concentration and the QCM signal (Passamano and Pighini 2006). Optimization of the immobilization conditions for the probe on the QCM chip has been described (Karamollaoğlu, Öktem, and Mutlu 2009), while a gold-based biosensor, again with probes for P35S and tNOS, has also been reported (Tichoniuk, Ligaj, and Filipiak 2008).

While they also rely on hybridization, in comparison to DNA microarrays electrochemical biosensors remain a largely undeveloped technology for GMO detection. Their capacity for direct electrical detection of targets and the fact that chips can be re-used could make them highly cost-effective. However, all the biosensor chips reported to date have only used a single probe; it remains unclear how practical it would be to produce a multiplex biosensor. Further studies are also required to determine the specificity and sensitivity of, for example, QCM chips when analyzing mixed samples. However, the potential utility of this kind of biosensor has been demonstrated in one study, in which the concentration of GMO RoundupReady Soybean was followed throughout an industrial food processing chain by applying samples from each stage to the same biosensor chip (Bogani et al. 2009).

## 6.3 TECHNICAL CONSIDERATIONS FOR A SUCCESSFUL MICROARRAY APPROACH

Technical details are important to the success of any DNA microarray experiment, but the specific requirements of GMO analysis introduce some additional considerations. Whereas most other microarrays are designed to evaluate a pure DNA/RNA sample, GMO screening requires the capacity to detect a small amount of the target DNA when mixed with an excess of non-GMO sample (e.g., ≥0.9 per cent of the total DNA, to comply with EU requirements). Furthermore, in order to quantify the detected GMOs, there must be a linear relationship between the starting concentration and the signal from the microarray. These requirements influence each stage of the experimental procedure.

### 6.3.1 Sample Preparation and Microarray Design

DNA samples for GMO analysis may come from a variety of sources ranging from seeds to lightly processed food products (e.g., flour) to heavily processed food products (e.g., baked goods, confectionery). The concentration and quality of DNA that can be isolated varies greatly with the sample, and no single extraction method is suitable for every sample type, as reported in many previous studies (Turkec et al. 2014, 2015). Furthermore, food products may contain other compounds such as polysaccharides, lipids, and small molecules that could inhibit enzymatic reactions and/or interfere with hybridization. For this reason, the majority of the microarray studies listed in Table 6.1 only used DNA extracted from seeds or certified reference materials, with a few cases also including food samples.

In principle, microarray hybridization ought to be more robust to DNA fragmentation during food production than, for example, PCR, as the target sequences can be relatively short (30–90 nt, depending on the probe length). However, the thermodynamics and kinetics of microarray hybridization are highly complex and can be altered by, for example, the relative concentration of target and non-target DNA fragments (Koltai and Weingarten-Baror 2008). Therefore, empirical optimization of the hybridization conditions is necessary to ensure that microarray data are reproducible.

An additional consideration is the design of microarray probes. Most of the studies described above found that oligomers of 15–30 nt in length provided sufficient specificity to discriminate between sequences. However, the Agilent platform uses 60-mer probes, which offer greater specificity when trying to detect sequences that are similar to those in the plant genome, or when screening for unknown GMOs (Tengs et al. 2010). In general, all probes on the same array should be the same length, have the same guanine-cytosine (GC) content, and be free of secondary structure so that they all hybridize with equal efficiency. One way to ensure this is to use a "universal array" spotted with "zipcode" probes that are thermodynamically equivalent to each other, but unrelated to the target sequence (Bordoni et al. 2005; Liu et al. 2016). In this instance, a secondary probe in the form of a labeled chimeric oligonucleotide is generated using a ligation detection reaction (LDR, see Section 6.3.3); this probe has sections complementary both to the target sequence and to a specific zipcode.

Even when the probes have identical physical characteristics, their specificity and sensitivity will be affected by the presence or absence of similar sequences in the plant genome. Turkec et al. (2016) tested probes covering the entirety of each GM sequence of interest at 5 nt intervals, and observed that some probes gave signals 10–100 fold stronger than others from within the same gene.

### 6.3.2 Target DNA Amplification

As noted above, GMO screening involves the detection of GM DNA at low concentrations. To add to the challenge, GM elements comprise a very small percentage of the plant genome—for example, ~10 kb in the 2.3 Gb maize genome. This means that 100 ng of maize genomic DNA from a mixture containing 1 per cent GMO will contain only ~400 copies of the GM target sequences. Therefore, it is not surprising that most GMO detection methods require an amplification step to achieve sufficient sensitivity, usually multiplex PCR. However, multiplex PCR is problematic in that it limits the number of elements that can be detected simultaneously, and different amplicons within the same reaction may amplify with different efficiency. Furthermore, the exponential nature of PCR amplification means that small differences in amplification efficiency between different amplicons can, after numerous cycles, result in large differences in the final concentration of PCR products; therefore, they cannot be used to quantify the starting material.

Several modifications and alternatives have been suggested to address these problems. In a 2-step PCR, the targets are amplified for only a few cycles using target-specific primer pairs, all of which are tagged with the same 5′ sequences (Rudi, Rud, and Holck 2003). In the second step, the amplicons are amplified in a single reaction with primers for the universal sequence, minimizing the variation in amplification efficiency between templates. Using this approach, Rudi et al. were able to demonstrate a dose–response relationship for GM targets in 7-plex and 12-plex PCRs, although the relationships were not linear for all targets. A similar 2-step amplification is used in the MACRO system (Shao et al. 2014), although in this case the first amplification is carried out as simplex, 25-cycle PCR reactions in separate microwells. The authors demonstrated the high sensitivity of this system (down to ~10 copies of target DNA in the original sample) but not whether it could be used for accurate quantification.

As variable amplification efficiency is an inherent weakness of PCR, some studies have used entirely different amplification methods. Nucleic acid sequence-based amplification (NASBA) is one such method, which mimics the replication machinery used by retroviruses, reviewed in (Deiman, van Aarle, and Sillekens 2002), and is most often used for detection and quantitation of viral RNA in clinical samples. However, it can also be modified to amplify DNA targets, as reported in the NASBA implemented microarray analysis (NAIMA) approach (Morisset et al. 2008). In this system, a single cycle of amplification with *Taq* polymerase and multiplex primers tailed at the 5′ end with binding sites for T7 and SP6 RNA polymerases was used to generate short dsDNA templates from the target regions. The templates were then incubated with T7 RNA polymerase, AMV reverse transcriptase and RNase H in the presence of universal primers, resulting in a cyclical amplification reaction via a ssRNA/ssDNA duplex intermediate. The end product was cRNA (ssRNA complementary to the original target sequence) that could be directly hybridized to a microarray. Using two different triplexes at the initial template generation step, NAIMA was shown to have faster kinetics and comparable sensitivity and specificity to real-time PCR; furthermore, the resulting fluorescence signal showed a tightly linear relationship with template copy number across a wide concentration range (0.1–25 per cent GMO). Therefore, NAIMA was the first truly quantitative multiplex GMO detection method (Dobnik, Morisset, and Gruden 2010), and NASBA seems to solve to problem of variable PCR amplification efficiency. However, it is more costly per reaction than PCR in terms of reagents and time; the authors calculated that a hexaplex NAIMA would be competitive in terms of resources used with singleplex real-time PCR. Also, it is not yet clear how far the multiplexing capacity of NASBA can be increased without loss of quantitative accuracy.

Another approach that shows promise for quantitative detection involves the use of "Padlock Probe Ligation," or PPL (Prins et al. 2008). Padlock probes are linear oligonucleotides, typically 100–140 nt in length, that include sections at their 5′ and 3′ ends that complement adjacent segments of the target sequence. On target binding, the ends of the probe are ligated together to produce a circular molecule. Ligated probes are then amplified by PCR across the joined ends. In the aforementioned study, asymmetric PCR was applied in which one of the primers was supplied in a limiting quantity; once this was exhausted, linear amplification from the remaining primer produced ssDNA products that could be hybridized to the microarray. The authors reported a limit of detection of 1–2.5 per cent for different targets in a 10-plex PPL amplification, and a close to linear relationship between end signal and initial concentration for those for which three or more concentration levels had been measured. The utility of this approach was further confirmed by (Ujhelyi et al. 2012), who compared five different ligation-based protocols and concluded that PPL gave the best overall results. They also tested two different 10-plex PPL reactions followed by microarray detection in two laboratories for three different complex GMO mixtures, and showed complete reproducibility of the results for 1 per cent GMO targets, and all but one of the targets at 0.1 per cent GMO concentration (Ujhelyi et al. 2012). These results suggest that PPL is robust enough for multiplex GMO detection, however further research is required to determine whether it is fully quantitative.

As both PCR and the alternative amplification methods summarized above have limited multiplexing capacity, is it possible to eliminate the amplification step altogether? In two studies focusing on the identification of unknown GMO contaminants (Tengs et al. 2007, 2010), it was demonstrated that non-amplified GMO DNA could be accurately identified using microarrays consisting of multiple overlapping probes covering the GM sequences, although only 100 per cent GMO samples were tested. Furthermore, in recent years "comparative genomic hybridization" (CGH) microarray platforms have been developed for several species, with which it is possible to identify unit changes in the copy number of specific sections of genomic DNA between different individuals (Baumbusch et al. 2008). Therefore, a CGH-like approach was tested to see whether it would be sensitive enough to detect GM insertions into the genome even at low concentrations (Turkec et al. 2016). In this study, the Agilent Custom CGH platform was used to design a microarray containing overlapping 60-mer probes covering the GM cassettes of 12 different GMOs. Using certified reference materials, it was demonstrated that 10/12 GMOs could be detected at <1 per cent GMO concentration without any amplification of the GM elements. Furthermore, a linear relationship between the hybridization signal and GMO concentration was demonstrated for several of the probes. The major disadvantage of the CGH-microarray approach for routine GMO screening is the relatively high cost and expertise required. However, the authors were able to identify a subset of 3–5 probes for each GMO of interest that gave optimal accuracy and sensitivity, which could form the basis of a more cost-effective detection solution.

### 6.3.3 Labeling and Detection

Tied to the question of sensitivity, and therefore the need for amplification prior to microarray hybridization, is the labeling of GM DNA fragments so that they can be detected once they are bound to the array. While the earliest microarrays utilized antibody-enzyme conjugates to catalyse a colorimetric reaction (Blais, Phillippe, and Vary 2002; Rudi, Rud, and Holck 2003), in the vast majority of subsequent studies the GM DNA fragments were fluorescently labeled (Table 6.1). Fluorophores such as the cyanine dyes Cy3 and Cy5 are small enough (590 and 762 Da respectively) to be covalently attached to DNA, and fluoresce brightly when excited with light of a specific wavelength, giving high sensitivity and specificity. Where a GMO-specific PCR amplification step is employed, this can incorporate fluorescent labeling, either by including a fluorophore-dNTP (Xu et al. 2006) or by including Cy3/Cy5-labeled primers (Germini et al. 2004) in the reaction mix. Alternatively, the PCR products can be labeled after amplification, for example using Cy3-ULS (universal linkage system), a platinum compound that reacts with purine nucleotides (Schmidt et al. 2008). Another post-amplification labeling method that provides an additional level of specificity is the LDR (Bordoni et al. 2005). In this approach, multiplex PCR products are incubated with DNA ligase in the presence of pairs of oligonucleotides that hybridize to adjacent sites in the GM target of interest; the first is labeled with Cy3, while the second includes a region complementary to a specific "zipcode" probe on a universal array. Only if the target sequence is present are the two oligos ligated together, to form a labeled product that will hybridize to the array.

When PCR amplification is not used, a separate labeling reaction is required. For example, in the NAIMA method the amplified cRNA was ligated to dendrimers containing the fluorescent dye Oyster-550 (Morisset et al. 2008). Similarly, when the GMO DNA is not amplified at all (Tengs et al. 2010; Turkec et al. 2016), it must first be fragmented, for example, by digestion with restriction enzymes, and then used as a template to synthesize short pieces of labeled ssDNA. In the Agilent protocol, this is carried out using random primers, DNA polymerase I (Klenow fragment) and Cy3/Cy5-dUTP to incorporate the fluorophore.

Fluorescent dyes are the preferred method for microarray labeling because they can be visualized directly without an additional detection reaction and because they generate a strong signal with little background, essential for distinguishing between the thousands of spots on a high-density microarray. However, scanning such microarrays requires expensive and specialist equipment: a modern microarray scanner includes laser(s) to excite the fluorophores, a high-resolution camera to photograph the fluorescing microarray, and data analysis software to extract the fluorescence signals from each spot and identify which probes they contain. Furthermore, the fluorophores themselves are relatively expensive and require careful handling, as they can be bleached by exposure to light and atmospheric ozone—in the case of Cy5, even at quite low levels (Fare et al. 2003). Many labs where routine GMO screening is carried out do not have the equipment or expertise for fluorescent microarray analysis. Therefore, when the commercial DualChip GMO screening kit was developed (Leimanis et al. 2008), a colorimetric labeling method based on silver staining was used instead (cf. Section 6.2.2). For rapid analysis, this still required a microarray scanner, albeit a much cheaper and simpler device than fluorescence scanners. However, this technology lacked the resolution to be used for high-density microarrays.

### 6.3.4 Remaining Technical Challenges

In summary, while a number of effective technologies for GMO microarray analysis have been described, there remain unresolved dilemmas that are barriers to development of a commercially viable screening solution. The first is between sensitivity vs. throughput vs. quantification. The major advantage of microarrays over real-time PCR is the capacity to screen for hundreds or thousands of GM elements simultaneously. However, in order to achieve the sensitivity required by regulatory authorities, 11/16 microarray methods reported to date (Table 6.1) used a multiplex-PCR amplification of the GM targets prior to hybridization, both limiting the breadth of the analysis to a few known targets and making it unsuitable for quantification. Other amplification methods such as PPL and NASBA are as sensitive as PCR and more quantitative, but currently have limited multiplexing capacity (Prins et al. 2010; Dobnik, Morisset, and Gruden 2010). The MACRO system has enough sensitivity to detect 91 GMO elements simultaneously

(Shao et al. 2014), but is not proven for quantification. Meanwhile, the direct hybridization strategy offers multiplex quantitative detection only limited by the number of probes on the microarray, but further optimization is required to achieve the desired sensitivity (Turkec et al. 2016).

The second dilemma is between effectiveness vs. cost/ease of use. While each of the newer technologies mentioned above is more powerful than standard PCR screening, they are also more expensive, more time-consuming, and require more technical expertise. To save time, methods in which target labeling is incorporated into the amplification step are preferable to those requiring two separate procedures. Most GMO microarray studies to date have used the cyanine dyes as they are readily available and well characterized; indeed, fluorescence detection is the only method suitable for scanning high-density microarrays, in spite of its high cost. However, there are many other fluorophores available, some of which are reportedly more stable and/or sensitive than Cy3/Cy5. These fluorophores should be explored for GMO analysis, as should lower cost alternatives to fluorescence.

## 6.4 FUTURE PROSPECTS FOR MICROARRAY-BASED GMO DETECTION

### 6.4.1 Detection of Unknown GMOs and Edited Genomes

All the methods currently used for routine GMO screening require prior knowledge of the sequence of the GM elements that are to be detected. With the growing distribution and variety of GM crops worldwide (cf Section 6.1), there is an increasing need for a tool that could be used to detect the presence of unknown or previously uncharacterized GMOs. The potential of high-density microarrays for this purpose has been uniquely demonstrated by Arne Holst-Jensen and colleagues at the National Veterinary Institute, Norway. They initially demonstrated that a microarray could be designed to include all probes for sequences of a given length that correspond to probable GMO inserts (Nesvold et al. 2005). Using the sequenced genome of *Arabidopsis thaliana* as an example, they started with all possible sequences of length $n$, then carried out three levels of complexity reduction:

i. All probes that could hybridize to the non-GM genome were eliminated.
ii. Sequences that are biologically unlikely (e.g., very high/low GC content, low complexity and repetitive sequences) were eliminated.
iii. Sequences that would perform poorly in standard hybridization conditions were eliminated.

Using these criteria, the authors showed that a DNA microarray of $10^6$ 15-mer probes would hybridize to >95 per cent of 85 reported GM insert sequences of 5–10 kb in length, in an arabidopsis background. However, this strategy requires complete knowledge of the target species genome sequence to eliminate false positives. Therefore, the authors developed an alternative design targeting the sequences of all publically available GM constructs (Tengs et al. 2007). This approach relied on the fact that many GMOs incorporate some of the same genetic elements, such as P35S and tNOS, reducing the total number of sequences to be represented. By tiling 25-mer probe sequences with an average of 15 nt overlap on both strands of the GM constructs, all could be covered on a 40,000 probe

Affymetrix microarray. This array was successful in detecting GM inserts in transgenic arabidopsis and rice lines. Improved performance and more comprehensive GMO coverage was obtained using an Agilent array containing 93,000 60-mer probes, tiled with an average of 53 nt overlap (Tengs et al. 2010). In both cases, false positive signals were observed from 0.5–4 per cent of probes during each hybridization, but these could largely eliminated by requiring a minimum window size of at least five overlapping probes (for the 60-mers; 30 for the 25-mers) to give a positive signal to determine a true positive. This latter array was able to correctly identify >90 per cent of the insert sequences in two known transgenic soya and maize lines, and was also able to characterize the majority of the GM elements present in soya GMO A5547-127, for which sequence information was not previously available.

These tiling arrays represent the first method to be described that could in practice identify any existing GMO in a single experiment. However, they do require 100 per cent GMO DNA, and rely on the unknown GMO containing at least some elements in common with those that have been described previously. While this is a reasonable assumption for conventional GMOs, a new generation of "genome edited" crops is now being developed, using the CRISPR/Cas9 system, reviewed in (Lucas, Türkeç, and Karlik 2016). These crop lines need not have any transgenic DNA inserted, as many desirable traits can be induced simply by deletion of a handful of bases in the host genome. While it is not yet clear whether regulatory bodies will require genome edited crops to be monitored in the same way as conventional GMOs, there is no doubt that none of the current GMO screening technologies, including microarrays, could reliably detect such small variations.

### 6.4.2 Where Next for GMO Microarray Analysis?

DNA microarray analysis is now a mature technology that over the last 15 years has proven to be a powerful research tool in a variety of fields. However, in spite of the significant effort put into developing GMO screening microarray platforms described in this review, only one (DualChip GMO) became a commercial product, and this is no longer in production (Section 6.2.2). In part, this is because of the technical challenges that remain unresolved in producing a GMO array platform that is comprehensive, sufficiently sensitive, and quantitative (Section 6.3.4). While qPCR analysis is increasingly inadequate for the task of screening the growing number of GMOs on the market, it is sensitive, quantitive, and relatively inexpensive. Meanwhile, high-throughput DNA sequencing can in principle completely describe the genome of a suspected GMO with no prior knowledge of its sequence, and has decreased in price to the point where the cost per sample may be cheaper than high-density microarray analysis.

So are GMO microarrays a good idea, but one that is now superseded by newer technologies? On the contrary, this author would argue that there is still a need for a platform that can screen a large number of GM elements in parallel on a large number of samples for moderate cost. Of the studies described in this chapter, the MACRO system (Shao et al. 2014) has potential in this respect. Alternatively, in order to detect both the increasing variety of conventional GMOs, and future genome edited crops, recent advances in single nucleotide polymorphism (SNP) genotyping arrays should be applied to the field. Both the Infinium BeadArray (Illumina) and Axiom Genotyping arrays (Affymetrix) can screen tens of thousands of SNPs for dozens or hundreds of samples in a single experiment. These platforms should be readily adaptable to GMO detection; however, development and production of specialized GMO arrays would require considerable initial investment. Nevertheless, if current and future requirements for GMO monitoring are to be met, this investment would be well justified.

## REFERENCES


Baumbusch, Lars Oliver, Jørgen Aarøe, Frederik -Ekeberg Johansen, James Hicks, HailingSun, Laura Bruhn, Kevin Gunderson, et al. 2008. "Comparison of the agilent, ROMA/NimbleGen and illumina platforms for classification of copy number alterations in human breast tumors." *BMC Genomics* 9 (1): 379. doi:10.1186/1471-2164-9-379.

Blais, Burton W., Lucille M. Phillippe, and Neil Vary. 2002. "Cloth-based hybridization array system for detection of transgenic soy and corn by multiplex polymerase chain reaction." *Biotechnology Letters* 24 (17): 1407–1411. doi:10.1023/A:1019894330731.

Bogani, Patrizia, Maria Minunni, Maria M. Spiriti, Michele Zavaglia, Sara Tombelli, Marcello Buiatti, and Marco Mascini. 2009. "Transgenes monitoring in an industrial soybean processing chain by DNA-based conventional approaches and biosensors." *Food Chemistry* 113 (2): 658–664. doi:10.1016/j.foodchem.2008.07.056.

Bordoni, Roberta, Andrea Germini, Alessandra Mezzelani, Rosangela Marchelli, and Gianluca De Bellis. 2005. "A microarray platform for parallel detection of five transgenic events in foods: A combined polymerase chain reaction-ligation detection reaction-universal array Method." *Journal of Agricultural and Food Chemistry* 53 (4): 912–918. doi:10.1021/jf0486949.

Bordoni, Roberta, Alessandra Mezzelani, Clarissa Consolandi, Andrea Frosini, Ermanno Rizzi, Bianca Castiglioni, Claudia Salati, et al. 2004. "Detection and quantitation of genetically modified maize (Bt-176 transgenic maize) by applying ligation detection reaction and universal array technology." *Journal of Agricultural and Food Chemistry* 52 (5): 1049–1054. doi:10.1021/jf034871e.

Deiman, Birgit, Pierre van Aarle, and Peter Sillekens. 2002. "Characteristics and applications of nucleic acid sequence-based amplification (NASBA)." *Molecular Biotechnology* 20 (2): 163–179. doi:10.1385/MB:20: 2: 163.

Dobnik, David, Dany Morisset, and Kristina Gruden. 2010. "NAIMA as a solution for future GMO diagnostics challenges." *Analytical and Bioanalytical Chemistry* 396 (6): 2229–2233. doi:10.1007/s00216-009-3197-7.

European Commission. 2003a. "Regulation (EC) No 1829/2003 of the European parliament." *Official Journal of the European Union* L268: 1–23. http://eur-lex.europa.eu/legal-content/EN/TXT/?uri=uriserv:OJ.L_.2003.268.01.0001.01.ENG.

European Commission. 2003b. "Regulation (EC) No 1830/2003 of the European Parliament." *Official Journal of the European Union* L268: 24–28. http://eur-lex.europa.eu/legal-content/EN/TXT/?uri=uriserv:OJ.L_.2003.268.01.0024.01.ENG.

Fare, Thomas L., Ernest M. Coffey, Hongyue Dai, Yudong D. He, Deborah A. Kessler, Kristopher A. Kilian, John E. Koch, et al. 2003. "Effects of atmospheric ozone on microarray data quality." *Analytical Chemistry* 75 (17): 4672–4675. doi:10.1021/ac034241b.

Germini, Andrea, Alessandra Mezzelani, Francesca Lesignoli, Roberto Corradini, Rosangela Marchelli, Roberta Bordoni, Clarissa Consolandi, and Gianluca De Bellis. 2004. "Detection of genetically modified soybean using peptide nucleic acids (PNAs) and microarray technology." *Journal of Agricultural and Food Chemistry* 52 (14): 4535–4540. doi:10.1021/jf035355r.

Germini, Andrea, Stefano Rossi, Alessandro Zanetti, Roberto Corradini, Corrado Fogher, and Rosangela Marchelli. 2005. "Development of a peptide nucleic acid array platform for the detection of genetically modified organisms in food." *Journal of Agricultural and Food Chemistry* 53 (10): 3958–3962. doi:10.1021/jf050016e.

Hamels, Sandrine, Thomas Glouden, Karine Gillard, Marco Mazzara, Frédéric Debode, Nicoletta Foti, Myriam Sneyers, et al. 2009. "A PCR-microarray method for the screening of genetically modified organisms." *European Food Research and Technology* 228 (4): 531–41. doi:10.1007/s00217-008-0960-5.

Karamollaoğlu, İrem, Hüseyin Avni Öktem, and Mehmet Mutlu. 2009. "QCM-based DNA biosensor for detection of genetically modified organisms (GMOs)." *Biochemical Engineering Journal* 44 (2–3): 142–150. doi:10.1016/j.bej.2008.11.011.

Kim, Jae Hwan, Su Youn Kim, Hyungjae Lee, Young Rok Kim, and Hae Yeong Kim. 2010. "An Event-Specific DNA Microarray to Identify Genetically Modified Organisms in Processed Foods." *Journal of Agricultural and Food Chemistry* 58 (10): 6018–6026. doi:10.1021/jf100351x.

Koltai, Hinanit, and Carmiya Weingarten-Baror. 2008. "Specificity of DNA microarray hybridization: Characterization, effectors and approaches for data correction." *Nucleic Acids Research* 36 (7): 2395–2405. Oxford University Press. doi:10.1093/nar/gkn087.

Leimanis, Serge, Sandrine Hamels, Florence Nazé, Guillaume Mbongolo Mbella, Myriam Sneyers, Rupert Hochegger, Hermann Broll, et al. 2008. "Validation of the performance of a GMO multiplex screening assay based on microarray detection." *European Food Research and Technology* 227 (6): 1621–1632. doi:10.1007/s00217-008-0886-y.

Leimanis, Serge, Marta Hernández, Sophie Fernández, Francine Boyer, Malcolm Burns, Shirin Bruderer, Thomas Glouden, et al. 2006. "A microarray-based detection system for genetically modified (GM) food ingredients." *Plant Molecular Biology* 61 (1–2): 123–139. doi:10.1007/s11103-005-6173-4.

Liu, Xiaolei, Shengying Qin, Hui Wang, and Yingying Le. 2016. "Monitoring genetically modified rice using multiplex PCR coupled with universal DNA microarray." *Journal of Nutrition & Health* 2 (2): 6. doi:10.13188/2469-4185.1000019.

Lucas, Stuart J., Aydin Türkeç, and Elif Karlik. 2016. "The future of GM foods or GM foods of the future: Where is the biotech revolution heading?" In *Food Toxicology*, edited by Debasis Bagchi, Anand Swaroop, and Sidney J. Stohs, 518–537. Boca Raton: CRC Press. doi:10.1201/9781315371443-26.

Mannelli, Ilaria, Maria Minunni, Sara Tombelli, and Marco Mascini. 2002. "Quartz crystal microbalance (QCM) Affinity biosensor for genetically modified organisms (GMOs) detection." *Biosensors and Bioelectronics* 18 (2–3): 129–140. doi:10.1016/S0956-5663(02)00166-5.

Morisset, Dany, David Dobnik, Sandrine Hamels, Jana Ẑel, and Kristina Gruden. 2008. "NAIMA: Target amplification strategy allowing quantitative on-chip detection of GMOs." *Nucleic Acids Research* 36 (18). doi:10.1093/nar/gkn524.

Nesvold, Håvard, Anja Bråthen Kristoffersen, Arne Holst-Jensen, and Knut G Berdal. 2005. "Design of a DNA chip for detection of unknown genetically modified organisms (GMOs)." *Bioinformatics (Oxford, England)* 21 (9): 1917–1926. doi:10.1093/bioinformatics/bti248.

Parisi, Claudia, Pascal Tillie, and Emilio Rodríguez-Cerezo. 2016. "The global pipeline of GM crops out to 2020." *Nature Biotechnology* 34 (1): 31–36. Nature Publishing Group. doi:10.1038/nbt.3449.

Passamano, Myriam, and Monica Pighini. 2006. "QCM DNA-sensor for GMOs detection." *Sensors and Actuators, B: Chemical* 118 (1–2): 177–181. doi:10.1016/j.snb.2006.04.012.

Prins, Theo W., Jeroen P. van Dijk, A. M. Angeline Van Hoef, Marleen M. Voorhuijzen, Sylvia Broeders, Stefanie Trapmann, Ralf Seyfarth, et al. 2010. "Towards a multiplex cereal traceability tool using padlock probe ligation on genomic DNA." *Food Chemistry* 118 (4): 966–973. doi:10.1016/j.foodchem.2008.10.085.

Prins, Theo W., Jeroen P. van Dijk, Henriek G. Beenen, A.M. Angeline Van Hoef, Marleen M. Voorhuijzen, Cor D. Schoen, Henk J.M. Aarts, and Esther J. Kok. 2008. "Optimised padlock probe ligation and microarray detection of multiple (non-authorised) GMOs in a single reaction." *BMC Genomics* 9 (1): 584. doi:10.1186/1471-2164-9-584.

Rudi, K., I. Rud, and A. Holck. 2003. "A novel multiplex quantitative DNA array based PCR (MQDA-PCR) for quantification of transgenic maize in food and feed." *Nucleic Acids Research* 31 (11): 62e–62. doi:10.1093/nar/gng061.

Schmidt, Anna Mary, Robert Sahota, Derek S. Pope, Tracy S. Lawrence, Mark P. Belton, and Michael E. Rott. 2008. "Detection of genetically modified canola using multiplex PCR coupled with oligonucleotide microarray hybridization." *Journal of Agricultural and Food Chemistry* 56 (16): 6791–6800. doi:10.1021/jf800137q.

Secretariat of the Convention on Biological Diversity. 2003. "Cartagena protocol on biosafety convention on biological diversity." *Biological Conservation* 114: 467. doi:10.1016/S0006-3207(03)00053-3.

Shao, Ning, Shi Meng Jiang, Miao Zhang, Jing Wang, Shu Juan Guo, Yang Li, He Wei Jiang, et al. 2014. "MACRO: A combined microchip-PCR and microarray system for high-throughput monitoring of genetically modified organisms." *Analytical Chemistry* 86 (2): 1269–1276. doi:10.1021/ac403630a.

Su, Wenijn, Siyang Song, Minnan Long, and Guangming Liu. 2003. "Multiplex polymerase chain reaction/membrane hybridization assay for detection of genetically modified organisms." *Journal of Biotechnology* 105 (3): 227–233. doi:10.1016/j.jbiotec.2003.07.001.

Sutandy, F., X. Reymond, Jiang Qian, Chien Sheng Chen, and Heng Zhu. 2013. "Overview of Protein Microarrays." *Current Protocols in Protein Science*, no. SUPPL.72. doi:10.1002/0471140864.ps2701s72.

Tengs, Torstein, Anja B Kristoffersen, Knut G Berdal, Tage Thorstensen, Melinka A Butenko, Håvard Nesvold, and Arne Holst-Jensen. 2007. "Microarray-based method for detection of unknown genetic modifications." *BMC Biotechnology* 7 (1): 91. doi:10.1186/1472-6750-7-91.

Tengs, Torstein, Anja Bråthen Kristoffersen, Haibo Zhang, Knut G. Berdal, Marie Løvoll, and Arne Holst-Jensen. 2010. "Non-prejudiced detection and characterization of genetic modifications." *Food Analytical Methods* 3 (2): 120–128. doi:10.1007/s12161-009-9111-2.

Tichoniuk, M, M Ligaj, and M Filipiak. 2008. "Application of DNA hybridization biosensor as a screening method for the detection of genetically modified food components." *Sensors* 8 (4): 2118–2135. doi:10.3390/S8042118.

Turkec, Aydin, Hande Kazan, Aykut Baykut, and Stuart J Lucas. 2015. "Evalution of DNA extraction methods in order to monitor genetically modified materials in soy foodstuffs and feeds commercialised in Turkey by multiplex real-time PCR." *Journal of the Science of Food and Agriculture* 95 (2): 386–392. doi:10.1002/jsfa.6731.

Turkec, Aydin, Hande Kazan, Burçin Karacanlı, and Stuart J. Lucas. 2014. "DNA Extraction Techniques Compared for Accurate Detection of Genetically Modified Organisms (GMOs) in Maize Food and Feed Products." *Journal of Food Science and Technology*. Springer India. doi:10.1007/s13197-014-1547-8 <http://dx.doi.org/10.1007/s13197-014-1547-8>.

Turkec, Aydin, Stuart J. Lucas, Burçin Karacanli, Aykut Baykut, and Hakki Yuksel. 2016. "Assessment of a direct hybridization microarray strategy for comprehensive monitoring of genetically modified organisms (GMOs)." *Food Chemistry* 194: 399–409. doi:10.1016/j.foodchem.2015.08.030.

Ujhelyi, Gabriella, Jeroen P van Dijk, Theo W Prins, Marleen M Voorhuijzen, AM Angeline Van Hoef, Henriek G Beenen, Dany Morisset, Kristina Gruden, and Esther J Kok. 2012. "Comparison and transfer testing of multiplex ligation detection methods for GM Plants." *BMC Biotechnology* 12 (1): 4. doi:10.1186/1472-6750-12-4.

Von Götz, Franz. 2010. "See what you eat-broad GMO screening with microarrays." *Analytical and Bioanalytical Chemistry* 396 (6): 1961–1967. doi:10.1007/s00216-009-3204-z.

Xu, Jia, Haizhen Miao, Houfei Wu, Wensheng Huang, Rong Tang, Minyan Qiu, Jianguo Wen, Shuifang Zhu, and Yao Li. 2006. "Screening genetically modified organisms using multiplex-PCR coupled with oligonucleotide microarray." *Biosensors and Bioelectronics* 22 (1): 71–77. doi:10.1016/j.bios.2005.12.001.

Xu, Jia, Shuifang Zhu, Haizhen Miao, Wensheng Huang, Minyan Qiu, Yan Huang, Xuping Fu, and Yao Li. 2007. "Event-specific detection of seven genetically modified soybean and maizes using multiplex-PCR coupled with oligonucleotide microarray." *Journal of Agricultural and Food Chemistry* 55 (14): 5575–5579. doi:10.1021/jf070433m.

Xu, Xiaodan, Yingcong Li, Heng Zhao, Si-yuan Wen, Sheng-qi Wang, Jian Huang, Kunlun Huang, and Yun-bo Luo. 2005. "Rapid and reliable detection and identification of GM events using multiplex PCR coupled with oligonucleotide microarray." *Journal of Agricultural and Food Chemistry* 53 (10): 3789–3794. doi:10.1021/jf048368t.

CHAPTER 7

# Recent Developments in Detection Methods of Genetically Modified Organisms

*Leo M.L. Nollet*
University College Ghent

CONTENTS



## 7.1 INTRODUCTION

In the following sections, the most prevalent detection methods of genetically modified organisms (GMOs) are discussed. Three interesting papers were recently published on these topics (1–3). Figure 7.1 (3) gives an overview of strategies in GMO detection.

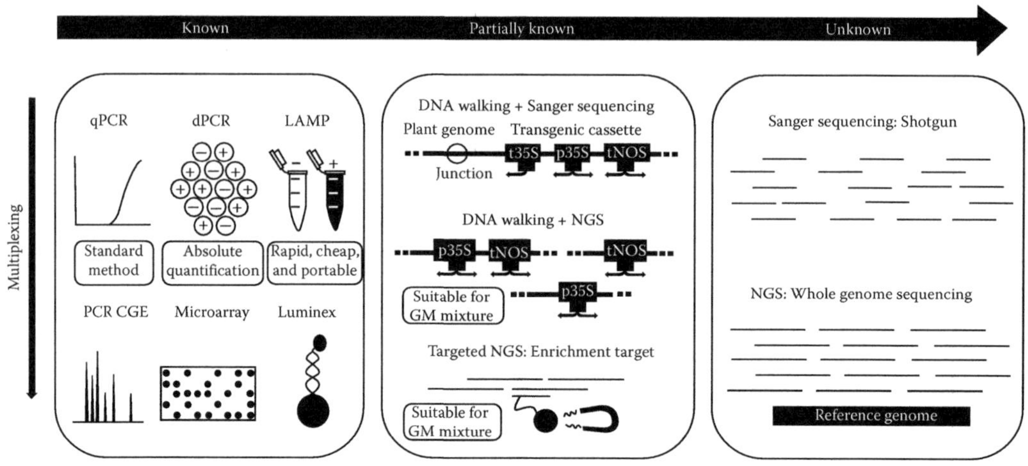


FIGURE 7.1 Suitable application of GMO detection approaches regarding the adopted strategy as well as available information about the sequences of tested GMO.

## 7.2 REAL-TIME POLYMERASE CHAIN REACTION MULTIPLEX STRATEGIES

Multiplex polymerase chain reaction (PCR) allows concurrent amplification of different targets in a single PCR tube. Multiplexing not only saves time, reagents, and samples but also makes simultaneous comparison of multiple amplicons possible.

A four duplex real-time assay system was used by Chaouachi et al. (4) to identify genetically modified (GM) maize lines (Bt11, Bt176, MON810, and T25). Park et al. (5) used three triplicate multiplex real-time PCR systems to enable the tracking of authorized and unauthorized GM (UGM) soybean events in food and feed.

Datukishvili et al. (6) present novel multiplex PCR methods. New designed PCR primers targeting four frequently used GMO-specific sequences permitted identification of new DNA markers, in particular 141 bp fragment of cauliflower mosaic virus (CaMV) 35S promoter, 224 bp fragment of *Agrobacterium tumefaciens* nopaline synthase (NOS) terminator, 256 bp fragment of 5-enolpyruvylshikimate-phosphate synthase (*epsps*) gene, and 258 bp fragment of Cry1Ab delta-endotoxin (*cry1Ab*) gene for GMO screening. The certified reference materials containing Roundup Ready soybean (RRS) and maize MON 810 were applied for the development and optimization of uniplex and multiplex PCR systems. Evaluation of amplification products by agarose gel electrophoresis using negative and positive controls confirmed high specificity and sensitivity at 0.1 per cent GMO for both RRS and MON 810. The fourplex PCR was developed and optimized that allows simultaneous detection of three common transgenic elements: CaMV 35S promoter, NOS terminator, and *epsps* gene together with soybean-specific *lectin* gene. The triplex PCR was developed that enables simultaneous identification of transgenic elements such as 35S promoter and *cry1Ab* gene together with maize zein gene.

Two novel multiplex real-time PCR systems were developed and validated (7). One system determines DNA contents from maize, soya, CaMV 35S promoter (P35S), and NOS terminator of *Agrobacterium tumefaciens* and CaMV, and the second PCR system simultaneously detects DNA sequences from figwort mosaic virus promoter, from bar gene of *Streptomyces hygroscopicus,* from gene coding for phosphinothricin acetyl-transferase, and from a DNA construct of EPSPS gene (CP4 EPSPS) and *Arabidopsis thaliana* (*CPT2*).

A specific and sensitive qPCR assay was developed for *vip3A* element detection based on the *vip3Aa20* coding sequences of the recently marketed MIR162 maize and COT102 cotton (8). Furthermore, SiteFinding-PCR in combination with Sanger, Illumina, or Pacific BioSciences (PacBio) sequencing was performed targeting the flanking DNA of the *vip3Aa20* element in MIR162. De novo assembly and basic local alignment search tool searches were used to mimic unauthorized GMO (UGMO) identification. PacBio data resulted in relatively long contigs in the upstream (1,326 nucleotides (nt); 95 per cent identity) and downstream (1,135 nt; 92 per cent identity) regions, whereas Illumina data resulted in two smaller contigs of 858 and 1,038 nt with higher sequence identity (>99 per cent identity). Both approaches outperformed Sanger sequencing, underlining the potential for next-generation sequencing in UGMO identification.

Noguchi et al. (9) developed a feasible qPCR method in which the GMO content is calculated based on the quantification of two herbicide-tolerant trait genes, 5-enolpyruvylshikimate-3-phosphate synthase from *Agrobacterium* sp. strain CP4 (*cp4-epsps*) and phosphinothricin *N*-acetyl-transferase from *Streptomyces viridochromogenes* (*pat*) to quantify the GMO content in ground grain samples containing stacked GM maize. The GMO contents of two genes were quantified using a plasmid calibrant and summed for quantification of total GMO content. The trait-specific method revealed lower biases for examination of test samples containing stacked GM maize compared with the event-specific method.

In order to control imports of maize products from retailers, efficient and reliable methods for the detection and quantification are a prerequisite. Actually, in the EU, more than 25 GM Maize traits were authorized and are allowed to be sold. To ensure correct labeling and exclude UGM traits from sale, five multiplex real-time PCR systems were developed and validated (10). These 20 systems for the most prevalent maize GM traits allow relative multiplex quantification and/or delta–delta Ct method quantification in routine in a reliable, cost- and time-efficient way.

Debode et al. (11) present the results of the inter-laboratory studies for the successful validation of qualitative real-time PCR methods for the detection of GMOs in food and feed. Two singleplex TaqMan methods were developed for the detection of the tE9 terminator present in several GM events and the detection of the endogenous *lectin* gene from pea; the tE9 terminator donor organism. In addition, a TaqMan duplex method was validated, which allows the simultaneous detection of the pat and bar elements.

The paper explains the different acceptance parameters used during the in-house validation, the method transferability study and finally the inter-laboratory validation, how this validation was conducted and the problems encountered. Statistical methods for the validation of the qualitative methods are also presented.

SYBR® Green I-based duplex and triplex real-time PCR assays targeting event-specific sequences of three GM maize events, namely Bt11, Bt176, and MON89034, and taxon-specific endogenous Adh1 gene were developed to simultaneously identify multiple events (12). Duplex real-time PCR assay based on TaqMan® chemistry targeting Bt176 event-specific sequence and Adh1 was also optimized for quantification purpose. Limit of detection of developed assays was up to 0.05 per cent and limit of quantification of the reported TaqMan-based real-time PCR was up to 0.5 per cent.

See for more papers reference 3.

## 7.3 PRE-SPOTTED REAL-TIME PCR PLATES

Ready-to-use multi-target PCR-based detection systems, such as pre-spotted plates (PSP), reduce analysis time while increasing capacity. Rosa et al. (13) describe the development and applicability to GMO testing of a screening strategy involving a PSP and its associated web-based decision support system. The screening PSP was developed to detect all GMOs authorized in the EU in one single PCR experiment, through the combination of 16 validated assays. The screening strategy was successfully challenged in a wide inter-laboratory study on real-life food/feed samples. The positive outcome of this study could result in the adoption of a PSP screening strategy across the EU; a step that would increase harmonization and quality of GMO testing in the EU. Furthermore, this system could represent a model for other official control areas where high-throughput DNA-based detection systems are needed.

Considering that the number of GMOs placed on the EU market is constantly growing, laboratories need to expand their capacity accordingly to be able to identify and, if necessary, quantify any GM material. To this purpose, a multi-target ready-to-use system, also known as a pre-spotted plate was developed (14), which allows the qualitative detection of up to 44 GM events in one single real-time PCR experiment. Should any event be detected, the laboratory would proceed with its quantification. This study evaluates the possibility to use the data generated by the PSP system in a semi-quantitative manner, allowing a categorization of the GM quantity in the sample. Six maize GM events frequently found in food and feed were selected for this evaluation (Bt11, MON810, MON88017, MON89034, NK603, and TC1507).

A platform based on the use of multiple singleplex assays, spotted into individual wells of a 96-well PCR plate, has been developed by the European Union Reference Laboratory for GM in Feed and Food (EU-RL GMFF) and used for routine screening purposes (15,16).

## 7.4 PCR CAPILLARY GEL ELECTROPHORESIS (PCR-CGE)

Capillary electrophoresis (CE) is emerging as an alternative to conventional techniques for the study and characterization of GMOs. Vega and Marina review (17) the most recent applications of CE for the analysis and characterization of transgenic cultivars in the last five years. Different strategies have been described depending on the level analyzed (DNA, proteins, or metabolites). Capillary gel electrophoresis (CGE) has shown to be particularly useful for the analysis of DNA fragments amplified by PCR. Metabolites and proteins have been mainly separated using capillary zone electrophoresis (CZE) using UV and MS detections. Electrophoretic chips have also proven their ability in the analysis of transgenic cultivars.

A qualitative method for detection of GMOs by combining PCR methodology with capillary gel electrophoresis (PCR-CGE) in a sequencing platform to detect *Bacillus thuringiensis* (Bt)-cotton (MON 531) and RRS (GTS 40–3-2) was developed (18). A sensitive duplex PCR-CGE method was developed in which target DNA sequences (*35S* and *Nos*) were separated both by size and color to detect 0.01 per cent *Cry1Ac* DNA (w/w) in Bt-cotton. A multiplex PCR-CGE method was developed to simultaneously detect four targets such as *Sad1, Cry1Ac, 35S,* and *Nos* in Bt-cotton. Four novel PCR primers were designed to customize amplicon size for multiplexing for better visualization of multiple peaks. The LOD for *Cry1Ac* DNA-specific PCR was 0.01 per cent for Bt-cotton. The

LOD for multiplex PCR assay was 0.05 per cent for Bt-cotton. A singleplex PCR-CGE method was developed to detect *Lec, 35S* and *Nos* in a trace sample of RR soybean grain powder (0.1 per cent, w/w).

An event-specific multiplex PCR system using microsatellite markers and fluorescently labeled primers to detect six different GM animal lines, including human lactoferrin GM cattle, human lysozyme GM cattle, human α-lactalbumin GM cattle, myostatin knockout pigs, phytase GM pigs, and ω-3 fatty acid desaturase gene GM pigs was established (19). Four different microsatellite loci for species identification, along with six GM animal-specific fragments, were selected as targets for primer design.

Liang and Zeng discuss alternative detection methods that utilize CE having the advantages of high efficiency, high throughput, high speed, and automation (20). These methods are coupled with various nucleic acid detection strategies to overcome the drawbacks of traditional identification methods, and to prevent false results. Therefore, this review focuses on the application of CE based on nucleic acid detection in food analysis and provides an introduction to the limitations, advantages, and future developments of this approach.

The study of Patwardhan et al. (21) aimed to develop a sensitive post-PCR detection method by using PCR-chip capillary electrophoresis (PCR-CCE) to detect and identify specific GMOs in their genomic DNA mixture by targeting event-specific nucleotide sequences. Using the PCR-CCE approach, novel multiplex methods were developed to detect MON531 cotton, EH 92–527-1 potato, Bt176 maize, GT73 canola, or GA21 maize simultaneously when their genomic DNAs in mixtures were amplified using their primer mixture. The repeatability relative standard deviation ($RSD_r$) of the peak migration time was 0.06 and 3.88 per cent for the MON531 and Bt176, respectively. The RSD ($RSD_r$) of the Cry1Ac peak ranged from 0.12 to 0.40 per cent in multiplex methods. The method was sensitive in resolving amplicon of size difference up to 4 bp.

## 7.5 DIGITAL PCR

Digital PCR (dPCR) is a novel method for precise quantification of nucleic acids. It uses similar assay reagents as used in standard analog measurements, but counts the total number of individual target molecules in a digital format, enabling many applications that require high sensitivity and have restricted sample availability.

Two approaches have been developed: microfluidic chamber dPCR (cdPCR) and droplet dPCR (ddPCR).

Several dPCR methods for the quantification of GM plant traits were set up by Köppel and Bucher (22). The focus during establishment was on rapidity in conjunction with flexibility leading to efficient duplex assays. The absolute quantification using a multitarget amplicon and verified accurate quantification by determination of certified reference material and comparing results from real-time PCR with results from droplet dPCR using the QX200 dPCR system from Bio-Rad were assessed.

Droplet dPCR platforms, which include two fluorescence filters, support at least duplex reactions, and with some developments and optimization, higher multiplexing is possible. The study of Dobnik et al. (23) not only shows a development of multiplex assays in droplet dPCR but also presents a first thorough evaluation of several parameters in such multiplex dPCR. Two 4-plex assays were developed for quantification of eight different DNA targets (seven GM maize events and maize endogene). Per assay, two of the targets were labeled with one fluorophore and two with another. As current analysis software does not support analysis of more than duplex, a new R- and Shiny-based web application analysis tool (24) was developed that automates the analysis of 4-plex results.

13 GMO traits which were predominantly detected in the past were chosen (25). The results showed that in the range of 1 per cent GMO content, the dPCR has a little superior performance compared to real-time PCR. In the range of the detection limit, measurement uncertainty remains comparable to real-time PCR. During validation, a conversion factor was determined for each trait suggesting that the calculation from % copies/copies to % weight/weight may be possible.

More examples of dPCR may found in references 26–32.

## 7.6 LOOP-MEDIATED ISOTHERMAL AMPLIFICATION

Loop-mediated isothermal amplification (LAMP) is a single tube technique for the amplification of DNA. In contrast to the PCR technology in which the reaction is carried out with a series of alternating temperature steps or cycles, isothermal amplification is carried out at a constant temperature, and does not require a thermal cycler. Numerous papers on LAMP can be found in the literature. Only a few examples are given in the texts that follow.

Takabatake et al. (33) developed new LAMP-based detection methods for the screening of GM maize and soybean events. The LAMP methods developed targeted seven sequences: cauliflower mosaic virus 35S promoter; *5-enolpyruvylshikimate-3-phosphate synthase gene from Agrobacterium tumefaciens* strain *CP4* (*cp4-epsps*); *phosphinothricin acetyltransferase*(*pat*) gene; mannose-6-phosphate isomerase gene; *Pisum sativum* ribulose 1, 5-bisphosphate carboxylase terminator; a common sequence between *cry1Ab* and *cry1Ac* genes; and a GA21 construct-specific sequence. New specific primer sets were developed for each target, and the limit of detection was evaluated using authorized GM maize and soybean events. LODs for each target were ≤0.5 per cent. To make the DNA extraction process simple and rapid, these authors also developed a direct LAMP detection scheme using crude cell lysates. The entire process, including pretreatments and detection, could be completed within 1 h.

Currently, 138 GM maize events have been authorized for commercial cultivation, comprising more than 65 per cent stacked events. With the increase in number of GM maize events globally, cost- and time-efficient diagnostics with on-site applicability are required to check for authorized GM events. Six GM maize events, namely, *Bt*11, GA21, MON810, MON89034, NK603, and TC1507, also present in 89 stacked events, are being widely commercialized in more than 17 countries. Visual and real-time LAMP assays targeting these six GM maize events are being reported (34). Specificity of the developed LAMP assays was confirmed using fourteen commercialized GM maize events. Limit of detection of visual and real-time LAMP assays targeting *Bt*11, GA21, MON810, MON89034, and TC1507 was up to 0.01 per cent, detecting eight target copies, and for NK603 event-specific assays, was up to 0.1 per cent, detecting 73 target copies. Practical applicability of developed LAMP assays was verified using a set of five stacked GM maize events—*Bt*11 × GA21, MON89034 × NK603, MON89034 × NK603 × TC1507, TC1507 × NK603, and TC1507 × MON810—and six powdered maize samples of proficiency testing.

An international collaborative ring trial was performed to validate gene-specific LAMP assays targeting four exogenous transgenes commonly utilized in the development of GM crops: *bar*, *pat*, *cp4-epsps*, and *Cry1Ac*, respectively (35). A total of 12 laboratories participated in the ring trial and returned their test results. Statistical analysis of the returned results showed high specificity and low limit of detection of the four LAMP assays. The LOD for *cp4-epsps, Cry1Ac, bar,* and *pat* genes assay was 5, 10, 20, and 20 haploid genome equivalents (HGEs), respectively. Furthermore, good performance of the four assays was further demonstrated in the analysis of practical samples in which all participating laboratories returned expected and accurate test results. Altogether, the ring trial results confirmed that the four gene-specific LAMP assays can be utilized for quick screening of transgenic traits in routine laboratory analysis.

To carry out the regulations of GMOs in China's inward and outward, environmental release and labeling, and to achieve effective management of GM soybean (*Glycine max*), LAMP primers were designed according to the flanking sequence of GM soybean DAS-81419-2, DP356043-5, A2704–12, FG72, BPS-CV127–9, and MON89788, separately (36). Through specificity, sensitivity, and limit of detection testing, a LAMP method for the inspection of GM soybean DAS-81419-2, DP356043-5, A2704–12, FG72, BPS-CV127–9, and MON89788 was developed. The results showed that this method could detect GM soybean DAS-81419-2, DP356043-5, A2704–12, FG72, BPS-CV127–9, and MON89788 specifically and stably with a low detection limit of 0.1 per cent (W/W). LAMP detection could be finished within 30 min and the results could be directly detected according to the color change produced by SYBR Green I dye with the naked eye.

## 7.7 LUMINEX TECHNOLOGY

Biotinylated targets amplified by single or multiplex PCR assays could be analyzed with the Luminex technology, potentially able to simultaneously detect up to 500 different targets in one sample using spectrally distinct sets of beads that are independently coupled to unique nucleic acid probes (3). After hybridization of biotinylated oligonucleotides to corresponding probe-bead complexes, the reader device individually analyzes each microsphere by flow cytometry in applying a laser excitation of 635 nm and 532 nm allowing, respectively, identifying the bead set and determining the presence or absence of the target. This technology was first assessed in GMO detection by Fantozzi et al., 2008. In this study, the p35S and EPSPS elements, earlier individually amplified by PCR from the GTS-40–3-2 soybean event, were simultaneously detected (37). Afterwards, the GM stacked LS28 × Cry1Ac rice and 281-24-236 × 3006–210–23 cotton events were identified on the Luminex platform using upstream, respectively, a pentaplex PCR or a hexaplex PCR (35,36). This technology was also used to detect ten GM maize events through four sets of multiplex PCR assays (38). Similarly, a liquid bead array approach allowing identifying thirteen GM maize was recently developed.

Due to its potential high throughput, the Luminex technology seems to be a promising alternative in GMO detection. Moreover, the liquid bead array is considered as more sensitive and faster than the microarray system (39). Nevertheless, the drawback linked to the PCR complicates the setting of a unique multiplex assay targeting simultaneously all GM events. Furthermore, as only few studies using this technology in GMO detection have been reported to date, experiments have still to be carried out in order to provide effective and validated systems.

For the purpose of GMO inspection, quarantaine, and manipulation, a high-throughput Bt-based GMOs screening method based on the liquid bead array was devised (40). This novel method is based on the direct competitive recognition between biotinylated antibodies and beads-coupled antigens, searching for Bt presence in samples if it contains Bt Cry1 Aa, Bt Cry1 Ab, Bt Cry1 Ac, Bt Cry1 Ah, Bt Cry1 B, Bt Cry1 C, Bt Cry1 F, Bt Cry2 A, Bt Cry3, or Bt Cry9 C. This method has a wide GMO species coverage, so that more than 90 per cent of the completely commercialized GMO species can be identified throughout the world. Based on optimization, specificity, sensitivity, repeatability, and availability validation, the method shows a high specificity and 10–50 ng/mL sensitivity of quantification. More than 1,800 samples in the field and food market were assesses to prove capacity of the method in performing a high throughput screening work for GMO manipulation.

## 7.8 MICROARRAY-BASED TECHNOLOGY

A multiplex amplification on a chip with readout on an oligo microarray (MACRO) system was developed, specifically for convenient GMO monitoring (41). This system is composed of a microchip for multiplex amplification and an oligo microarray for the readout of multiple amplicons, containing a total of 91 targets (18 universal elements, 20 exogenous genes, 45 events, and 8 endogenous reference genes) that covers 97.1 per cent of all GM events that have been commercialized up to 2012. It was demonstrated that the specificity of MACRO is ~100 per cent, with a limit of detection that is suitable for real-world applications. Moreover, the results obtained of simulated complex samples and blind samples with MACRO were 100 per cent consistent with expectations and the results of independently performed real-time PCRs, respectively.

In the study of Turkec et al. (42), the suitability of a high-density oligonucleotide microarray platform for direct, quantitative detection of GMOs found in the Turkish feed market was tested. 1830 different 60 nt probes designed to cover the GM cassettes from 12 different GM cultivars (3 soya, 9 maize) were tested, as well as plant species-specific and contamination controls, and a data analysis method aiming to provide maximum throughput and sensitivity was developed. The system was able specifically to identify each cultivar, and in 10/12 cases was sensitive enough to detect GMO DNA at concentrations of ≤1 per cent. These GMOs could also be quantified using the microarray, as their fluorescence signals increased linearly with GMO concentration.

## 7.9 DNA SEQUENCING-BASED APPROACHES

In Sanger sequencing, the target DNA is copied many times, making fragments of different lengths. Fluorescent "chain terminator" nucleotides mark the ends of the fragments and allow the sequence to be determined (52).

Next-generation sequencing techniques are new, large-scale approaches that increase the speed and reduce the cost of DNA sequencing. The most recent set of DNA sequencing technologies are collectively referred to as next-generation sequencing.

There are a variety of next-generation sequencing techniques that use different technologies. However, most share a common set of features that distinguish them from Sanger sequencing:

- Highly parallel: many sequencing reactions take place at the same time;
- Micro scale: reactions are tiny and many can be done at once on a chip;
- Fast: because reactions are done in parallel, results are ready much faster;

- Low-cost: sequencing a genome is cheaper than with Sanger sequencing; and
- Shorter length: reads typically range from 50–700 nucleotides in length (53).

See also reference 50.

### 7.9.1 Pyrosequencing

A portable bioluminescence analyzer for detecting the DNA sequence of GMOs was developed by using a photodiode array (43). Pyrosequencing on eight genes (zSSIIb, Bt11, and Bt176 gene of GM maize; lectin, 35S-CTP4, CP4 EPSPS, CaMV35S promoter, and NOS terminator of the GM RRS) was successfully detected with this instrument. The corresponding limit of detection was 0.01 per cent with 35 PCR cycles. The maize and soya available from three different provenances in China were detected.

The presence of GMOs in food and feed is mainly detected by the use of targets focusing on promoters and terminators. As some genes are frequently used in GM construction, they also constitute excellent screening elements and their use is increasing. A new target for the detection of *cry1Ab* and *cry1Ac* genes by real-time PCR and pyrosequencing was proposed (44). The specificity, sensitivity, and robustness of the real-time PCR method were tested following the recommendations of international guidelines, and the method met the expected performance criteria. How the robustness testing was assessed was explained. This new *cry1Ab/Ac* method can provide a positive signal with a larger number of GM events than do the other existing methods using double dye-probes. The method permits the analysis of results with less ambiguity than the SYBRGreen method recommended by the EU-RL GMFF. A pyrosequencing method was also developed to gain additional information thanks to the sequence of the amplicon. This method of sequencing-by-synthesis can determine the sequence between the primers used for PCR. Pyrosequencing showed that the sequences internal to the primers present differences following the GM events considered and three different sequences were observed. The sensitivity of the pyrosequencing was tested on reference flours with a low percentage GM content and different copy numbers. Improvements in the pyrosequencing protocol provided correct sequences with 50 copies of the target. Below this copy number, the quality of the sequence was more random.

The study of Shang et al. (45) described a novel multiplex qualitative detection method using pyrosequencing. Based on the principle of the universal primer-multiplex-PCR, only one sequencing primer was employed to realize the detection of the multiple targets. Samples containing three GM crops in different proportions were used to validate the method. The dNTP dispensing order was designed based on the product sequences. Only 12 rounds (ATCTGATCGACT) of dNTPs addition and, often, as few as three rounds (CAT) under ideal conditions, were required to detect the GM events qualitatively, and sensitivity was as low as 1 per cent of a mixture. However, when considering a mixture, calculating signal values allowed the proportion of each GM to be estimated.

### 7.9.2 DNA Walking

The specific identification of unknown nucleotide sequences adjacent to known DNA regions in the given genome using specific primers for a known sequence is referred to as DNA walking.

A strategy to identify UGMOs containing a pCAMBIA family vector, frequently present in transgenic plants was developed (54). This integrated approach is performed in two successive steps on Bt rice grains. First, the potential presence of UGMOs is assessed by the qPCR SYBR®Green technology targeting the terminator 35S pCAMBIA element. Second, its presence is confirmed via the characterization of the junction between the transgenic cassette and the rice genome. To this end, a DNA walking strategy is applied using a first reverse primer followed by two semi-nested PCR rounds using primers that are each time nested to the previous reverse primer. This approach allows to rapidly identify the transgene flanking region and can easily be implemented by the enforcement laboratories.

To identify UGMOs in food and feed matrices, an integrated approach has recently been developed targeting pCAMBIA family vectors, highly present in transgenic plants (54). Their presence is first assessed by qPCR screening and is subsequently confirmed by characterizing the transgene flanking regions, using DNA walking. Here, the DNA walking performance has been thoroughly tested for the first time, regarding the targeted DNA quality and quantity. Several assays, on model food matrices mimicking common rice products, have allowed to determine the limit of detection as well as the potential effects of food mixture and processing. This detection system allows the identification of transgenic insertions as low as 10 HGEs and was not affected by the presence of untargeted DNA. Moreover, despite the clear impact of food processing on DNA quality, this method was able to cope with degraded DNA. Given its specificity, sensitivity, reliability, applicability, and practicability, the proposed approach is a key detection tool, easily implementable in enforcement laboratories.

In order to provide a system fully integrated with qPCR screening, usually used in GMO routine analysis, as well as being able to detect, characterize, and identify a broad spectrum of GMOs in food/feed matrices, two bidirectional DNA walking methods targeting p35S or tNOS, the most common transgenic elements found in GM crops, were developed (55). These newly developed DNA walking methods are completing the previously implemented DNA walking method targeting the t35S pCAMBIA element.

First, the newly developed DNA walking methods, anchored on the sequences used for the p35S or tNOS qPCR screening, were tested on Bt rice that contains these two transgenic elements. Second, the methods were assessed on a maize sample containing a low amount of the GM MON863 event, representing a more complex matrix in terms of genome size and sensitivity. Finally, to illustrate its applicability in GMO routine analysis by enforcement laboratories, the entire workflow of the integrated strategy, including qPCR screening to detect the potential presence of GMOs and the subsequent DNA walking methods to characterize and identify the detected GMOs, was applied on a GeMMA Scheme Proficiency Test matrix. Via the characterization of the transgene flanking region between the transgenic cassette and the plant genome as well as of a part of the transgenic cassette, the presence of GMOs was properly confirmed or infirmed in all tested samples.

### 7.9.3 Next-Generation Sequencing

Current GMO detection systems have limited abilities to detect UGMOs. A new workflow, based on next-generation sequencing technology, to overcome this problem was proposed (46). In providing information about DNA sequences, this high-throughput workflow can distinguish authorized GMOs and UGMOs by strengthening the tools commonly used by enforcement laboratories with the help of NGS technology. In addition, thanks to its massive sequencing capacity, this workflow could be used to monitor GMOs present in the food and feed chain.

The detection of T-DNA from a GM flaxseed line (FP967, formally CDC Triffid) in a shipment of Canadian flaxseed exported to Europe resulted in a large decrease in the amount of flax planted in Canada (47). The Canadian flaxseed industry undertook major changes to ensure the removal of FP967 from the supply chain. This study aimed to resolve the genetics and structure of the FP967 transfer DNA (T-DNA).

The FP967 T-DNA is thought to be inserted in at single genomic locus. The junction between the T-DNA and genomic DNA consisted of two inverted Right Borders with no Left Border (LB) flanking genomic DNA sequences recovered. This information was used to develop an event-specific quantitative PCR (qPCR) assay. This assay and an existing assay specific to the T-DNA construct were used to determine the genetics and prevalence of the FP967 T-DNA. These data supported the hypothesis that the T-DNA is present at a single location in the genome.

The FP967 T-DNA is present at a low level (between 0.01 and 0.1 per cent) in breeder seed lots from 2009 and 2010. None of the 11,000 and 16,000 lines selected for advancement through the Flax Breeding Program in 2010 and 2011, respectively, tested positive for the FP967 T-DNA, however.

Most of the FP967 T-DNA sequence was resolved via PCR cloning and next-generation sequencing. A 3,720 bp duplication of an internal portion of the T-DNA (including a Right Border) was discovered between the flanking genomic DNA and the LB. An event-specific assay, SAT2-LB, was developed for the junction between this repeat and the LB.

Next-generation sequencing as an alternative to qPCR, its practical use has not been assessed for routine analysis. In the study of Willems et al. (48), a statistical framework was developed to predict the number of NGS reads needed to detect transgene sequences, to prove their integration into the host genome, and to identify the specific transgene event in a sample with known composition. This framework was validated by applying it to experimental data from food matrices composed of pure GM rice, processed GM rice (noodles) or a 10 per cent GM/non-GM rice mixture, revealing some influential factors. Finally, feasibility of NGS for routine analysis of GM crops was investigated by applying the framework to samples commonly encountered in routine analysis of GM crops.

### 7.9.4 Whole Genome Sequencing

A whole genome sequencing approach allows the characterization of samples to be performed without the requirement for any prior knowledge of the transgene inserts that may be present. With this sequencing strategy a DNA library is first constructed from sheared genomic DNA extracted from the sample, which is then sequenced in its entirely. The sequencing reads are initially assembled in order to generate contig scaffolds, and then analyzed using bioinformatics tools based on prior knowledge of currently characterized GMOs as an aid in confirming the identity of any GMOs.

The emergence of high-throughput, massive or next-generation sequencing technologies has created a completely new foundation for molecular analyses. Various selective enrichment processes are commonly applied to facilitate detection of predefined (known) targets. Such approaches, however, inevitably introduce a bias and are prone to miss unknown targets. The application of high-throughput sequencing technologies and the preparation of fit-for-purpose whole genome shotgun sequencing libraries for the detection and characterization of GM and derived products were reviewed (49). The potential impact of these new sequencing technologies for the characterization, breeding selection, risk assessment, and traceability of GMOs and genetically modified products is yet to be fully acknowledged. The published literature is reviewed, and the prospects for future developments and use of the new sequencing technologies for these purposes are discussed.

Identification of transgenic sequences in an unknown GM papaya (*Carica papaya* L.) by whole genome sequence analysis was demonstrated (5). Whole genome sequence data were generated for a GM-positive fresh papaya fruit commodity detected in monitoring using real-time PCR. The sequences obtained were mapped against an open database for papaya genome sequence. Transgenic construct- and event-specific sequences were identified as a GM papaya developed to resist infection from a *Papaya ringspot virus*. Based on the transgenic sequences, a specific real-time PCR detection method for GM papaya applicable to various food commodities was developed. Whole genome sequence analysis enabled identifying unknown transgenic construct- and event-specific sequences in GM papaya and development of a reliable method for detecting them in papaya food commodities.

As more and more new developed GM crops including new plant breeding technology (NPBT) generated crops are in the pipeline for commercialization, alternative "-omics" approaches, particularly next-generation sequencing, have been developed for molecular characterization of authorized or UGM crops. The review of R. Li et al. (51) summarizes first those methods, addresses their challenges, and discusses possible strategies for molecular characterization of engineered crops generated by NPBT, highlighting needs for a global information-sharing database and cost-effective, accurate, and comprehensive molecular characterization approaches.

## 7.10 SENSORS

Food regulations attempt to offer a high level of protection and to guarantee transparent information to the consumers. The availability of analytical methods is essential to comply these requirements. Protein-based strategies are usually employed for this purpose, but present some limitations. Because DNA is a more stable molecule, present in most tissues, and can be amplified, there has been an increasing interest in developing DNA-based approaches (PCR, microarrays, and genosensors). In this regard, electrochemical genosensors may play a major role in fulfilling the needs of food industry, such as reliable, portable, and affordable devices. Begoña Martín-Fernández et al. (57) review the achievements of this technology applied to allergen detection, species identification, and GMOs testing. They summarized the legislative framework, current design strategies in sensor development, their analytical characteristics, and future prospects.

For further information on sensors, the reader is directed to Chapter 6 of this book.

## 7.11 OTHER DETECTION METHODS

### 7.11.1 Chromatography and Mass Spectrometry

A few methods by these techniques on the detection of GMOs appeared recently in the literature. A study was focused on distinguishing of GMO (Monsanto 89788 variety) and conventional soybeans by employing high-resolution mass spectrometry techniques for non-target screening of sample extracts (58). Two hyphenated instrumental platforms represented by (i) ultrahigh-performance liquid chromatography coupled to quadrupole/time of flight and (ii) ambient mass spectrometry with direct analysis in real time ion source-coupled OrbitrapMS were used. The statistical processing of generated data (metabolomic fingerprints) was performed by multivariate data analysis; principal component analysis (PCA) and orthogonal partial least squares regression discriminant analysis (PLS-DA) showed that both employed techniques enabled correct classification of GM and conventional soybeans.

Stable-isotope dimethyl labeling was applied to the quantification of GM soya (59). The herbicide-resistant gene-related protein 5-enolpyruvylshikimate-3-phosphate synthase (CP4 EPSPS) was labeled using a dimethyl labeling reagent, formaldehyde-$H_2$ or -$D_2$. The identification and quantification of CP4 EPSPS was performed using matrix-assisted laser desorption/ionization mass spectrometry (MALDI-MS). The CP4 EPSPS protein was separated from high abundance proteins using strong anion exchange chromatography and sodium dodecyl sulfate-polyacrylamide gel electrophoresis. Then, the tryptic peptides from the samples and reference were labeled with formaldehyde-$H_2$ and formaldehyde-$D_2$, respectively. The two labeled pools were mixed and analyzed using MALDI-MS. The data showed a good correlation between the peak ratio of the H- and D-labeled peptides and the GM soya percentages at 0.5, 1, 3, and 5 per cent, with $R^2$ of 0.99. The labeling reagents are readily available. The labeling experiments and the detection procedures are simple. The approach is useful for the quantification of GM soya at a level as low as 0.5 per cent.

GC-MS-based metabolomics of GM rice varieties are widely reported but involves tedious derivatization processes. Broad-scale LC-MS-based metabolomics are lacking or limited to targeted analyses. In the study of Akram et al. (60), metabolite diversity in natural rice variants including basmati and non-basmati rice varieties was investigated using polymeric hydrophilic interaction chromatography coupled to an Orbitrap mass analyzer. Identification was performed using exact mass and standard retention times. A total of 329 metabolites were selected using IDEOM (identification of metabolites) software. Statistical tests were used to filter out top 50 rice varieties discriminating metabolites. Several up- or down-regulated metabolites were observed in rice varieties and can be used as biomarker compounds to differentiate between rice varieties. The developed method and generated data can be used for the comparison of GM rice varieties with natural ones.

GMOs express one or more exogenous genes inserted through genetic engineering resulting in the production of novel protein(s). Agencies responsible for deregulating GMOs require that levels of the newly expressed protein(s) be characterized.

Targeted protein quantitation may be performed using enzyme-linked immunosorbent assay (ELISA) with commercial kits or specially produced and validated antibodies. Proteins may also be quantitated by liquid chromatography coupled to tandem mass spectrometry (LC-MS/MS) (61). Although some scientific guidance exists for validation of ELISA, the need remains for a harmonized set of protocols for protein quantitation in testing of GMOs, particularly for LC-MS/MS. Current practices for assay linearity, accuracy, and precision; assay specificity; detection limits; and methods to assess analyte stability for both ELISA and LC-MS/MS were surveyed. The survey results were compared with assay criteria suggested in the literature and governmental guidance documents.

### 7.11.2 Near Infrared Spectroscopy

Near-infrared reflectance spectroscopy (NIRS), a non-destructive measurement technique, was combined with PLS-DA to discriminate the transgenic (TCTP and mi166) and wild type (Zhonghua 11) rice (62). Furthermore, rice lines transformed with protein gene (*OsTCTP*) and regulation gene (*Osmi166*) were also discriminated by the NIRS method. The performances of PLS-DA in spectral ranges of 4,000–8,000 $cm^{-1}$ and 4,000–10,000 $cm^{-1}$ were compared to obtain the optimal spectral range. As a result, the transgenic and wild type rice were distinguished from each other in the range of 4,000–10,000 $cm^{-1}$, and the correct classification rate was 100 per cent in the validation test. The transgenic rice TCTP and mi166 were also distinguished from each other in the range of 4,000–10,000 $cm^{-1}$, and the correct classification rate was also 100 per cent.

A comparison of various spectroscopic techniques for identifying GMOs was performed, including Fourier transform near-infrared (FT-NIR), visible near-infrared (VIS-NIR), mid-infrared (MIR), and Raman spectroscopy (63). Transgenic rice (Huahui-1) and its parent (Minghui 63) were chosen as subjects in this study. The obtained spectra were analyzed using three common chemometrics methods: PCA, PLS-DA, and discriminant analysis (DA). The highest classification accuracy (100 per cent) was obtained using Raman (applying PLSDA model) and VIS-NIR (applying DA and PLSDA model) spectroscopy. The accuracies obtained by MIR and FT-NIR reached 96.7 per cent (using DA model) and 95.7 per cent (using PLSDA model), respectively. These results indicate that FT-NIR, VIS-NIR, Raman, and MIR spectroscopy together with chemometrics methods could be effective in differentiating transgenic rice.

### 7.11.3 Terahertz Spectroscopy

An approach for the identification of terahertz (THz) spectral of GMOs based on active learning affinity propagation clustering algorithm (ALAP) combined with support vector machine (SVM), and THz transmittance spectra of some typical GM cotton samples were investigated to prove its feasibility (64). First, PCA was applied to extract features of the spectrum data. Second, instead of the original spectrum data, the feature signals were fed into the ALAP–SVM pattern recognition, where an improved active learning ALAP was applied to SVM. The experimental results show that THz spectroscopy combined with ALAP–SVM can be effectively utilized for identification of different GM cottons.

Terahertz spectroscopy combined with chemometrics techniques for discrimination of GM and non-GM sugar beets was applied (65). THz spectra of 84 sugar beet samples (36 GM sugar beets and 48 non-GM ones) were obtained by using terahertz time-domain spectroscopy (THz–TDS) system in the frequency range from 0.2 to 1.2 THz. Three chemometrics methods, PCA, DA, and discriminant partial least squares (DPLS), were employed to classify sugar beet samples into two groups: GMOs and non-GMOs. The DPLS method yielded the best classification result, and the percentages of successful classification for GM and non-GM sugar beets were both 100 per cent.

The feasibility of a non-destructive discrimination of transgenic rice seeds from its non-transgenic counterparts was examined by terahertz spectroscopy imaging system combined with chemometrics (66). PCA, least squares SVM (LS-SVM), PCA-back propagation neural network, and random forest (RF) models with the first and second derivative and standard normal variate transformation pretreatments were applied to classify rice seeds based on genotype. The results demonstrated that differences between non-transgenic and transgenic rice seeds did exist, and an excellent classification (accuracy was 96.67 per cent in the prediction set) could be achieved using the RF model combined with the first derivative pretreatment.

Due to the parameters of traditional support vector machine are difficult to determine in huge information data, so it is seriously limiting its application field (67). On the basis of classical particle swarm optimization algorithm, an adaptive particle swarm optimization algorithm which can filter the redundant information and adaptive to choose the best parameters in the process of training support vector machine, and the support vector machine using the optimal parameter to establish identification model, was proposed. It was found that different insect-resistant genes (Bt-Cry2, Bt-Cry4, Bt-Cry10) were recognized by using this optimization model.

## REFERENCES


1. M. Kamle, P. Kumar, J. Kumar Patra, V.K. Bajpai. Current perspectives on genetically modified crops and detection methods. *Biotechnology*, 7, 2017, 219.
2. T. Wilkes, G. Nixon, M. Burns. Recent developments in DNA-based screening approaches for detection of GMO's. *Journal of the Association of Public Analysis*, 44, 2016, 40–50.
3. M.A. Fraiture, P. Herman, I. Taverniers, M. De Loose, D. Deforce, N.H. Roosens. Current and new approaches in GMO detection: Challenges and solutions. *BioMed Research International*, 2015, 2015, 1–22.
4. M. Chaouachi, M.S. Zellama, N. Nabi, A.B. Hafsa, K. Saïd. Molecular identification of four genetically modified maize (Bt11, Bt176, Mon810 and T25) by duplex quantitative real-time PCR. *Food Analytical Methods*, 7 (1), 2014, 224–233.
5. S.B. Park, H.Y. Kim, J.H. Kim, Multiplex PCR system to track authorized and unauthorized genetically modified sobean events in food and feed. *Food Control*, 54, 2015, 47–52.
6. N. Datukishvili, T. Kutateladze, I. Gabriadze, K. Bitskinashvili, B. Vishnepolsky. New multiplex PCR methods for rapid screening of genetically modified organisms in foods. *Frontiers in Microbiology*, 6, 2015, 757.
7. R.A. Köppel, A. Sendic, H.U. Waiblinger. Two quantitative multiplex real-time PCR systems for the efficient GMO screening of food products. *European Food Research and Technology*, 239 (4), 2014, 653–659.
8. C. Liang, J.P. van Dijk, I.M.J. Scholtens, M. Staats, T.W. Prins, M.M. Voorhuijzen, A.M. da Silva, A.C. Maisonnave Arisi, J.T. den Dunnen, E.J. Kok. Detecting authorized and unauthorized genetically modified organisms containing vip3A by real-time PCR and next-generation sequencing. *Analytical and Bioanalytical Chemistry*, 406 (11), 2014, 2603–2611.
9. A. Noguchi, H. Akiyama, K. Nakamura, K. Sakata, Y. Minegishi, J. Mano, R. Takabatake, S. Futo, K. Kitta, R. Teshima, K. Kondo, T. Nishimaki-Mogami. A novel trait-specific real-time PCR method enables quantification of genetically modified (GM) maize content in ground grain samples containing stacked GM maize. *European Food Research and Technology*, 240 (2), 2015, 413–422.
10. R. Köppel, A. Ganeshan, F. van Velsen, T. Bucher. Five pentaplex real-time PCR systems for the efficient determination of 20 genetically modified maize traits in food. *European Food Research and Technology*, 243 (2), 2017, 215–225.
11. F. Debode, I. Huber, R. Macarthur, P.E. Rischitor, M. Mazzara, V. Herau, D. Sebah, D. Dobnik, S. Broeders, N.H. Roosens, U. Busch, G. Berben, D. Morisset, J. Zel. Interlaboratory studies for the validation of two singleplex (tE9 and pea lectin) and one duplex (pat/bar) real-time PCR methods for GMO detection. *Food Control*, 73, Part B, 2017, 452–461.
12. R.K. Bhoge, R. Chhabra, M. Singh, M. Sathiyabama, G. Randhawa. Multiplex real-time PCR-based detection and quantification of genetically modified maize events employing SYBR Green I and TaqMan chemistries. *Current Science*, 110 (8), 2016, 1446–1451.

13. S.F. Rosa, F. Gatto, A. Angers-Loustau, M. Petrillo, J. Kreysa, M. Querci. Development and applicability of a ready-to-use PCR system for GMO screening. *Food Chemistry*, 201, 2016, 110–119.
14. F. Gatto, N. Bassani, S.F. Rosa, A. Lievens, R. Brustio, J. Kreysa, M. Querci. Semi-quantification of GM maize using ready-to-use RTi-PCR plates. *Food Analytical Methods*, 10 (2), 2017, 549–558.
15. M. Querci, G. Kleter, J.-P. Malingreau, H. Broll, G. Van den Eede. Scientific and technical contribution to the development of an overall health strategy in the area of GMOs, 2008, JRC Reference Reports.
16. L. Kluga, M. Van den Bulcke, S. Folloni, J.-M. Gineste, T. Weber, N. Foti, M. Mazzari, G. Van den Eede, M. Querci. A ready-to-use multi-target analytical system for GM soy and maize detection for enforcement laboratories. 2011. INTECH. Open Access.
17. E. Domínguez Vega, M.L. Marina. Characterization and study of transgenic cultivars by capillary and microchip electrophoresis. *International Journal of Molecular Sciences*, 15 (12), 2014, 23851–23877.
18. S. Basak, N.Z. Ehtesham, B. Sesikeran, S. Ghosh. Detection and identification of transgenic elements by fluorescent-PCR-based capillary gel electrophoresis in genetically modified cotton and soybean. *Journal of AOAC International*, 97 (1), 2014, 159–165.
19. X. Liu, X.S. Qiu, X. Li, D. Liu, H. Jing, Q. Wang, X. Lin, D. Pan, N. Shi. Establishment of a decaplex PCR-capillary gel electrophoresis method for the simultaneous detection of six kinds of genetically modified animals. *Journal of AOAC International*, 2017.
20. H. Liang, H.-S. Zeng. Capillary electrophoresis based on nucleic acid detection as used in food analysis. *Comprehensive Reviews in Food Science and Food Safety*, 16 (6), 2017, 1281–1295.
21. S. Patwardhan, S. Dasari, K. Bhagavatula, S. Mueller, S.A. Deepak, S. Ghosh, S. Basak. Simultaneous detection of genetically modified organisms in a mixture by multiplex PCR-chip capillary electrophoresis. *Journal of AOAC International*, 98 (5), 2015, 1366–1374.
22. R. Köppel, T. Bucher. Rapid establishment of droplet digital PCR for quantitative GMO analysis. *European Food Research and Technology*, 241, 2015, 427–439.
23. D. Dobnik, D. Štebih, A. Blejec, D. Morisset, J. Žel. Multiplex quantification of four DNA targets in one reaction with Bio-Rad droplet digital PCR system for GMO detection. *Scientific Reports*, 6, 2016, Article number: 35451.
24. http://bit.ly/ddPCRmulti.
25. R. Köppel, T. Bucher, D. Bär, F. van Velsen, A. Ganeshan. Validation of 13 duplex droplet digital PCR systems for quantitative GMO analysis of most prevalent GMO traits. *European Food Research and Technology*, 244, 2018, 313–321.
26. B.K.M. Jacobs, E. Goetghebeur, J. Vandesompele, A. De Ganck, N. Nijs, A. Beckers, N. Papazova, N.H. Roosens, L. Clement. Model-based classification for digital PCR: Your umbrella for rain. *Analytical Chemistry*, 89 (8), 2017, 4461–4467.
27. A. Iwobi, L. Gerdes, U. Busch, S. Pecoraro. Droplet digital PCR for routine analysis of genetically modified foods (GMO)–A comparison with real-time quantitative PCR. *Food Control*, 69, 2016, 205–213.
28. D. Dobnik, T. Demšar, I. Huber, L. Gerdes, S. Broeders, N. Roosens, F. Debode, G. Berben, J. Zel. Inter-laboratory analysis of selected genetically modified plant reference materials with digital PCR. *Analytical and Bioanalytical Chemistry*, 410 (1), 2018, 211–221.
29. R. Köppel, V. Peterseil, E. Dagand, E. Schütz, N. Kolberg, M. Milavec, D. Moor. Collaborative trial to assess the performance of digital PCR in the field of GMO analysis using an artificial sample material. *European Food Research and Technology*, 243 (6), 2017, 1091–1096.
30. P. Zhu, C. Wang, K. Huang, Y. Luo, W. Xu. A novel pretreatment-free duplex chamber digital PCR detection system for the absolute quantitation of GMO samples. *International Journal of Molecular Sciences*, 17 (3), 2016, 402.

31. W. Fu, P. Zhu, C. Wang, K. Huang, Z. Du, W. Tian, Q. Wan, H. Wang, W. Xu, S. Zhu. A highly sensitive and specific method for the screening detection of genetically modified organisms based on digital PCR without pretreatment. *Scientific Reports*, 5, 2015, 12715.
32. R. Köppel, T. Bucher, A. Frei, H.U. Waiblinger. Droplet digital PCR versus multiplex real-time PCR method for the detection and quantification of DNA from the four transgenic oy traits MON87769, MON87708, MON87705 and FG72, and lectin. *European Food Research and Technology*, 241 (4), 2015, 521–527.
33. R. Takabatake, Y. Kagiya, Y. Minegishi, S. Yeasmin, S. Futo, A. Noguchi, K. Kondo, J. Mano, K. Kitta. Development and evaluation of rapid screening detection methods for genetically modified crops using loop-mediated isothermal amplification. *Food Chemistry*, In Press.
34. R.K. Bhoge, R. Chhabra, G. Randhawa, M. Sathiyabama, M. Singh. Event-specific analytical methods for six genetically modified maize events using visual and real-time loop-mediated isothermal amplification. *Food Control*, 55, 2015, 18–30.
35. R. Li, J. Shi, B. Liu, D. Zhang, X. Zhao, L. Yang. International collaborative ring trial of four gene-specific loop-mediated isothermal amplification assays in GMO analysis. *Food Control*, 84, 2018, 278–283.
36. Z. Jie, H.W. Sheng, D.T. Ting, W.Y. Jun, H.Q. Hui, C. Ying. Detection of six kinds of genetically modified soybean (*Glycine max*) by LAMP method. *Journal of Agricultural Biotechnology*, 25 (2), 2017, 335–344.
37. A. Fantozzi, M. Ermolli, M. Marini, B. Balla, M. Querci, G. Van den Eede. Innovative application of fluorescent microsphere based assay for multiple GMO detection. *Food Analytical Methods*, 1 (1), 2008, 10–17.
38. X. Han, H. Wang, H. Chen, L. Mei, S. Wu, G. Jia, T. Cheng, S. Zhu, X. Lin. Development and primary application of a fluorescent liquid bead array for the simultaneous identification of multiple genetically modified maize. *Biosensors and Bioelectronics*, 49, 2013, 360–366.
39. S.H. Choi, Y.T. Oh, J.Y. Kwon, S.N. Lee, B.D. Han, K.H. Ryu. Development of detection system using multiplex PCR and liquid bead array for stacked genetically modified rice event (LS28×Cry1Ac). *Journal of the Korean Society for Applied Biological Chemistry*, 53 (5), 2010, 639–646.
40. W. Fu, H. Wang, C. Wang, L. Mei, X. Lin, X. Han, S. Zhu. A high-throughput liquid bead array-based screening technology for Bt presence in GMO manipulation. *Biosensors and Bioelectronics*, 77, 2016, 702–708.
41. N. Shao, S.-M. Jiang, M. Zhang, J. Wang, S.-J. Guo, Y. Li, H.-W. Jiang, C.X. Liu, D.-B. Zhang, L.-T. Yang, S.-C. Tao. MACRO: A combined microchip-PCR and microarray system for high-throughput monitoring of genetically modified organisms. *Analytical Chemistry*, 86 (2), 2014, 1269–1276.
42. A. Turkec, S.J. Lucas, B. Karancanli, A. Baykut, H. Yuksel. Assessment of a direct hybridization microarray strategy for comprehensive monitoring of genetically modified organisms (GMOs). *Food Chemistry*, 194, 2016, 399–409.
43. Q. Song, G. Wei, G. Zhou. Analysis of genetically modified organisms by pyrosequencing on a portable photodiode-based bioluminescence sequencer. *Food Chemistry*, 154 (1), 2014, 78–83.
44. F. Debode, E. Janssen, C. Bragard, G. Berben. Detection by real-time PCR and pyrosequencing of the cry1Ab and cry1Ac genes introduced in genetically modified (GM) constructs. *Food Additives & Contaminants: Part A*, 34 (8), 2017, 1398–1409.
45. Y. Shang, W. Xu, Y. Wang, Y. Xu, K. Huang. Novel multiplex qualitative detection using universal primer-multiplex-PCR combined with pyrosequencing. *Food Chemistry*, 237, 2017, 773–778.
46. M.-A. Fraiture, P. Herman, M. De Loose, F. Debode, N.H. Roosens. How can we better detect unauthorized GMOs in food and feed chains? *Trends in Biotechnology*, 35 (6), 2017, 508–517.

47. L. Young, J. Hammerlindl, V. Babic, J. McLeod, A. Sharpe, C., Matsalla, F. Bekkaoui, L. Marquess, H.M. Booker. Genetics, structure, and prevalence of FP967 (CDC Triffid) T-DNA in flax. *SpringerPlus*, 4, 2015, 146.
48. S. Willems, M.-A. Fraiture, D. Deforce, S.C.J. De Keersmaecker, M. De Loose, T. Ruttink, P. Herman, F. Van Nieuwerburg, N. Roossens. Statistical framework for detection of genetically modified organisms based on next generation sequencing. *Food Chemistry*, 192, 2016, 788–798.
49. A. Holst-Jensen, B. Spilsberg, A.J. Arulandhu, E. Kok, J. Shi, J. Zel. Application of whole genome shotgun sequencing for detection and characterization of genetically modified organisms and derived products. *Analytical and Bioanalytical Chemistry*, 408 (17), 2016, 4595–4614.
50. K. Nakamura, K. Kondo, H. Akiyama, T. Shigaki, A. Noguchi, H. Katsuma, K. Takasaki, S. Futo, K. Sakata, N. Fukuda, J. Mano, K. Kitta, H. Tanaka, R. Akashi, T. Nishimaki-Mogami. Whole genome sequence analysis of unidentified genetically modified papaya for development of a specific detection method. *Food Chemistry*, 205, 2016, 272–279.
51. R. Li, S. Quan, X. Yan, S. Biswas, D. Zhang, J. Shi. Molecular characterization of genetically-modified crops: Challenges and strategies. *Biotechnology Advances*, 35 (2), 2017, 302–309.
52. J.M. Heather, B. Chain. The sequence of sequencers: The history of sequencing DNA. *Genomics*, 107, 2016, 1–8.
53. https://www.khanacademy.org/science/biology/biotech-dna-technology/dna-sequencing-pcr-electrophoresis/a/dna-sequencing.
54. M.-A. Fraiture, P. Herman, I. Taverniers, M. De Loose, D. Deforce, N.H. Roosens. An innovative and integrated approach based on DNA walking to identify unauthorised GMOs. *Food Chemistry*, 147, 2014, 60–69.
55. M.-A. Fraiture, P. Herman, I. Taverniers, M. De Loose, F. Van Nieuwerburg, D. Deforce, N. H. Roosens. Validation of a sensitive DNA walking strategy to characterise unauthorised GMOs using model food matrices mimicking common rice products. *Food Chemistry*, 173, 2015, 1259–1265.
56. M.-A. Fraiture, P. Herman, L. Lefèvre, I. Taverniers, M. De Loose, D. Deforce, N.H. Roosens. Integrated DNA walking system to characterize a broad spectrum of GMOs in food/feed matrices. *BMC Biotechnology*, 15, 2015, 76.
57. B. Martín-Fernández, C.L. Manzanares-Palenzuela, M. Sánchez-Paniagua, L.N. de-los-Santos-Álvarez, B. López-Ruiz. Electrochemical genosensors in food safety assessment. *Critical Reviews in Food Science and Nutrition*, 57 (13), 2017, 2758–2774.
58. V. Hrbek, V. Krtkova, J. Rupert, H. Chmelarova, K. Demnerova, J. Ovesna, J. Hajslova. Metabolomic strategies based on high-resolution mass spectrometry as a tool for recognition of GMO (MON 89788 variety) and non-GMO soybean: A critical assessment of two complementary methods. *Food Analytical Methods*, 10 (11), 2017, 3723–3737.
59. P.-C. Chang, P.M. Reddy, Y.-P. Ho. Quantification of genetically modified soya using strong anion exchange chromatography and time-of-flight mass spectrometry. *Analytical and Bioanalytical Chemistry*, 406 (22), 2014, 5339–5346.
60. M.I. Akram, I.M. Vincent, A.J. Siddiqui, G. Musharraf. Polymeric hydrophilic interaction liquid chromatography coupled with Orbitrap mass spectrometry and chemometric analysis for untargeted metabolite profiling of natural rice variants. *Journal of Cereal Science*, 73, 2017, 165–173.
61. S.B. Settlage, J.E. Eble, J.K. Bhanushali, M.L. Cheever, A.-G. Gao, D.A. Goldstrohm, R. Hill, T.X. Hu, C.R. Powley, A. Unger, G. Shan. Validation parameters for quantitating specific proteins using ELISA or LC-MS/MS: Survey results. *Food Analytical Methods*, 10 (5), 2017, 1339–1348.
62. L. Zhang, S.-S. Wang, Y.-F. Ding, J. Pan, C. Zhu. Discrimination of transgenic rice based on near infrared reflectance spectroscopy and partial least squares regression discriminant analysis. *Rice Science*, 22 (5), 2015, 245–249.

63. W. Xu, X. Liu, L. Xie, Y. Ying. Comparison of fourier transform near-infrared, visible near-infrared, mid-infrared, and Raman spectroscopy as non-invasive tools for transgenic rice discrimination. *Transactions of the ASABE*, 57 (1), 2014, 141–150.
64. J. Liu, Z. Li, F. Hu, T. Chen, Y. Du, H. Xin. Identification of GMOs by terahertz spectroscopy and ALAP–SVM. *Optical and Quantum Electronics*, 47 (3), 2015, 685–695.
65. T. Chen, Z. Li, X. Yin, F. Hu, C. Hu. Discrimination of genetically modified sugar beets based on terahertz spectroscopy. *Spectrochimica Acta Part A: Molecular and Biomolecular Spectroscopy*, 153, 2016, 586–590.
66. W. Liu, C. Liu, X. Hu, J. Yang, L. Zheng. Application of terahertz spectroscopy imaging for discrimination of transgenic rice seeds with chemometrics. *Food Chemistry*, 210, November 1, 2016, 415–421.
67. J. Liu, L. Mao, J. Ki, J. He, L. Fan. THz spectroscopy detection method for GMOs based on adaptive particle swarm optimization. *Optical and Quantum Electronics*, 48, 2016, 167–176.

## SECTION 4

# Validation and Standardization of Methods

# CHAPTER 8

# Verification of Analytical Methods for GMO Testing When Implementing Interlaboratory Validated Methods

*Lotte Hougs, Francesco Gatto, O. Goerlich, Lutz Grohmann, K. Lieske, Marco Mazzara, Frank Narendja, J. Ovesna, Nina Papazova, I.M.J. Scholtens, and Jana Zel*
Joint Research Centre

CONTENTS

## 8.1 INTRODUCTION

Regulation (EC) No 882/2004[1] provides that official laboratories shall be accredited according to the ISO 17025[2] standard. An ISO 17025 accreditation, under a fixed or flexible scope, implies that "the laboratory shall confirm that it can properly operate standard methods before introducing the tests or calibrations." If the standard method changes, the confirmation shall be repeated (ISO 17025:2005 Section 5.4.2).

In turn, still according to the same Regulation (EC) No 882/2004[1], it is the task of the European Union Reference Laboratory for Genetically Modified Food and Feed (EU-RL GMFF) to provide national reference laboratories with details of analytical methods, including reference methods.

Note: In November 2010, the ENGL and the EU-RL GMFF have published a "Compendium of reference methods for GMO analysis," which includes 79 DNA-based detection methods that have been validated through a collaborative trial according to ISO5725 and/or the IUPAC protocol.

A new method evolves through a number of steps. After the initial development and optimization phases, the developing laboratory performs an in-house validation on the method to ensure that the method is fit for the intended purpose. Before the method can be accepted as an International Standard, it needs to be validated in a number of laboratories[3,4].

In the EU, method validation is an essential part of the process that regulates the introduction of new GMOs as food and/or feed into the market. The European Regulation laying down the methods of sampling and analysis for the official control of feed as regards the presence of genetically modified material for which an authorization procedure is pending or the authorization of which has expired [so-called low level presence (LLP) regulation] that was adopted in February 2011 also confirms that event-specific quantitative detection methods that are validated by the EU-RL GMFF need to be used.

When this interlaboratory validation study is completed, the method is ready to be implemented in routine testing laboratories. When implementing the new method, the laboratory has to verify that the method can be used for its intended purpose (method verification). The scope of this chapter is to provide guidance on how to carry out the method verification.

In GMO detection laboratories, qualitative and quantitative methods with different levels of specificity are used (e.g., genetic element-, construct-, or event-specific). For the detection of GMOs in food and feed products, the event-specific detection methods provided in applications for authorization in the frame of Regulation (EC) No 1829/2003 are validated by the EU-RL GMFF in collaboration with the ENGL. The validation is performed according to internationally recognized guidelines(3,4) through collaborative studies. Data from the interlaboratory validation process are evaluated according to the document *Definition of Minimum Performance Requirements for Analytical Methods of GMO Testing*(5) (MPR).

Despite the fact that several guidelines on method verification have been published(6,7), no specific guidelines are available for GMO detection. Peer-reviewed papers have been published on verification of GMO detection methods in accredited laboratories(8–10). The aim of this guidance document is to harmonize the in-house verification of interlaboratory validated methods for the qualitative and quantitative detection of GMOs, including element-, construct-, and event-specific methods.

Considering that the polymerase chain reaction (PCR) is the method of choice in the EU for the identification and quantification of GMOs, this document refers exclusively to real-time PCR. However, if novel methods are subsequently developed that fulfill legal requirements, then this document will be amended accordingly.

The interlaboratory validation of methods is not within the scope of this document.

The principles of the modular approach(11) have been taken into account in this document.

Procedures for the calculation of measurement uncertainty are explained in the guidance document on measurement uncertainty for GMO testing laboratories(12) and will not be included further in this document.

## 8.2 TERMINOLOGY

### 8.2.1 Validation of Method

Validation is the confirmation by examination and provision of objective evidence that the particular requirements for a specific intended use are fulfilled (ISO 17025 Section 5.4.5.1).

### 8.2.2 Verification of Method

Verification is the confirmation, through the provision of objective evidence, that specified requirements have been fulfilled (ISO 9000:2000 Section 3.8.4). Verification that a laboratory can adequately operate a standard method requires that the laboratory provides objective evidence that the performance parameters specified in the test method have been met for the sample matrices to which the method is being applied. Most often, the critical requirements are the trueness (generally expressed in terms of bias)(3) and the precision (generally accepted as repeatability and reproducibility), which are reflected in the measurement uncertainty. The objective evidences are the trueness and precision obtained from actual laboratory data(7).

### 8.2.3 Precision—Relative Repeatability Standard Deviation (RSDr)

The relative standard deviation of test results obtained under repeatability conditions. Repeatability conditions are conditions where test results are obtained with the same method on identical test items in the same laboratory by the same operator using the same equipment within short intervals of time.

### 8.2.4 Laboratory Sample (see also Fig. 1)

Sample as prepared for sending to the laboratory and intended for inspection or testing [(13)].

### 8.2.5 Analytical Sample

Sample prepared from the laboratory sample by grinding, if necessary, and homogenization[(14)].

### 8.2.6 Test Portion

Sample, as prepared for testing or analysis, the whole quantity being used for analyte extraction at one time[(13)].

### 8.2.7 Test Result

A test result is a Ct value or copy number originating from a PCR replicate.

### 8.2.8 DNA Extraction Replicates (as Used in this Chapter)

DNA extracted from different test portions from the same analytical sample.

### 8.2.9 PCR Replicates (as Used in this Chapter)

PCR performed on the same DNA extraction replicate analyzed in different reaction wells.

### 8.2.10 Working Dilution

The highest DNA concentration intended to be used in the subsequent PCR method.

### 8.2.11 Limit of Quantification (LOQ[(5)])

LOQ is the lowest amount or concentration of analyte in a sample, which can be reliably quantified with an acceptable level of precision and trueness.

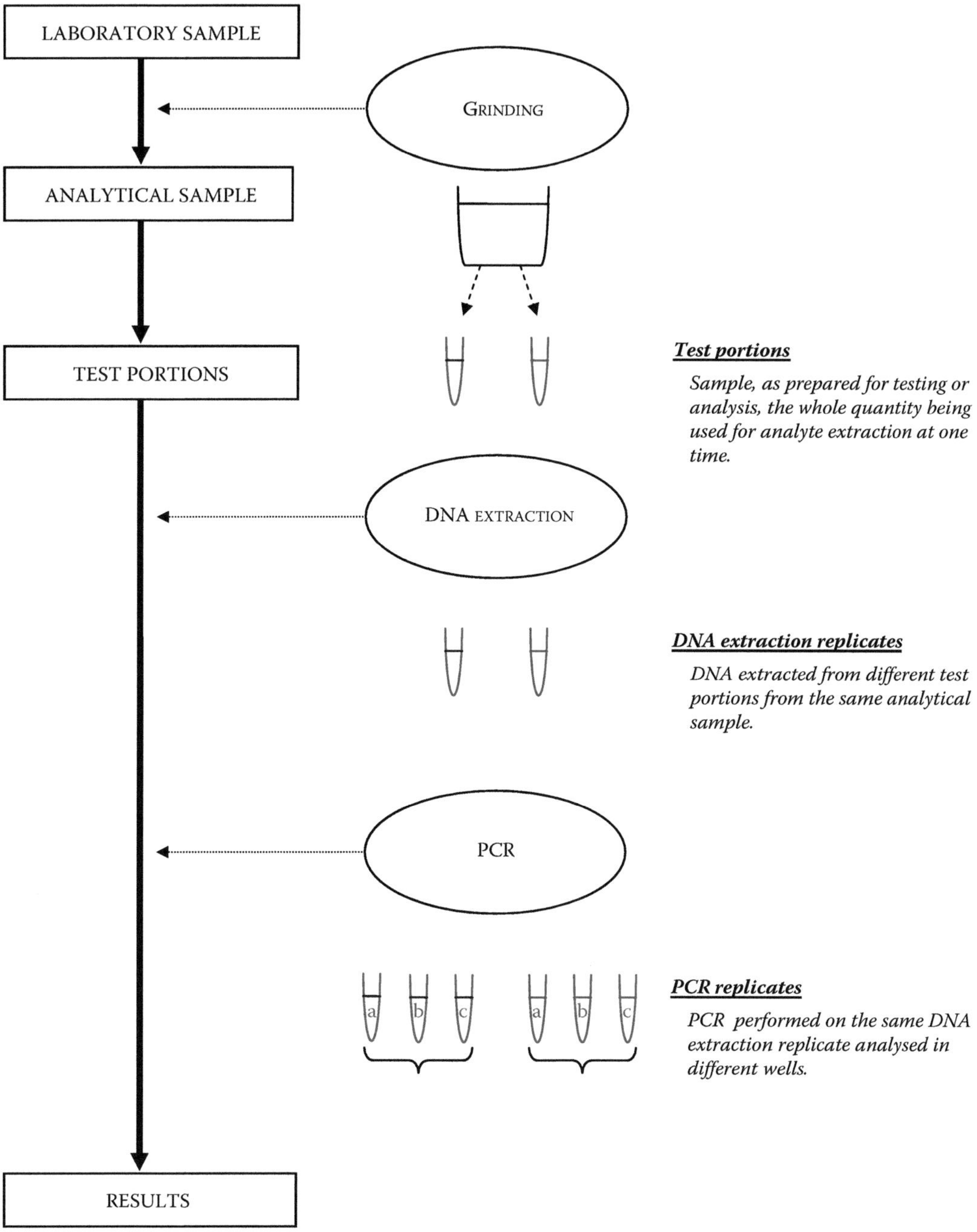


FIGURE 8.1 Illustration of replicates terminology.

### 8.2.12 Practical Limit of Quantification (Practical LOQ)

The practical LOQ is the lowest relative quantity of the target DNA that can be reliably quantified, given a known (determined/estimated) number of target taxon genome copies[(13)].

### 8.2.13 Limit of Detection[5]

Limit of detection (LOD) is the lowest amount or concentration of analyte in a sample, which can be reliably detected but not necessarily quantified. Experimentally, methods should detect the presence of the analyte at least 95 per cent of the times at the LOD, ensuring ≤5 per cent false negative results.

### 8.2.14 Practical Limit of Detection (Practical LOD)

The practical LOD is the lowest relative quantity of the target DNA that can be reliably (e.g., with ≥95 per cent probability) detected, given a known (determined/estimated) number of target taxon genome copies[13].

### 8.2.15 Specificity[5]

The property of the method to respond exclusively to the characteristic or the analyte of interest.

### 8.2.16 Dynamic Range[5]

The range of concentrations over which the method performs in a linear manner with an acceptable level of trueness and precision.

### 8.2.17 Trueness[5]

The closeness of agreement between the average value obtained from a large series of test results and an accepted reference value. The measure of trueness is usually expressed in terms of bias.

### 8.2.18 Amplification Efficiency[5]

The rate of PCR amplification that leads to a theoretical slope of –3.32 with an efficiency of 100 per cent in each cycle. The efficiency (in percentage) can be calculated by the following equation:

$$Efficiency = \left(10^{(-1/slope)} - 1\right) \times 100$$

### 8.2.19 $R^2$ Coefficient[5]

$R^2$ is the coefficient of determination, which is calculated as the square of the correlation coefficient (between the measured Ct-value and the logarithm of the concentration) of a standard curve obtained by linear regression analysis.

### 8.2.20 Robustness[5]

The robustness of a method is a measure of its capacity to remain unaffected by small, but deliberate deviations from the experimental conditions described in the procedure (Figure 8.1).

## 8.3 GENERAL CONSIDERATIONS

An accredited laboratory shall have a management system in place to provide objective evidence that the personnel is adequately qualified and regularly trained to perform the analysis (ISO/IEC 17025:2005 Section 5.2). In addition, a metrology system shall ensure that the equipment used is periodically calibrated (ISO/IEC 17025:2005 Section 5.5). When an interlaboratory validated method is used by an accredited laboratory, the laboratory must, prior to its use, ensure that the chosen method shows performance characteristics similar to those assessed in the interlaboratory study. The verification process must be documented and recorded in the quality system.

The laboratory must record the procedure used, the results obtained, and a statement as to whether the method is fit for the intended use. For example:

- Design and planning of the verification;
- Description of the method;
- Acceptance criteria and performance requirements, as decided by the laboratory;
- Test records;
- Approval of the method.

As interlaboratory validated event-specific methods are assessed according to the acceptance criteria and performance requirements described in the document MPR[5]. This document can be more generally used as a basis for assessing the results of a method in a verification process. The methods are available in the JRC reference report *Compendium of Reference Methods for GMO Analysis*[15] as well as on: http://gmo-crl.jrc.ec.europa.eu/. The following sections describe the parameters to be studied for the verification of validated methods for the detection of GMOs. During the verification process, a laboratory should ensure compliance to the requirements described in the following standards: ISO 24276[13], ISO 21568[14], ISO 21570[16], ISO 21569[17], and ISO 21571[18].

As a matter of principle, a method should be implemented as validated in interlaboratory trial, without introducing modifications. If single elements like, for example, the brand of ready-to-use reaction mix or *Taq* polymerase, the PCR reaction volume, the primer and probe concentrations, and/or PCR cycling parameters are modified, additional parameters should be experimentally assessed (e.g., specificity and robustness).

When the method is only qualitative, or employed as qualitative determination, it is not necessary to verify the LOQ, trueness, or precision.

## 8.4 DNA EXTRACTION AND PURIFICATION

The DNA isolation method should provide DNA of suitable quality and quantity for subsequent analysis. Although this document focuses on the verification of PCR methods, the evaluation of DNA extraction methods is a crucial step, as the quality and quantity of DNA extracted may significantly affect the final result.

Methods for DNA extraction can be interlaboratory validated methods, single-laboratory validated methods, standardized methods (e.g., ISO) and/or other available methods.

*Procedure*: If the DNA extraction method was previously validated, the DNA extraction is carried out at least twice (tree times recommended) each time on two test portions, if possible on different days and with different operators. The DNA extractions have to meet the acceptance criteria for DNA concentration and quality (e.g., by controlling amplification efficiency and presence of inhibitors by real-time PCR, see Appendix B).

DNA extraction methods applied to one matrix may not be suitable for other matrices. This procedure may need to be carried out on different matrices. For the verification of a DNA extraction method the tested matrix does not necessarily have to contain GMO.

### 8.4.1 DNA Concentration

*Procedure:* The concentration of the DNA extracts should be measured by the method applied to the routine samples.

*Acceptance criterion*: In the verification process, when a DNA extraction method is applied to the same matrix of the validation study, the yield should be comparable to the results obtained in that study. The method should provide DNA in an appropriate yield for the intended analysis (at least enough to meet the desired practical LOD/LOQ).

If a DNA extraction method does not give an appropriate yield for the intended analysis on a particular matrix, the practical LOD will be affected (Appendix A).

### 8.4.2 Absence of Inhibitors in the DNA Extracts

*Procedure:* Each DNA extraction replicate is diluted to a working dilution (e.g., 40 ng/µL). From this working dilution, a dilution series of, for example, four points are analyzed using real-time PCR (at least two PCR replicates per dilution). A calibration curve is obtained from these four dilutions.

The preferred PCR assay for the inhibition test is the reference gene assay (e.g., the taxon-specific reference system). The total DNA amount in the working dilution should be at least the same as the total DNA amount intended to be used in the verification process and in routine analysis (e.g., the DNA amount indicated in the PCR protocol of the taxon-specific reference system).

*Acceptance criterion*: The average difference ($\Delta$Ct) between the measured Ct value and the extrapolated Ct value of the working dilution should be <0.5 [(Measured Ct – extrapolated Ct) <0.5] and the slope of the inhibition curve should lie between –3.6 and –3.1.[5]

An example for an inhibition assay is given in Appendix B.

If the extracted DNA contains inhibitors, the DNA has to be further purified or diluted to the level where no inhibition of PCR reaction is observed, before it is used for real-time PCR.

## 8.5 SPECIFICITY

Specificity should already have been investigated in the context of method validation. Therefore, the specificity does not need to be re-investigated in a verification study.

In the case of screening methods targeting genetic elements common to several GM events, the method should be tested in-house (if this validation data are not available) for cross-reactivity with new GMO events placed on the market after the method has been taken into use. This can only be done when positive control materials are available for the new GMO events.

## 8.6 DYNAMIC RANGE, $R^2$ COEFFICIENT, AND AMPLIFICATION EFFICIENCY

*Procedure*: Dynamic range, $R^2$ coefficient, and amplification efficiency are verified simultaneously from standard curves when testing other parameters, such as trueness and precision. The average values of at least two standard curves should be taken (see Table 8.1 for details).

*Acceptance criterion for dynamic range*: The dynamic range must cover the values corresponding to the expected use. This can be expressed as GMO per cent or copy number range.

*Example*: 0.09 and 4.5 per cent for a 0.9 per cent GMO target concentration or 50 and 2500 genome copies if the target is 500 copies.

*Acceptance criterion for amplification efficiency*: For both, qualitative and quantitative methods, the average value of the slope of the standard curve shall be in the range of $-3.6 \leq \text{slope} \leq -3.1$[5], corresponding to an amplification efficiency of 90–110 per cent.

*Acceptance criterion for $R^2$ coefficient*: the average value of $R^2$ shall be $\geq 0.98$.

## 8.7 TRUENESS

*Procedure:* The trueness should be determined at a level close to the level set in legislation (e.g., 0.9 per cent threshold), or according to the intended use of the method, and additionally at a level close to the LOQ. The trueness can be measured using certified reference material(s) (CRM), with at least two concentrations (e.g., 0.1 and 1 per cent) and if possible a third one at the upper end of the dynamic range (e.g., 5 per cent). Alternatively, a reference sample (e.g., 1 per cent) can be made from a higher percentage CRM. Appendix C provides a guideline for the preparation of such a reference sample.

Testing conditions (reaction volume, PCR machine, etc.) should be the same as during routine testing of samples. At least results from 16 PCR replicates should be obtained. Examples for possible test designs are shown in Table 8.1 and Figures 8.2 and 8.3.

Appendix D provides guidelines for the calculation of mean, standard deviation and relative repeatability standard deviation of GMO-content of related and unrelated real-time PCR replicates.

If CRMs for estimating the trueness are not available, a proficiency test material can be used or a Z- score in a proficiency test can provide an indication of the trueness of the method.

*Acceptance criterion*: The trueness shall be within ±25 per cent of the accepted reference value or a Z-score within the range of 2 and –2 should be obtained.

## 8.8 RSDR

*Procedure*: Repeatability can be determined in a similar way as described under Trueness. It is calculated from PCR replicates run under repeatability conditions (see Terminology). Repeatability should be available for all tested GM-levels.

Testing conditions (reaction volume, PCR machine, etc.) should be the same as during routine testing of samples. At least 16 single test results should be obtained. Examples for possible test designs are shown in Table 8.1 and Figures 8.2 and 8.3.

Appendix D provides guidelines for the calculation of standard deviation and relative repeatability standard deviation of GMO-content of related and unrelated real-time PCR replicates.

*Acceptance criterion*: The relative repeatability standard deviation should be ≤25 per cent, over the dynamic range of the method.

## 8.9 ESTIMATION OF THE LOQ

Relative LOQ (in percentage) and/or absolute LOQ (in copy numbers) can be determined.

*Procedure for Relative LOQ* ($LOQ_{rel}$): A positive control material of 0.1 per cent can be analyzed in 10 PCR replicates of the GM target and 10 replicates of the reference gene target. The RSD of the $LOQ_{rel}$ should be below 25 per cent. To establish the true $LOQ_{rel}$, it will be necessary to make dilutions with a lower GM percentage.

*Procedure for Absolute LOQ* ($LOQ_{abs}$): A dilution series of a known amount of a positive control material of 1 per cent can be measured in 10 PCR replicates (e.g., 80, 60, 40, 20, 10, 5, and 1 copies). The $LOQ_{abs}$ can be estimated as the last dilution in a series where the RSD of the measurements is below 25 per cent. The standard curve should cover the value of $LOQ_{abs}$.

The probability distribution suggests that 1 copy should give approximately 30 per cent negative results. Therefore, as a requirement to verify that the copy numbers of the dilution series are approximately correct, at least one replicate has to be negative for the one copy dilution.

The mean of the ten PCR replicates may be a part of the standard curve as long as the standard curve still meets the acceptance criterion for $R^2$ and slope/efficiency. The rest of the standard curve only needs to have two PCR replicates per point.

*Acceptance criterion*: Whenever validation data are available, the LOQ should be in line with (or better than) those data.

## 8.10 ESTIMATION OF LIMIT OF DETECTION (LOD)

Relative LOD (in per cent) and/or absolute LOD (in copy number) can be determined.

*Procedure for Relative LOD* ($LOD_{rel}$): A positive control material of low GM concentration can be measured in ten PCR replicates, and if all replicates are positive, this infers that the $LOD_{rel}$ is below or equal to the positive control material level.

TABLE 8.1 Example of Practical Settings for the Verification of a Quantitative Real-Time PCR Method

| | |
|---|---|
| 1. Optional: Preliminary test to define appropriate DNA concentrations | Test at least three target concentrations in the range of 300 ng–0.1 ng (dependent on plant species)(19).<br>For example, 300 ng maize DNA corresponds to approx. 110,000 endogenes gene copies, whereas 0.1 ng corresponds to approximately 37 copies. |
| 2. Dynamic range, $R^2$ coefficient, and amplification efficiency | Example 1: Two calibration curves:<br>Minimum requirements: Five calibration points with three PCR replicates each (triplicates);<br>All slopes should be in the range of $-3.6 \leq$ slope $\leq -3.1$ and all $R^2$ values should be $\geq 0.98$.<br>Example 2: Four calibration curves:<br>Five calibration points with two PCR replicates each (duplicates); average of four slopes and $R^2$ are used to verify the acceptance.<br>Example 3: Two calibration curves:<br>Eight calibration points with five PCR replicates (pentaplicates) also covering the low concentrations for LOD and LOQ. Average of the part above LOQ for slope and $R^2$ are used to verify the acceptance. |
| 3. Trueness, precision, $RSD_r$ | At least two GM levels (one around labeling threshold and one around LOQ, a third recommended to the upper part of the dynamic range)<br>Example 1: Two DNA extraction replicates per GM level, two PCR replicates per extraction/plate, four plates resulting in 16 test results and 8 GM—estimations per GM level[a] (Figure 8.2)<br>Example 2: Two DNA extraction replicates per GM level, 4 PCR replicates per extraction/plate, 2 plates resulting in 16 test results and 4 GM—estimations per GM level[a] (Figure 8.3)<br>For the estimation of intermediate precision, PCR runs are carried out at least on two different days by the same operator or, if possible, by an additional operator. |
| 4. LOQ, LOD | LOQ: Ten PCR replicates at a low concentration (e.g., 80, 60, 40, 20, 10, 5, and 1 copies). LOQ is the lowest concentration of a series where RSD of the copy number measurements are below 25 per cent, and the point is covered by the standard curve.<br>LOD: 10 PCR replicates at a low concentration (e.g., 20, 10, 5, and 1 copies). LOD is then the lowest concentration in a series where all replicates are positive. |

[a] If based on experience, the laboratory can prove that the repeatability between two experienced operators is the same as the repeatability among repetitions of one person, it is not necessary to have the repetition done by another operator.

*Procedure for Absolute LOD* ($LOD_{abs}$): To calculate the $LOD_{abs}$ of a method with 95 per cent confidence, it is necessary to analyze 60 PCR replicates for each tested concentration. As this may not be a practical approach, it is proposed to calculate the false negative rate on a lower number of replicates, for example, ten replicates. The false negative rate has to be below 5 per cent (i.e., all ten PCR replicates have to be positive). This approach allows an approximate estimation of the $LOD_{abs}$.

The definition of false negative rate is the probability that a known positive test sample is classified as negative by the method. An increase in the false negative rate is observed when the amount of analyte approaches the LOD of the method. The dilution series should

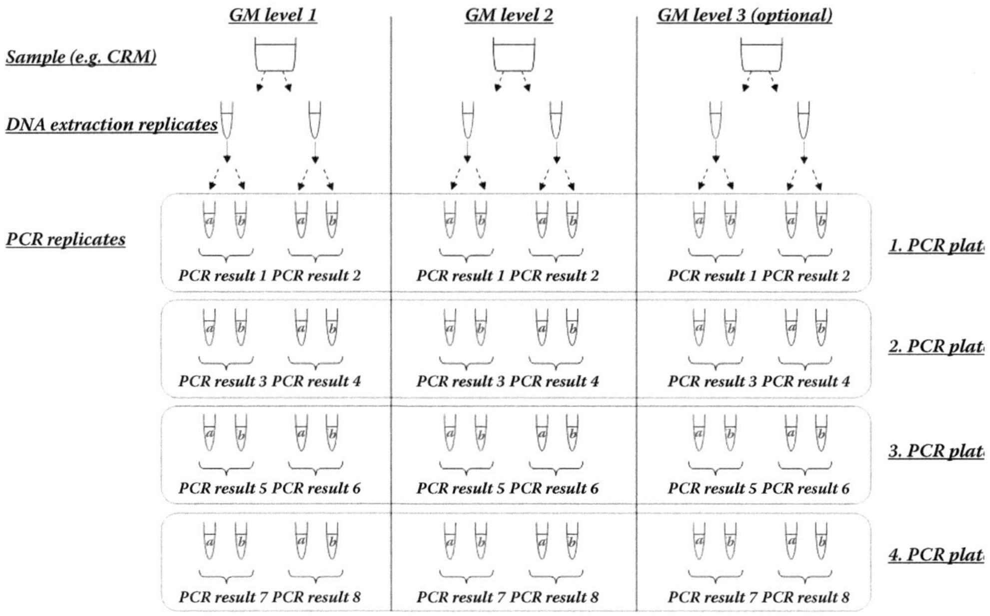


FIGURE 8.2 Experimental design for trueness/precision (Example 1).

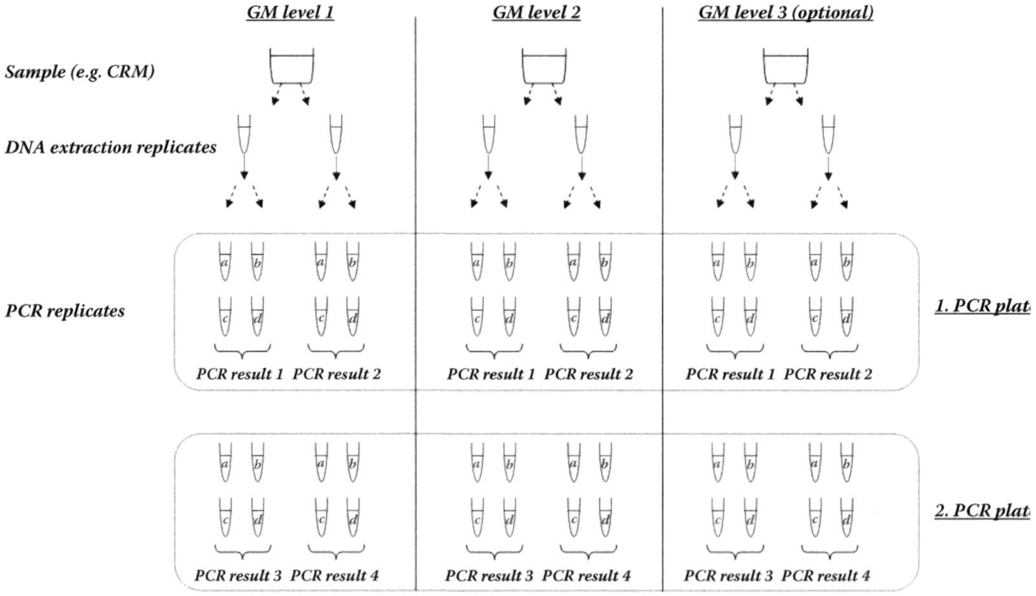


FIGURE 8.3 Experimental design for trueness/precision (Example 2).

be chosen so that it represents an interval above and below the expected $LOD_{abs}$ based on prior knowledge of the performance of that method (e.g., 20, 10, 5, and 1 copies). The lowest concentration where all 10 replicates are positive is the estimated $LOD_{abs}$. The probability distribution suggest that one copy should give approximately 30 per cent negatives.

Therefore, as a requirement to verify that the copy numbers of the dilution series are approximately correct, at least one replicate has to be negative for the one copy dilution. See also Table 8.1 for details.

*Acceptance criterion*: Whenever validation data are available, the LOD should be in line with those data.

The practical LOD ($LOD_{prac}$) is out of the scope of this document because it is sample and not method dependent. However, the $LOD_{prac}$ should be determined for each individual sample tested[13].

## 8.11 ROBUSTNESS

Robustness should have been investigated previously during method development/optimization, before the method was subjected to a collaborative trial. Therefore, the robustness does not need to be re-evaluated in a verification study.

## 8.12 RELEVANT SAMPLES

Laboratories would like to remain informed of methods for new GMOs becoming available on the market. However, at the time of the method verification usually only CRMs are available. Therefore, the verification process is usually conducted on CRMs. If these are not available, other GM positive material can be used. It can also be useful to additionally test a routine sample alone or spiked with reference material.

Note: It may be feasible to assess some of the parameters simultaneously in Table 8.1.

Note: For a single assay, the standard curve and the samples have to be on the same plate. Two assays (e.g., endogene and transgene assay) can be performed on two different plates using the same dilutions of the samples and having a standard curve on each plate.

## APPENDIX A: EFFECT OF DNA CONTENT ON THE PRACTICAL LOD

As shown in Table A.1, in a 0.1 per cent GM sample there are 1000 times more copies of the target-taxon specific sequence than of the GMO target. This implies that for an absolute LOD of the method of 10 copies, it is necessary to load in PCR 10,000 copies of the taxon-specific sequence to have a practical LOD of 0.1 per cent. If the absolute LOD is 10 copies and 100,000 copies are loaded in the PCR reaction, then the practical LOD is 0.01 per cent (see Table A.1). The practical LOD should be calculated for each individual sample[13].

TABLE A.1 Example of the Effect of DNA Content on the Practical LOD

| Copies of taxon-specific gene | Absolute LOD (copies of GMO target) | Practical LOD (%) |
|---|---|---|
| 100,000 | 10 | 0.01 |
| 10,000 | 10 | 0.1 |
| 1,000 | 10 | 1 |

# APPENDIX B: EVALUATION OF DNA—EXTRACTION METHOD (INHIBITION TEST)

## BACKGROUND

Substances known to inhibit the PCR reaction components affect the efficiency of target DNA amplification by interacting with the DNA template, by interfering with the DNA polymerase activity or decreasing the efficiency of enzymatic cofactors ($Mg^{2+}$). DNA extraction procedures eliminate or reduce considerably the amount of PCR-inhibiting substances. However, the final amount of inhibitors in a sample depends very much on the sample nature. The more the sample has been processed, the more likely the DNA will be fragmented. Plant DNA can also be affected by the presence of secondary metabolites such as polyphenols, oils, and polysaccharides, which can form complexes with DNA strands. Inhibitors can be added by the DNA isolation procedure: KCl and NaCl, ionic detergents, ethanol, isopropanol, and phenol, among others.

Different strategies can be adopted to test DNA preparations for presence of PCR inhibitory compounds. This appendix illustrates the application of the ENGL acceptance criteria to evaluate reaction efficiency (slope and $R^2$) of serially diluted samples from an undiluted source with the ability to test for presence of PCR inhibitors in the undiluted sample intended for the PCR analyses.

Basically, the inhibition depends on the concentration of the inhibitors. When DNA is diluted, the effect of inhibitors is often reduced or eliminated at lower DNA concentrations. Evaluation of the reaction efficiency on the diluted series and comparison of the theoretical Ct (threshold cycle) of a non-inhibited undiluted sample with its measured Ct, discloses information for the assessment of DNA quality for PCR applications. In case only the highest DNA concentration shows inhibition a lower DNA concentration can be used for quantification, but this will affect the practical LOD and LOQ.

However, in certain cases inhibitor compounds attached to DNA fragments may not be eliminated by sample dilution, thus resulting in less DNA copies available for amplification than expected from the nominal DNA concentration in a sample.

## PROCEDURE

DNA quality (relative absence of PCR inhibitors) can be demonstrated by analyzing two PCR replicates using four points of a four-fold serial dilutions (1:4, 1:16, 1:64, and 1:256) of each DNA extraction replicate (inhibition runs) using the taxon-specific reference system. The DNA extract is first brought to a level corresponding to the highest DNA concentration intended to be used in the subsequent PCR method, the so-called "undiluted" sample (working dilution). From this first sample, a fourfold dilution series is prepared (from 1:4 to 1:256). To assess the presence of inhibitors, the Ct values of the four serially diluted samples are plotted against the logarithm of the dilution factor and an equation is calculated by linear regression. The Ct value of the "undiluted" sample extrapolated from the linear regression is compared with the Ct measured from the same sample. To accept DNA extracts, three conditions should be met: the slope of the regression line must be between –3.6 and –3.1; the coefficient of determination ($R^2$) is equal to or above 0.98; and the difference between the measured Ct and the extrapolated Ct value ($\Delta$Ct) is below 0.5.

The Ct values from two PCR replicates from each dilution are needed for the calculation sheet illustrated below.

## EVALUATION OF DNA QUALITY

In the figures below, the wording "working dilution" in the blue cell reflects the term "undiluted sample."

Example A: Acceptable DNA quality: all criteria met.

**Sample code :**

| Dilution factor | Measured Ct | Ct Mean | ΔCt | Expected ΔCt | Logarithm |
|---|---|---|---|---|---|
| 1 : 4 | 24 | | | | -0.6021 |
| | 24 | 24.00 | 2.00 | 2 | -0.6021 |
| 1 : 16 | 26 | | | | -1.2041 |
| | 26 | 26.00 | 2.00 | 2 | -1.2041 |
| 1 : 64 | 28 | | | | |
| | 28 | 28.00 | 2.00 | 2 | -1.8062 |
| 1 : 256 | 30 | | | | -2.4082 |
| | 30 | 30.00 | 2.00 | 2 | -2.4082 |

| | Measured Ct | Ct Mean | Extrapol. Ct | Extrapol. - Mean Ct | |
|---|---|---|---|---|---|
| | 22 | | | | |
| Working dilution | 22 | 22.00 | 22.00 | 0.00 | Ok |

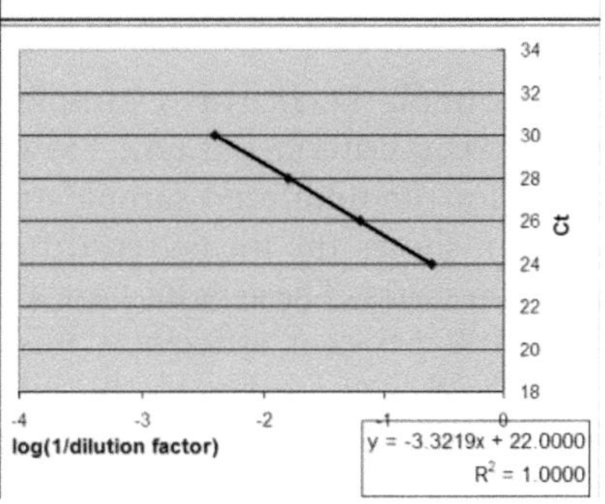


Example B: DNA inhibited. Even though the ΔCt does not exceed the limit of 0.5 (although it is close to this value) the underperforming DNA quality is demonstrated by the delay in reaction onset (Cts) for the undiluted sample and the 1:4 diluted sample. The latter affects the slope expressed by the serial dilution, which appears flatter than acceptable (−3.0).

**Sample code :**

| Dilution factor | Measured Ct | Ct Mean | ΔCt | Expected ΔCt | Logarithm |
|---|---|---|---|---|---|
| 1 : 4 | 24.5 | | | | -0.6021 |
| | 24.6 | 24.55 | 1.55 | 2 | -0.6021 |
| 1 : 16 | 26 | | | | -1.2041 |
| | 26.1 | 26.05 | 1.50 | 2 | -1.2041 |
| 1 : 64 | 28.1 | | | | |
| | 28 | 28.05 | 2.00 | 2 | -1.8062 |
| 1 : 256 | 30.2 | | | | -2.4082 |
| | 29.8 | 30.00 | 1.95 | 2 | -2.4082 |

| | Measured Ct | Ct Mean | Extrapol. Ct | Extrapol. - Mean Ct | |
|---|---|---|---|---|---|
| | 23 | | | | Out of |
| Working dilution | 23 | 23.00 | 22.58 | 0.43 | A.C. |

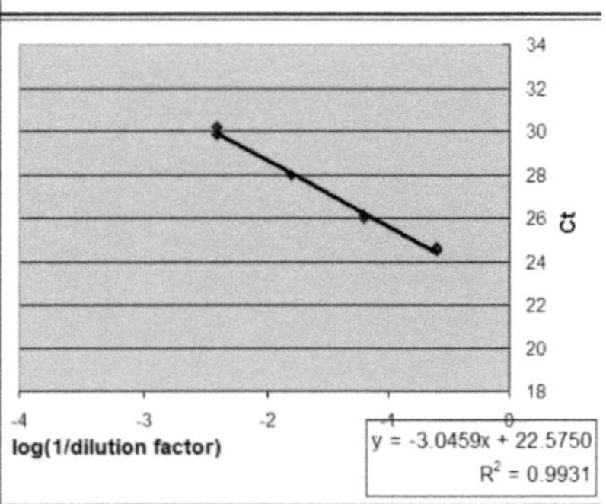


Example C: DNA inhibited. This is another occurrence of low quality associated with the DNA extract. The slope of the dilution series is within the acceptance range; however, the extrapolated Ct for the undiluted sample (22.48), based on the four-point straight line should be lower than measured (23). This indicates a delay in onset for the undiluted sample, which is less evident on the subsequent diluted sample 1:4. Therefore, while the slope of the linear regression falls within the range from −3.6 to −3.1, the ΔCt demonstrated co-extraction of compounds inhibiting DNA amplification.

**Sample code :**

| Dilution factor | Measured Ct | Ct Mean | ΔCt | Expected ΔCt | Logarithm |
|---|---|---|---|---|---|
| 1 : 4 | 24.8 | | | | -0.6021 |
| | 24.6 | 24.70 | 1.70 | 2 | -0.6021 |
| 1 : 16 | 25.8 | | | | -1.2041 |
| | 26.1 | 25.95 | 1.25 | 2 | -1.2041 |
| 1 : 64 | 28.2 | | | | |
| | 28.6 | 28.40 | 2.45 | 2 | -1.8062 |
| 1 : 256 | 30.5 | | | | -2.4082 |
| | 30.3 | 30.40 | 2.00 | 2 | -2.4082 |
| | **Measured Ct** | **Ct Mean** | **Extrapol. Ct** | **Extrapol. - Mean Ct** | |
| | 23 | | | | Out of |
| Working dilution | 23 | 23.00 | 22.48 | 0.52 | A.C. |

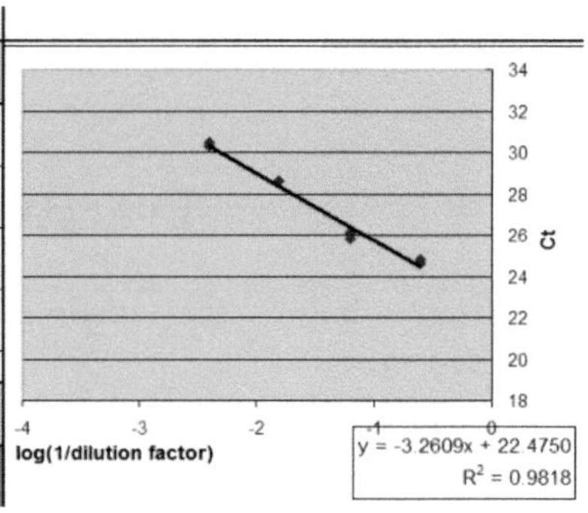


Example D: In this example, the slope of the regression line is out of the ENGL acceptance criteria (–3.66). However, contrary to Example B, there is no delay in Ct onset for the undiluted sample and in the first samples of the dilution series. The "ΔCt" column shows the measured difference in Ct values between subsequent samples of the dilution series. These values are always greater than the expected value of 2 for a reaction with 100 per cent efficiency. Basically, the dilution series behaves as if less DNA than calculated was present in the diluted samples. Therefore, we do not expect to classify this sample as affected by the presence of inhibitory compounds. However, if technical mistakes are ruled out (pipetting errors) and no other reasons are clearly identified, the possibility of inhibitors attached to DNA targets should not be discarded a priori.

**Sample code :**

| Dilution factor | Measured Ct | Ct Mean | ΔCt | Expected ΔCt | Logarithm |
|---|---|---|---|---|---|
| 1 : 4 | 24.2 | | | | -0.6021 |
| | 24.3 | 24.25 | 2.25 | 2 | -0.6021 |
| 1 : 16 | 26.5 | | | | -1.2041 |
| | 26.5 | 26.50 | 2.25 | 2 | -1.2041 |
| 1 : 64 | 28.6 | | | | |
| | 28.8 | 28.70 | 2.20 | 2 | -1.8062 |
| 1 : 256 | 30.8 | | | | -2.4082 |
| | 30.9 | 30.85 | 2.15 | 2 | -2.4082 |
| | **Measured Ct** | **Ct Mean** | **Extrapol. Ct** | **Extrapol. - Mean Ct** | |
| | 22 | | | | Out of |
| Working dilution | 22 | 22.00 | 22.08 | 0.08 | A.C. |

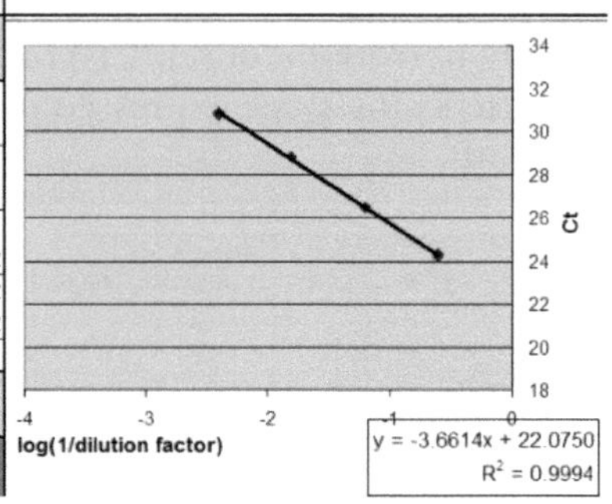


## APPENDIX C: PRODUCTION OF INTERMEDIATE CONCENTRATIONS OF POSITIVE MATERIAL

Some of the reference materials are only available in one or a few limited GM concentrations. It may be necessary to mix the positive material with non-GM material to produce other GM concentrations, for example, for determining the relative LOQ and LOD.

This can be done by measuring the content of the reference gene for the GM positive and a GM negative DNA preparation on the same plate with the same standard curve. Following this, the dilution factor for the two DNA preparations can be calculated using the following formula:

$$X = (A/B)*(Y-1)+1$$

X = the practical dilution factor (how much the GM material has to be diluted compensated for difference in concentration)

A = copy number of reference gene for the GM positive DNA preparation

B = copy number of the reference gene for the GM negative DNA preparation Y = the theoretical dilution factor, for example, from 10% GM to 0.1% GM = 100x

Example:

DNA A = 100% GMO, DNA B = 0%

5 μL DNA is added per PCR well for A and B

Quantification as unknown sample on reference gene calibration curve result:

A (from DNA A): 10 copies/5 μL

B (from DNA B): 8 copies/5 μL

To make 10 per cent GMO from 100 per cent GM corresponds to 10 times dilution (theoretically Y = 10). X has to be used like Y in calculating the volumes to be mixed. If X = 12.25, then practical dilution factor X: (10/8)*(10 – 1) + 1 = ((10/8) * 9) + 1 = 90/8 + 1 = 11.25 + 1 = 12.25, so 1 μl A has to be mixed with 11.25 μl B.

After adding together the two DNA preparations, the DNA solution has to be mixed thoroughly. The trueness of the mixtures can be analyzed using the 100 per cent mixture for standard curve and analyzing three samples in triplicates on three different days.

## APPENDIX D: ESTIMATION OF THE MEAN, STANDARD DEVIATION AND RELATIVE REPEATABILITY STANDARD DEVIATION OF GM-CONTENT FROM REAL-TIME PCR

The correct calculation of GM content and its standard deviation from PCR assays is in most experimental designs a two-step process combining mean values that are calculated in two different ways. The procedure outlined in detail below starts from the measured values of the copy numbers of target and reference genes. From these test results, an estimate of GM-content and a standard deviation is calculated. Most experimental procedures provide several such values (e.g., from runs on the same or different plates) of GM content and standard deviation. These estimates can, if needed and appropriate, be combined in a standard way, for example by taking the arithmetic mean in case of the GM-content.

*Estimation of GM-content from copy numbers of target and reference genes*

Two assays are required to estimate the percentage of GM-DNA from samples using real-time PCR: one assay is used to detect the copy number of the GM target DNA sequence ($X$), the other is used to determine the copy number of the endogenous reference gene DNA sequence ($Y$). The estimate of the percentage of GM content is obtained using the following ratio of

$$\%GM = \frac{\text{target DNA copy number}}{\text{reference DNA copy number}}100 = \frac{X}{Y}100. \qquad (1)$$

Both $X$ and $Y$ are random variables.* It is standard practice to run assays for the target and the reference genes in duplicates, triplicates etc. This results in 2, 3, etc. test results for the GM target DNA sequence and 2, 3, etc. test results for the reference gene DNA

* A random variable can be thought of as a quantity whose value is not fixed, but which can take on different values according to a probability distribution (which may be determined by, e.g., measurement uncertainty). It is common to use the capital letter for a random variable (i.e., $X$ for target DNA concentration) and small letters for an actual value (i.e., a measurement result).

target sequence, and what is required is the calculation of an average GM-percentage from these two sets of test results. There are unfortunately no exact formula for the mean and variance of the ratio of random variables, but approximations do exist[(20)]. The mean, denoted by E[·], and the variance of a ratio of independent random variables are approximated by

$$E\left[\frac{X}{Y}\right] \approx \frac{\bar{x}}{\bar{y}} + \frac{\bar{x}}{\bar{y}^3} Var(y) \tag{2}$$

and

$$Var\left[\frac{X}{Y}\right] \approx \left(\frac{\bar{x}}{\bar{y}}\right)^2 \left(\frac{Var(x)}{\bar{x}^2} + \frac{Var(y)}{\bar{y}^2}\right), \tag{3}$$

where $x$ is the arithmetic mean of the target GM DNA copy numbers and $y$ is the arithmetic mean of the reference DNA copy numbers.

These approximations assume that there is no correlation between $X$ and $Y$. The standard deviation is given by $sd[X/Y] = \sqrt{Var[X/Y]}$. Relative repeatability standard deviation $RSD_r$ is calculated at the end of the procedure from the component standard deviations; the details of how to calculate $RSD_r$ are outlined in the examples below.

All these calculation can be implemented in Excel.

**Examples**

In the examples, we use $x$ for the copy number of the GM target gene and $y$ for the copy number of the reference gene. These examples correspond to the examples given in Table 8.1, demonstrate in detail the calculations needed for one plate, and then describe how the calculation results from several plates are combined.

***Example 1: Two DNA Extractions; for Each Extraction, Both GM Target and Reference Genes are Tested in Two PCR Replicates on Four Plates***

This design provides two GM-estimates and standard deviations for each plate and thus eight GM-estimates ($GM_{1-8}$) and eight standard deviations ($sd_{1-8}$) in total. Each of these eight GM-estimates and standard deviations is derived using Equations (1) and (2) from two test results each of the target gene copy number and the reference gene copy number. If the mean of all 8 GM-estimates is taken, this average value depends on 16 test results of the target gene copy number and 16 test results of the reference gene copy number; this also applies of course to the combined standard deviation.

EXTRACTION 1:

| GM Target Gene | | Reference Gene | |
|---|---|---|---|
| Ct | Copy Number | Ct | Copy Number |
| 24.41 | 16119 | 21.30 | 156758 |
| 24.61 | 13954 | 21.18 | 171196 |

Thus, $x = 15036.97$, $y = 163977$, $\mathrm{Var}(x) = 2343612.5$, and $\mathrm{Var}(y) = 104227922$. Putting the appropriate values into Equation (2) gives a mean $GM_1$ of 0.092 or 9.2 per cent; using Equation (3) with the above values and taking the square root gives a standard deviation $sd_1$ of 0.010943.

EXTRACTION 2:

| GM Target Gene | | Reference Gene | |
|---|---|---|---|
| Ct | Copy Number | Ct | Copy Number |
| 25.50 | 13405 | 21.10 | 172089 |
| 25.44 | 14000 | 21.19 | 160907 |

Here, $x = 13702.5$, $y = 166498$, $\mathrm{Var}(x) = 177012.5$ and $\mathrm{Var}(y) = 62518562$. With the appropriate values, Equation (2) gives a mean $GM_2$ of 0.082 or 8.2 per cent; using Equation (3) and taking the square root gives a standard deviation $sd_2$ of 0.004654.

### Combining the Plates

This entire procedure is repeated on four different plates, giving in addition to $GM_1$, $GM_2$, $sd_1$ and $sd_2$ the means $GM_3$, $GM_4$, ..., $GM_8$ and the standard deviations $sd_3$, $sd_4$, ..., $sd_8$.

The overall mean of the sample $GM$ can then be calculated by taking the arithmetic mean of $GM_1$–$GM_8$, i.e., $\overline{GM} = \sum_{i=1}^{8} GM_i/8$. Using $n$ as the number of replicates per extraction ($n = 2$, in this example) and $k$ as the number of separate standard deviations to be pooled ($k = 8$, here), the standard deviation of the overall mean $sd_{GM} = \sqrt{\sum_{i=1}^{8}(n_i - 1)sd_i^2 \Big/ \left(\sum_{i=1}^{8} n_i - k\right)}$; the term in the denominator is $16 - 8 = 8$ in this example. The relative repeatability standard deviation $RSD_r = \frac{sd_{GM}}{\overline{GM}}100$.

### *Example 2: Two DNA Extractions; Both GM Target and Reference Genes are Tested in Four PCR Replicates on Two Plates*

This design provides two GM-estimates and standard deviations for each plate and thus four GM-estimates ($GM_{1-4}$) and four standard deviations ($sd_{1-4}$) in total. Each of these four GM-estimates and standard deviations is derived using Equations (1) and (2) from four test results each of the target gene copy number and the reference gene copy number. If the mean of all four GM-estimates is taken, the average value depends—as in Example 1—on 16 test results of the target gene copy number and 16 test results of the reference gene copy number; this also applies of course to the combined standard deviation.

EXTRACTION 1:

| GM Target Gene | | Reference Gene | |
|---|---|---|---|
| Ct | Copy Number | Ct | Copy Number |
| 24.41 | 16119 | 21.30 | 156758 |
| 24.61 | 13954 | 21.18 | 171196 |
| 25.50 | 13405 | 21.10 | 172089 |
| 25.44 | 14000 | 21.19 | 160907 |

Here, $x$ = 14369.5, $y$ = 165237.5, Var($x$) = 1433394 and Var($y$) = 57700642. Applying Equation (2) gives a mean $GM_1$of 0.087 or 8.7 per cent; using Equation (3) and taking the square root gives a standard deviation $sd_1$ of 0.00828.

**EXTRACTION 2:**

| GM Target Gene | | Reference Gene | |
|---|---|---|---|
| Ct | Copy Number | Ct | Copy Number |
| 26.21 | 14826.97 | 21.09 | 165248 |
| 26.30 | 13885.92 | 21.09 | 165248 |
| 26.38 | 13099.69 | 21.20 | 152168 |
| 26.20 | 14935.39 | 21.25 | 146569 |

Here, $x$ = 14187, $y$ = 157308, Var($x$) = 747515 and Var($y$) = 89272181. Applying Equation (2) gives a mean $GM_2$ of 0.091 or 9.1 per cent; using Equation (3) and taking the square root gives a standard deviation $sd_2$ of 0.0077.

**Combining the Plates**

This entire procedure is repeated on two different plates, giving in addition to $GM_1$, $GM_2$, $sd_1$, and $sd_2$, the means $GM_3$ and $GM_4$ and the standard deviations $sd_3$ and $sd_4$.

The overall mean of the sample $GM$ can then be calculated by taking the arithmetic mean of $GM_1$–$GM_8$, i.e., $\overline{GM} = \sum_{i=1}^{4} GM_i / 4$. Using $n$ as the number of replicates per extraction ($n$ = 4, in this example) and $k$ as the number of separate standard deviations to be pooled ($k$ = 4, here), the standard deviation of the overall mean $sd_{GM} = \sqrt{\sum_{i=1}^{4} (n_i - 1) sd_i^2 \Big/ \left(\sum_{i=1}^{4} n_i - k\right)}$; the term in the denominator is 16 – 4 = 12 in this example. The relative repeatability standard deviation $RSD_r = \frac{sd_{GM}}{\overline{GM}} 100$.

## REFERENCES


1. Commission Regulation (EC) No 882/2004 of the European Parliament and Council of 29 April 2004 on official controls performed to ensure the verification of compliance with feed and food law, animal health and animal welfare rules.
2. International Standard (ISO) 17025, *General Requirements for the Competence of Testing and Calibration Laboratories.* International Organisation for Standardisation, Geneve, Switzerland, 2005.
3. International Standard (ISO) 5725, *Accuracy (Trueness and Precision) of Measurement Methods and Results.* International Organisation for Standardisation, Geneve, Swizerland, 1994.
4. Horwitz W., Protocol for the design, conduct and interpretation of method performance studies. *Pure and Applied Chemistry.* 67: 331–343, 1995.
5. Definition of minimum performance requirements for analytical methods of GMO testing. European Network of GMO Laboratories (ENGL), 2008, http://gmo-crl.jrc.ec.europa.eu/guidancedocs.htm.
6. Thompson M., Ellison S.L.R., Wood R. Harmonised guidelines for single-laboratory validation of methods of analysis. *Pure and Applied Chemistry* 74: 835–855, 2002.

7. ALACC guide, How to meet ISO 17025 requirements for method verification, 2007.
8. Žel J., Mazzara M., Savini C., Cordeil S., Camloh M., Štebih D., Cankar K., Gruden K., Morisset D., Van den Eede G. Method validation and quality management in the flexible scope of accreditation: An example of laboratories testing for genetically modified organisms. *Food Analytical Methods* 1 (2): 61–72, 2008.
9. Scholtens I.M.J., Kok E.J., Hougs L., Molenaar B., Thissen J.T.N.M., van der Voet H. Increased efficacy for in-house validation of real-time PCR GMO detection methods. *Analytical and Bioanalytical Chemistry* 396 (6): 2213–2227, 2010.
10. Ciabatti I., Froiio A., Gatto F., Amaddeo D., Marchesi U. In-house validation and quality control of real-time PCR methods for GMO detection: A practical approach. *Developments in Biologicals* 126: 79–86; discussion 324, 2006.
11. Holst-Jensen A., Berdal K.G. The modular analytical procedure and validation approach and the units of measurement for genetically modified materials in foods and feeds. *Journal of AOAC International* 87 (4): 927–936, 2004.
12. Trapmann S., Burns M., Broll H., Macarthur R., Wood R., Zel J., Guidance document on measurement uncertainty for GMO testing laboratories. EUR - Scientific and Technical Research series, EUR 22756 EN/2, DOI:10.2787/18988, 2009, http://irmm.jrc.ec.europa.eu/html/reference_materials_catalogue/user_support/EUR22756EN.pdf.
13. International standard (ISO) 24276, *Foodstuffs. Methods of Analysis for the Detection of Genetically Modified Organisms and Derived Products—General Requirements.* International Organisation for Standardisation, Geneve, Switzerland, 2006.
14. EN/TS 21568, *Foodstuffs. Methods of Analysis for the Detection of Genetically Modified Organisms and Derived Products. Sampling Strategies.* European Committee for Standardisation, Brussels, Belgium, 2006.
15. European Union reference laboratory for GM food and feed (EURL-GMFF), European Network of GMO Laboratories (ENGL), Compendium of reference methods for GMO analysis, JRC reference reports, EUR-Scientifical and Technical Research series, EUR 24596 EN, 2010, http://ec.europa.eu/dgs/jrc/downloads/jrc_reference_report_2010_11_gmo_analysis_compendium.pdf.
16. International standard (ISO) 21570, *Foodstuffs. Methods of Analysis for the Detection of Genetically Modified Organisms and Derived Products—Quantitative Nucleic Acid Based Methods.* International Organisation for Standardisation, Geneve, Switzerland, 2006.
17. International standard (ISO) 21569, *Foodstuffs. Methods of Analysis for the Detection of Genetically Modified Organisms and Derived Products—Qualitative Nucleic Acid Based Methods.* International Organisation for Standardisation, Geneve, Switzerland, 2006.
18. International standard (ISO) 21571, *Foodstuffs. Methods of Analysis for the Detection of Genetically Modified Organisms and Derived Products – Nucleic Acid Extraction.* International Organisation for Standardisation, Geneve, Switzerland, 2006.
19. Hübner P., Waiblinger H-U., Pietsch P., Brodmann P. Validation of PCR methods for quantification of genetically modified plants in food. *Journal of AOAC International* 84 (6): 1855–1864, 2001.
20. Rinne H. *Handbuch der Statistik.* Frankfurt am Main, Harri Deutsch Verlag, 2008.

# CHAPTER 9

# Reference Materials for GMO Analysis

*Leo M.L. Nollet*
University College Ghent

CONTENTS



Most of the text in the following sections is taken from the webpage of the European Commission on *Reference Materials for GMO analysis* (1).

The use of genetically modified organisms (GMOs) as food/feed needs to be authorized in Europe. Food/feed products containing more than 0.9 per cent of GMOs have to be labeled (2). This labeling threshold applies for adventitiously added GMOs, while GMOs added on purpose always need to be labeled. GMOs for which an authorization procedure is pending or for which the authorization has expired are allowed in European feed products up to a level of 0.1 per cent (3).

Quantification of GMOs is required for the implementation of both regulations; consequently, they explicitly demand the availability of validated methods and of reference materials. The Joint Research Centre—Institute for Reference Materials and Measurements (JRC-IRMM) develops and produces the required reference materials, while the Joint Research Centre—Institute for Health and Consumer Protection (JRC-IHCP) hosts the European Reference Laboratory for GM Food and Feed (EU-RL GMFF) (4) where the method validation is carried out. Validated methods and reference materials are important for the standardization and ensure that the measurement results of laboratories quantifying GMOs are comparable.

## 9.1 GMO REFERENCE MATERIALS

For the implementation of the European legislation that regulates the authorization and the labeling of GMOs, the JRC-IRMM develops, produces, and distributes certified reference materials (CRMs). These CRMs are used for the calibration or quality control of GMO quantification measurements, typically carried out by quantitative real-time polymerase chain reaction (qPCR). Numerous sets of reference materials for different GM events in maize, soybean, potato, sugar beet, and cotton are offered to testing and control laboratories worldwide. Research activities are ongoing to develop further GMO CRMs, including CRMs for new plant species.

## 9.2 AVAILABLE GMO REFERENCE MATERIALS

The majority of CRMs intended for the quantification of GMOs are powders produced from seeds or vegetables. These so-called matrix materials are mixtures of non-GMO materials with GMO materials, which have gravimetrically been certified for their mass fraction (expressed in g/kg) of a specific GMO event. The available concentrations differ for the individual GMO event (and the set of CRM) and range from nominal 0 to 1,000 g/kg.

Available sets of GMO CRMs are available in the online reference materials catalog (5–6).

## 9.3 DEVELOPMENT OF GMO REFERENCE MATERIALS

The development of CRMs for GMO analysis requires research. Investigations have resulted in major improvements, for instance the possibility to produce powders with a homogenous and sufficiently small particle size using cryo-grinding techniques. Another example is the application of a dry-mixing technique, specifically developed to avoid DNA degradation during the production of a powder CRM. Ongoing research investigates production tools for stable and homogenous GMO CRMs for further plant species.

IRMM also offers to the Biotech Industry a service to develop GMO reference materials (7).

## 9.4 USE OF GMO REFERENCE MATERIALS

The majority of GMO CRMs are powder (matrix) materials and are intended to be used for the calibration or quality control for GMO quantification measurements (CRM code ERM-BF). A few GMO CRMs that exist are limited to the calibration of GMO measurements (CRM code ERM-AD).

Reference material in general contributes to the standardization of measurements and ensures that measurement results are comparable. GMO CRMs are commonly used for the calibration or quality control of GMO quantification measurements based on quantitative real-time qPCR. Additionally, they are well suited for the validation and verification of GMO quantification methods. Their use is recommended in ISO/IEC 17025 (8), while official GMO control laboratories are required to be accredited according to ISO/IEC 17025 (Regulation (EC) No 882/2004) (9).

The JRC has issued a number of application notes (10) dedicated to the proper use of Reference Materials. The application notes of interest for GMO testing laboratories are as follows:

ERM application note 1: Comparison of a measurement result with the certified value.
ERM application note 4: Use of CRMs for the quantification of GMO in food and feed.
ERM application note 5: Use of CRMs for the quantification of GMO in DNA copy number ratio.

Guidance on the estimation of measurement uncertainty (MU) in the area of GMO quantification is provided in the guidance document on MU for GMO testing laboratories (11).

## 9.5 WHO DOES WHAT ON GMOs IN THE JRC?

- JRC-IRMM—development, production, and distribution of CRMs for analysis of GMOs;
- JRC-IHCP—EU-RL GMFF, including the validation of GMO quantification methods;
- JRC's Institute for Prospective Technological Studies (JRC-IPTS)—European Coexistence Bureau, including the evaluation of co-existence measures.

## 9.6 REQUEST FOR THE DEVELOPMENT OF A SET OF GMO CRMs

The JRC in Geel, Belgium, has a long proven expertise in the production of CRMs for the quantification of GMOs. The Reference Materials Unit of the JRC offers to biotech companies to develop GMO CRMs as required according to Regulation (EC) No 1829/2003 (2) and Regulation (EU) No 619/2011 (3). A set of GMO CRMs is typically composed of CRMs with a GMO mass fraction of nominal 0, 0.1, 1, 10, and 100 (m/m) per cent.

Due to intellectual property rights, a material transfer agreement (MTA) is required for each GMO event for which GMO CRMs shall be developed. For the latter reason, JRC developed a MTA template. Changes to this MTA need to be agreed with the legal service of the JRC. Further, the JRC and the biotech company need to agree on the type, amount and delivery date of the required raw materials for the CRM production.

Typically, these are 10 kg of untreated seeds of the GMO event (including information about the zygosity) and 30 kg of untreated non-GMO seeds (preferable of a near isogenic parental line).

All seed materials need to be of seed quality (proven purity of >99 per cent), clean from any harvest debris and preferably of the same size. They need to be accompanied by a phytosanitary certificate (alternatively a letter confirming the origin of the material and an analysis certificate stating the purity and the methods used to establish the purity).

The raw materials need to be shipped by the biotech company to the JRC site in Geel within an agreed time frame, following IATA rules and providing the airway bill number in a timely manner to the JRC for custom clearance.

Additionally, the biotech company needs to provide to the JRC in Geel, the event-specific quantification method that was already submitted (or is intended to be submitted) for validation to the EU-RL GMFF. The method will be treated confidentially until published by the EU-RL GMFF.

Provided that no unforeseen complications arise, the JRC can offer to produce sets of GMO CRMs within an estimated time frame of 14 months for matrices such as soya, maize, rapeseed, and cottonseed seeds, as well as sugar beets and potato tubers. For other matrices, longer development times are required and need to be negotiated with the JRC.

## 9.7 AMERICAN OIL CHEMISTS' SOCIETY AND FLUKA/SIGMA-ALDRICH

As stated in previous paragraphs, The European Commission has mandated that as of 2004, a validated published method for detecting a new genetically modified event and a CRM must be available before the EC will authorize a new crop. Several nations outside of Europe require grain and ingredients to be labeled as genetically modified when trait levels exceed mandated thresholds. AOCS (American Oil Chemists' Society) CRMs are used by labs that perform those analyses (12).

This program is A2LA accredited to ISO Guide 17034:2016 (13). These CRMs are intended for use as quality control materials or calibrants in methods for the detection, identification, and/or quantification of genetically modified events.

CRMs can be purchased directly from Fluka/Sigma-Aldrich (14). The available reference material is listed in the product catalog under *GMO Reference Materials, Qualitative* (15).

## 9.8 U.S. FOOD AND DRUG ADMINISTRATION

The U.S. Food and Drug Administration regulates the safety of food for humans and animals, including foods produced from genetically engineered (GE) plants. Foods from GE plants must meet the same food safety requirements as foods derived from traditionally bred plants (16).

## REFERENCES

1. https://ec.europa.eu/jrc/en/research-topic/reference-materials-gmo-analysis.
2. Regulation (EC) No 1829/2003—http://eur-lex.europa.eu/legal-content/EN/TXT/?qid=1430223289654&uri=CELEX:32003R1829.
3. Regulation (EC) No 619/2011—http://eur-lex.europa.eu/legal-content/EN/TXT/?qid=1396874179317&uri=CELEX:32011R0619.
4. https://ec.europa.eu/jrc/en/network-bureau/european-union-reference-laboratory-genetically-modified-food-and-feed.
5. https://ec.europa.eu/jrc/en/reference-materials/catalogue.
6. https://crm.jrc.ec.europa.eu.
7. https://ec.europa.eu/jrc/en/reference-materials/development/gmo.
8. https://www.iso.org/standard/66912.html.
9. http://eur-lex.europa.eu/legal-content/EN/TXT/?qid=1396874941750&uri=CELEX:02004R0882-20120101.

10. https://ec.europa.eu/jrc/en/reference-materials/application-notes.
11. https://ec.europa.eu/jrc/en/publication/eur-scientific-and-technical-research-reports/guidance-document-measurement-uncertainty-gmo-testing-laboratories.
12. https://www.aocs.org/crm.
13. https://www.iso.org/standard/29357.html.
14. https://www.sigmaaldrich.com/.
15. https://www.sigmaaldrich.com/analytical-chromatography/analytical-products.html?TablePage=9641474.
16. https://www.fda.gov/Food/IngredientsPackagingLabeling/GEPlants/default.htm.

CHAPTER 10

# ISO (International Organization for Standardization)

*Leo M.L. Nollet*
University College Ghent

## CONTENTS



ISO, the International Organization for Standardization, develops and publishes International Standards (1).

**ISO 21569:2005**—Foodstuffs—Methods of analysis for the detection of genetically modified organisms and derived products—Qualitative nucleic acid based methods.

ISO 21569:2005 (2) describes the procedure to qualitatively detect genetically modified organisms (GMOs) and derived products by analyzing the nucleic acids extracted from the sample under study. The main focus is on polymerase chain reaction (PCR)-based amplification methods.

It gives general requirements for the specific detection and identification of target nucleic acid sequences (DNA) and for the confirmation of the identity of the amplified DNA sequence.

Guidelines, minimum requirements, and performance criteria laid down in ISO 21569:2005 are intended to ensure that comparable, accurate, and reproducible results are obtained in different laboratories.

ISO 21569:2005 has been established for food matrices, but could also be applied to other matrices (e.g., feed and plant samples from the environment).

This standard was last reviewed and confirmed in 2014. Therefore, this version remains current.

**ISO/TS 21569-2:2012**—Horizontal methods for molecular biomarker analysis—Methods of analysis for the detection of genetically modified organisms and derived products—Part 2: Construct-specific real-time PCR method for detection of event FP967 in linseed and linseed products.

This standard (3) was last reviewed and confirmed in 2016. Therefore, this version remains current.

**ISO/TS 21569-3:2015**—Horizontal methods for molecular biomarker analysis—Methods of analysis for the detection of genetically modified organisms and derived products—Part 3: Construct-specific real-time PCR method for detection of P35S-pat-sequence for screening genetically modified organisms.

ISO/TS 21569-3:2015 (4) describes a procedure for the detection of the DNA transition sequence between the 35S promotor (*P35S*) from cauliflower mosaic virus and a modified phosphinothricin-acetyltransferase gene (*pat*) from *Streptomyces viridochromogenes.*

ISO/TS 21569-3:2015 is applicable for the analysis of DNA extracted from foodstuffs. It may also be suitable for the analysis of DNA extracted from other products such as feedstuffs and seeds.

**ISO/TS 21569-4:2016**—Horizontal methods for molecular biomarker analysis—Methods of analysis for the detection of genetically modified organisms and derived products—Part 4: Real-time PCR-based screening methods for the detection of the *P-nos* and *P-nos-nptII* DNA sequences.

ISO/TS 21569-4:2016 (5) specifies a procedure for the detection of a DNA sequence of the promoter region of the nopaline synthase gene (*P-nos*) from *Agrobacterium tumefaciens* and a procedure for the detection of the DNA transition sequence between *P-nos* and the neomycin-phosphotransferase gene (*nptII)* from the Tn5 transposon of *Escherichia coli* K12. The *nos*-promoter and the *P-nos-nptII*-construct are frequently found in genetically modified plants. The *P-nos-* and *P-nos-nptII*-specific methods are based on real-time PCR and can be used for qualitative screening purposes. For identification and quantification of a specific genetically modified plant (event), a follow-up analysis has to be carried out.

The methods described are applicable for the analysis of DNA extracted from foodstuffs. They may also be suitable for the analysis of DNA extracted from other products such as feedstuffs and seeds. The application of these methods requires the extraction of an adequate amount of amplifiable DNA from the relevant matrix.

The DNA sequence amplified by the *P-nos* element-specific method can be detected in samples that contain DNA of the naturally occurring Ti-plasmid of *A. tumefaciens.* For this reason, it is necessary to confirm a positive screening result. Further analyses are required using construct-specific or event-specific methods.

ISO/TS 21569-5:2016—Horizontal methods for molecular biomarker analysis—Methods of analysis for the detection of genetically modified organisms and derived products—Part 5: Real-time PCR-based screening method for the detection of the FMV promoter (P-FMV) DNA sequence.

ISO/TS 21569-5:2016 (6) specifies a procedure for the detection of a DNA sequence used in genetically modified plants by means of a real-time PCR. The method detects a 78 base pairs long segment of the figwort mosaic virus 34S promoter DNA sequence. This segment in some GM plants is indicated as FMV promoter (P-FMV) and in other GM plants as FMV enhancer (E-FMV).

The method was developed and validated for the analysis of DNA extracted from foodstuffs. It may also be suitable for the analysis of other products such as feedstuffs and seeds. The procedure requires the extraction of an adequate quantity and quality of amplifiable DNA from the test sample.

The DNA sequence amplified by the P-FMV element-specific method can be detected in samples, which contain DNA of the naturally occurring figwort mosaic virus. For this reason, it is necessary to confirm a positive screening result. Further analyses are required using construct-specific or event specific methods.

**ISO/TS 21569-6:2016**—Horizontal methods for molecular biomarker analysis—Methods of analysis for the detection of genetically modified organisms and derived products—Part 6: Real-time PCR-based screening methods for the detection of *cry1Ab/Ac* and Pubi-cry DNA sequences.

ISO/TS 21569-6:2016 (7) specifies a procedure for the detection of a DNA sequence of the modified *cry1Ab/Ac* gene and a procedure for the detection of the DNA transition sequence between the maize ubiquitin promoter (*Pubi*) and the *cry1Ab/Ac* gene. The modified *cry1Ab/Ac* gene and the *Pubi-cry* construct are frequently found in genetically modified Bt plants. Both detection methods are based on real-time PCR and can be used for qualitative screening purposes. For identification and quantification of a specific genetically modified plant (event), a follow-up analysis has to be carried out.

ISO/TS 21569-6:2016 is applicable for the analysis of DNA extracted from foodstuffs. It may also be suitable for the analysis of DNA extracted from other products such as feedstuffs and seeds. The application of these methods requires the extraction of an adequate amount of amplifiable DNA from the relevant matrix.

**ISO/TS 21098:2005**—Foodstuffs—Nucleic acid based methods of analysis of genetically modified organisms and derived products—Information to be supplied and procedure for the addition of methods to ISO 21569, ISO 21570 or ISO 21571.

ISO/TS 21098:2005 (8) defines the principles and specifies the nature of the information to be supplied for acceptance of a method as an annex to ISO 21569, ISO 21570, or ISO 21571. It also specifies the process for adding, amending, and retaining methods annexed to these standards. ISO/TS 21098:2005 is necessary in order to attain consistency in methods that are to be employed as part of the standards. It does not cover the specifics of the development of a method or laboratory set-up.

The current status: withdrawn.

**ISO 21570:2005**—Foodstuffs—Methods of analysis for the detection of genetically modified organisms and derived products—Quantitative nucleic acid based methods

ISO 21570:2005 (9) provides the overall framework of quantitative methods for the detection of GMOs in foodstuffs, using the PCR.

It defines general requirements for the specific amplification of DNA target sequences in order to quantify the relative GMO-derived DNA content and to confirm the identity of the amplified DNA sequence.

Guidelines, minimum requirements, and performance criteria laid down in ISO 21570:2005 are intended to ensure that comparable, accurate and reproducible results are obtained in different laboratories.

ISO 21570:2005 has been established for food matrices, but is also applicable to other matrices, for example, feed and plant samples from the environment.

This standard was last reviewed and confirmed in 2015. Therefore, this version remains current.

**ISO 21571:2005**—Foodstuffs—Methods of analysis for the detection of genetically modified organisms and derived products—Nucleic acid extraction.

ISO 21571:2005 (10) provides general requirements and specific methods for DNA extraction/purification and quantification. These methods are described in Annexes A and B.

ISO 21571:2005 has been established for food matrices, but could also be applicable to other matrices, such as grains and feed.

It has been designed as an integral part of nucleic-acid-based analytical methods, in particular ISO 21569 on qualitative analytical methods, and ISO 21570 on quantitative analytical methods.

This standard was last reviewed and confirmed in 2015. Therefore, this version remains current.

**ISO 21572:2013**—Foodstuffs—Molecular biomarker analysis—Protein-based methods.

ISO 21572:2013 (11) provides general guidelines and performance criteria for methods for the detection and/or quantification of specific proteins or protein(s) of interest [POI(s)] in a specified matrix.

These general guidelines address existing antibody based methods. The same criteria as outlined in ISO 21572:2013 apply generally.

ISO/AWI 22753—Molecular biomarker analysis—Methods of analysis for the detection of genetically modified organisms. Semi-quantitative method for the statistical evaluation of weight/weight GMO content in seeds and grains.

The current status of this standard: under development (12).

**ISO 24276:2006**—Foodstuffs—Methods of analysis for the detection of genetically modified organisms and derived products—General requirements and definitions.

ISO 24276:2006 (13) specifies how to use the standards for sampling strategies (EN/TS 21568), nucleic acid extraction (ISO 21571), qualitative nucleic acid analysis (ISO 21569) and quantitative nucleic acid analysis (ISO 21570), and their relationship in the analysis of GMOs in foodstuffs, and contains general definitions, requirements and guidelines for laboratory set-up, method validation requirements, description of methods and test reports.

It has been established for food matrices, but could also be applied to other matrices (e.g., seeds, feed and plant samples from the environment).

This standard was last reviewed and confirmed in 2015. Therefore, this version remains current.

**ISO 24333:2009**—Cereals and cereal products—Sampling.

ISO 24333:2009 (14) specifies requirements for the dynamic or static sampling, by manual or mechanical means, of cereals and cereal products, for assessment of their quality and condition.

It is applicable to sampling for the determination of heterogeneously distributed contaminants, undesirable substances, and parameters usually homogeneously distributed like those used to assess quality or compliance with specification.

It can be used to determine insects in a grain lot.

It is applicable to sampling for assessment of the quality and condition of lots of GMOs but is inappropriate for the determination of the presence of adventitious genetically modified material in non-GM product.

It is not applicable to seed grain.

## REFERENCES

1. https://www.iso.org/home.html
2. https://www.iso.org/standard/34614.html
3. https://www.iso.org/standard/60166.html
4. https://www.iso.org/standard/63468.html
5. https://www.iso.org/standard/69339.html
6. https://www.iso.org/standard/69340.html
7. https://www.iso.org/standard/69356.html
8. https://www.iso.org/standard/40004.html
9. https://www.iso.org/standard/34615.html
10. https://www.iso.org/standard/34616.html
11. https://www.iso.org/standard/51005.html
12. https://www.iso.org/standard/73822.html
13. https://www.iso.org/standard/37125.html
14. https://www.iso.org/standard/42165.html

CHAPTER 11

# Reference Methods for GMO Analysis

*Leo M.L. Nollet*
University College Ghent

CONTENTS



## 11.1 EU DATABASE OF REFERENCE METHODS FOR GMO ANALYSIS

This EU Database of Reference Methods for GMO Analysis has been developed by the Joint Research Centre as European Union Reference Laboratory for GM Food and Feed (EU-RL GMFF) (1) in collaboration with the European Network of GMO Laboratories (ENGL) (2).

It aims at providing a list of reference methods for GMO analysis that have been:

- validated in a collaborative trial, according to the principles and requirements of ISO 5725 (3) and/or IUPAC protocol (4).
    or
- verified by the EU-RL GMFF in the context of compliance with an EU legislative act.

All efforts have been made to ensure that the information provided is accurate and correct but no responsibility can be taken for the data and information reported in the method validation publication.

The JRC does not own any intellectual property on the data and information reported in the method validation publication. Such data and information are owned by method developers. Some legal provisions on confidentiality and data protection are provided in article 30 and article 31, respectively, of Regulation (EC) No 1829/2003 (5).

The European Union disclaims all implied representations and warranties, including any warranty of merchantability and fitness, for a particular purpose. The entire risk as to the use, interpretation, and fitness for a particular concrete purpose is with the user. Under no circumstance, the European Union, the European Commission, and/or any natural person acting on behalf of these entities shall be liable for any incidental, consequential, direct, or indirect damages including, but not limited to, structural failure, lost, of profits, or any other financial loss arising from the use of, or inability to use, the data or any other matter relating to the service.

An event-specific detection searches for the presence of a DNA sequence unique to a certain GMO, usually the junction between the transgene and the organism's original DNA. This approach is ideal to precisely identify a GMO, yet highly similar GMOs will pass completely unnoticed. Event-specific detection is PCR based.

The construct-specific detection methods (DMs) can either be DNA or protein based. DNA-based detection looks for a part of the foreign DNA inserted in a GMO. For technical reasons, certain DNA sequences are shared by several GMOs. Protein-based methods detect the product of the transgene, for example, the Bt toxin. Since different GMOs may produce the same protein, construct-specific detection can test a sample for several GMOs in one step, but is unable to tell precisely which of the similar GMOs are present. Especially, in the United States, protein-based detection is used for the construct-specific approach.

In the database, one can search on terms or one can search via the following links:

- Quantitative GMO detection PCR methods
    - GMO-specific
        - Event-specific
            - Maize
            - Soybean
            - Cotton
            - Oilseed rape
            - Papaya
            - Potato
            - Rice
            - Sugar beet
            - Construct-specific
            - Element-specific
    - Taxon-specific
        - Validated independently
        - Validated in combination with other method(s)
- Qualitative GMO detection PCR methods
    - GMO-specific
        - Event-specific
        - Construct-specific
        - Element-specific
            - Cauliflower mosaic virus 35S promoter (CaMV P-35S)
            - *CP4-EPSPS* gene (*CP4-EPSPS*)
            - *Cry1Ab/Ac* gene (*cry1Ab/Ac*)
            - *Cry1A(b)* gene (*cry1A(b)*)
            - Figwort mosaic virus 35S promoter (P-FMV)
            - Neomycin phosphotransferase II gene (nptII)

- Nopaline synthase promoter (P-nos)
- Nopaline synthase terminator (T-nos)
- Phosphinothricin *N*-acetyltransferase gene (bar)
- Phosphinothricin *N*-acetyltransferase gene (pat)

- Taxon-specific
  - Validated independently
  - Validated in combination with other method(s)
  - Plant-specific

In order to provide reliable and harmonized information on methods for genetically modified organism (GMO) analysis, Bonfini et al. (6) have published a database called "GMOMETHODS" that supplies information on PCR assays validated according to the principles and requirements of ISO 5725 and/or the International Union of Pure and Applied Chemistry protocol. In addition, the database contains methods that have been verified by the EU-RL GMFF in the context of compliance with a European Union legislative act. The web application provides search capabilities to retrieve primers and probes sequence information on the available methods. It further supplies core data required by analytical labs to carry out GM tests and comprises information on the applied reference material and plasmid standards. The GMOMETHODS database currently contains 118 different PCR methods, allowing identification of 51 single GM events and 18 taxon-specific genes in a sample. It also provides screening assays for detection of eight different genetic elements commonly used for the development of GMOs. The application is referred to by the Biosafety Clearing House, a global mechanism set up by the Cartagena Protocol on Biosafety to facilitate the exchange of information on Living Modified Organisms. The publication of the GMOMETHODS database can be considered an important step toward worldwide standardization and harmonization in GMO analysis.

## 11.2 SUBMISSION OF METHOD FOR VALIDATION TO ENGL ADVISORY GROUP

Objective of the advisory group is to complete the portfolio of available methods and make the European system able to cope with the new developments in GMOs. High priority should be given to methods closing an analytical gap or anticipating future GM global developments potentially entering the European market, offering an added value (e.g., cost/time efficiency, performance, etc.) in comparison to previously adopted strategies, and complying with ENGL methods acceptance criteria as specified in the document definition of minimum performance requirements for analytical methods of GMO testing (7).

For each proposed method, a form has to be filled and sent by e-mail to the secretariat of ENGL.

## 11.3 GMO DETECTION METHOD DATABASE

This GMO detection method database (GMDD) is being set up by GMO Detection Laboratory in Shanghai Jiao Tong University (GMODL-SJTU) in collaboration with RIKILT, Shanghai Academy of Agricultural Sciences, Shanghai Food and Drug

Administration, Shanghai Entry-Exit Inspection and Quarantine Bureau, and Shanghai University Bioinformation Center. This platform is funded by Science and Technology Commission of Shanghai Municipality, Chinese Ministry of Science and Technology (8).

The aim of the database is to provide detailed information of GMO DMs, and also information of gene insert. These information will be very useful in the development and standardization of GMO DMs.

## 11.4 GMOFINDER

The aim of the study of Gerdes et al. (9,10) was the development of the GMOfinder, a database for collection and interpretation of information related to the screening for GMO. Different genetic elements (e.g., promoters, terminators, structural genes) are artificially introduced into plants to establish new genetic modifications. The introduced elements may vary between GMO events, depending on the intended trait(s). Screening for such inserted elements with (real-time) PCR is a common first step to analyze samples for the presence of any genetical modification. From the pattern of detectable and non-detectable elements, valuable conclusions about the identity of putative present GMO event(s) can be drawn with the GMOfinder. Information about selected genetic elements from the literature, applications for authorization and other (web) sources were systematically integrated in a tabular matrix format. Special care was taken to additionally record the sources of the information, thus facilitating evaluation of screening results, and tracing of possible errors in the matrix. The GMOfinder accesses data from the element matrix with implemented algorithms and facilitates to interpret the outcome of screenings. Such a pre-selection helps to systematically narrow down the candidates for subsequent identification reactions. Optional display of events with potentially masked elements completes the included features.

## 11.5 JRC GMO-MATRIX APPLICATION

The GMOseek matrix was built as a comprehensive, online open-access tabulated database which provides a reliable, comprehensive and user-friendly overview of more than 32 GMO events and more than 240 different genetic elements (10–13). The GMOseek matrix is aiming to facilitate GMO detection from plant origin at different phases of the analysis. It assists in selecting the targets for a screening analysis, interpreting the screening results, checking the occurrence of a screening element in a group of selected GMOs, identifying gaps in the available pool of GMO DMs, and designing a decision tree. The GMOseek matrix is an independent database with effective functionalities in a format facilitating transferability to other platforms. Data were collected from all available sources and experimentally tested where DMs and certified reference materials were available.

The GMOseek matrix is currently a unique and very valuable tool with reliable information on GMOs from plant origin and their present genetic elements that enables further development of appropriate strategies for GMO detection. It is flexible enough to be further updated with new information and integrated in different applications and platforms.

The JRC GMO-Matrix is an application that takes advantage of the GMO sequence information found in the Central Core DNA Sequence Information System (CCSIS) (14), which are received from companies as part of their legal obligations or extracted from nucleotide / patent sequences databases, as well as the primers and probes sequences of the existing DMs compiled in the GMOMETHODS database to perform in silico simulations of PCR amplification and, when applicable, probe binding using bioinformatics tools, such as re-PCR and matcher.

JRC GMO-Matrix application relies on a relational database that contains pre-computed values corresponding to the extent of matching between the methods primers and probe and each GMO sequence. Those pre-calculated values represent the results of in silico simulations of the detection of each GMO by each PCR-based detection method and form the core data used by the application for its different case uses. The current version of the JRC GMO-Matrix application contains a set interfaces available to the user, which is expected to grow based on the feedback that will be received.

GMDD is one part of Shanghai GMO platform and it provides the following services (8):

- GMDD is a database of GMO DMs, which provide detailed information of nucleic acid-based methods and protein-based methods, including primer sequences, amplicon length, endogenous reference gene primers, validation information, PCR programs, and references. Besides, the database also contains information on GMO insertion sequences and certified reference materials.

Recently, a novel bioinformatics method called *TranSeq* employing the power of NGS technology to investigate the GM events was established. The comprehensive molecular characteristics of two GM events were revealed with additional unintended insertions comparing with the results from PCR and Southern blotting.

By registration, users can submit their own methods and GMO inserted sequences to GMDD.

- GMO Detection Services

In China, this platform also provides services for GMO content detection, new method validation, and detection technique training.

## 11.6 THE CROPLIFE INTERNATIONAL DETECTION METHODS DATABASE

Reliable DMs to test for the presence of agricultural biotechnology products are critical to help ensure smooth international trade transactions.

The plant biotechnology industry is committed to doing its part to support smooth trade transactions in the global agricultural community. As part of this commitment, CropLife International and its members have made their DMs for commercialized biotech-derived products—and related materials and information—available in an online and searchable database (15).

Current and future biotech traits in the marketplace are increasingly complex and require specialized and accurate DMs. Today, more than ever, reliable, validated, and internationally-accepted DMs are critical to facilitate seamless global trade. The DMs available have been developed and validated by the technology providers for their own proprietary technologies and products. The plant biotechnology industry believes that sharing industry-developed DMs can assist in achieving global harmonization of testing efforts.

The CropLife International Detection Methods Database is the definitive online global source for testing information for the majority of commercialized biotech-derived plant products (16). It makes the most authoritative testing methods, which have been developed by the same technology companies that deliver biotech traits to the market, readily available.

The database was created primarily for use by regulators and policy makers seeking valid DMs and reference materials. It is updated frequently and includes commercialized products developed by the six major private plant biotechnology developers (BASF, Bayer, Dow AgroSciences, DuPont, Monsanto, and Syngenta).

The database is continuously being refined to respond to user recommendations and needs.

## REFERENCES

1. http://gmo-crl.jrc.ec.europa.eu/gmomethods/.
2. http://gmo-crl.jrc.ec.europa.eu/ENGL/ENGL.html.
3. https://www.iso.org/obp/ui/#iso:std:iso:5725:-1:en.
4. https://iupac.org/.
5. http://eur-lex.europa.eu/legal-content/en/ALL/?uri=CELEX%3A32003R1829.
6. L. Bonfini, M.H. van den Bulcke, M.B.E. Mazzara, A. Patak. GMOMETHODS: The European union database of reference methods for GMO analysis. *Journal of AOAC International*, 95(6), 2012, 1713–1719.
7. http://gmo-crl.jrc.ec.europa.eu/doc/Min_Perf_Requirements_Analytical_methods.pdf.
8. http://gmdd.sjtu.edu.cn/.
9. L. Gerdes, U. Busch, S. Pecoraro. GMOfinder—A GMO screening database. *Food Analytical Methods*, 5(6), 2012, 1368–1376.
10. http://gmo-crl.jrc.ec.europa.eu/jrcgmomatrix/matrices/event_finder.
11. http://gmo-crl.jrc.ec.europa.eu/jrcgmomatrix/.
12. A. Angers-Loustau, M. Petrillo, L. Bonfini, F. Gatto, S. Rosa, A. Patak, J. Kreysa. JRC GMO-Matrix: A web application to support genetically modified organisms detection strategies. *BMC Bioinformatics*, 15, 2014, 417–426.
13. A. Block, F. Debode, L. Grohmaan, J. Hulin, I. Taverniers, L. Kluga, E. Barbau-Piednoir, S. Broeders, I. Huber, M. Van den Bulcke, P. Heinze, G. Berben, U. Busch, N. Roosens, E. Janssen, J. Zel, K. Gruden, D. Morisset. The GMOseek matrix: A decision support tool for optimizing the detection of genetically modified plants. *BMC Bioinformatics*, 14, 2013, 256–270.
14. https://ec.europa.eu/jrc/en/research-topic/bioinformatics.
15. http://www.detection-methods.com/.
16. http://www.detection-methods.com/database-overview/.

# Index